Essential Clinical Procedures

Essential Clinical Procedures

Second Edition

Richard W. Dehn, MPA, PA-C
Clinical Professor and Assistant Director
Physician Assistant Program
The University of Iowa Carver College of Medicine
Iowa City, Iowa

David P. Asprey, PhD, PA-C
Associate Professor and Program Director
Physician Assistant Program
The University of Iowa Carver College of Medicine
Iowa City, Iowa

SAUNDERS

ELSEVIER

1600 John F. Kennedy Blvd.
Ste 1800
Philadelphia, PA 19103-2899

ESSENTIAL CLINICAL PROCEDURES

ISBN-13: 978-1-4160-3001-0
ISBN-10: 1-4160-3001-8

Notice

Knowledge and best practice in General and Internal Medicine are constantly changing. As new research and experience broaden our knowledge, changes in practice, treatment, and drug therapy may become necessary or appropriate. Readers are advised to check the most current information provided (i) on procedures featured or (ii) by the manufacturer of each product to be administered, to verify the recommended dose or formula, the method and duration of administration, and contraindications. It is the responsibility of the practitioner, relying on their own experience and knowledge of the patient, to make diagnoses, to determine dosages and the best treatment for each individual patient, and to take all appropriate safety precautions. To the fullest extent of the law, neither the Publisher nor the Editors assume any liability for any injury and/or damage to persons or property arising out of or related to any use of the material contained in this book.   The Publisher

---

Previous edition copyrighted 2002

Library of Congress Cataloging-in-Publication Data
Essential clinical procedures / [edited by] Richard W. Dehn, David P. Asprey––2nd ed.
    p. ; cm.
    Rev. ed. of: Clinical procedures for physician assistants. c2002.
    Includes bibliographical references and index.
    ISBN-13: 978-1-4160-3001-0   ISBN-10: 1-4160-3001-8
  1. Physicians' assistants.   I. Dehn, Richard W.   II. Asprey, David P.   III. Clinical procedures for physician assistants.
    [DNLM: 1. Diagnostic Techniques and Procedures.   2. Physician Assistants.   WB 141 E776 2006]

R697.P45C56 2006
610.73'72069––dc22

2006028605

Acquisitions Editor: Rolla Couchman
Editorial Assistant: Dylan Parker
Publishing Services Manager: Frank Polizzano
Project Manager: Michael H. Goldberg
Design Direction: Steven Stave

Printed in China

Last digit is the print number: 9 8 7 6 5 4

This book is dedicated to all physician assistants who are learning the science and art of practicing medicine as a physician assistant. While working on this edition, my father, Frank W. Dehn, suddenly contracted leukemia and died on October 3, 2005, at the age of 85, and I would also like to dedicate this book in loving memory of him. Additionally, I would like to thank my wife Elizabeth, and my children Jonathan, Michael, Clare, and Kelley, without whose support I could not have finished this project.

—RWD

To my wife Jill and my children Laura, Nolan, and Caleb thank you for supporting me in each of my endeavors and for the sacrifices that each of you has made to help me complete this text. I dedicate this edition of the text to my brother Randy Asprey, who died on July 17, 2006, at age 38 after a long and valiant battle with colon cancer. The courage and love you demonstrated as a husband, father, son, brother, and friend in the midst of this trial was truly remarkable and you will be greatly missed.

—DPA

David P. Asprey, PhD, PA-C
Associate Professor and Program Director, Physician Assistant Program,
  University of Iowa Carver College of Medicine, Iowa City, Iowa
  Documentation

Patrick C. Auth, PhD, PA-C
Program Director and Assistant Professor, Drexel University Hahnemann
  Physician Assistant Program, Philadelphia, Pennsylvania
  Incision and Drainage of an Abscess

Salah Ayachi, PhD, PA-C
Associate Professor and Associate Director, Physician Assistant Studies,
  School of Allied Health Sciences, University of Texas Medical Branch,
  Galveston, Texas
  Recording an Electrocardiogram

George S. Bottomley, DVM, PA-C
Associate Professor and Program Director, Physician Assistant Program,
  Pennsylvania College of Optometry, Elkins Park, Pennsylvania
  Incision and Drainage of an Abscess

Anthony Brenneman, MPAS, PA-C
Assistant Clinical Professor and Director of Clinical Education, Physician
  Assistant Program, University of Iowa Carver College of Medicine, Iowa
  City, Iowa
  Procedural Sedation

Darwin Brown, MPH, PA-C
Assistant Professor, Physician Assistant Program, University of Nebraska
  Medical Center, Omaha, Nebraska
  Obtaining Blood Cultures; Draining Subungual Hematomas

Lynn E. Caton, MPAS, PA-C
Assistant Professor of Family Medicine/PA Education and Associate
  Director for Clinical Education, Oregon Health & Science University
  School of Medicine, Physician Assistant Program, Portland, Oregon
  Outpatient Coding

L. Gail Curtis, MPAS, PA-C
Assistant Professor, Wake Forest University School of Medicine,
  Department of Family and Community Medicine, Winston-Salem, North
  Carolina
  The Pelvic Examination and Obtaining a Routine Papanicolaou Smear

Randy Danielsen, PhD, PA-C
Professor and Dean, Arizona School of Health Sciences, A.T. Still University,
Mesa, Arizona
Blood Pressure Measurement

Ellen Davis-Hall, PhD, PA-C
Academic Coordinator and Associate Professor, Department of Pediatrics,
University of Colorado Health Sciences Center, Child Health Associate
Physician Assistant Program, Aurora, Colorado
Inserting Intravenous Catheters

Richard W. Dehn, MPA, PA-C
Clinical Professor and Assistant Director, Physician Assistant Program,
University of Iowa Carver College of Medicine, Iowa City, Iowa
Examination of the Male Genitalia

Michelle DiBaise, MPAS, PA-C
Adjunct Assistant Professor, Arizona School of the Health Sciences,
A.T. Still University, Mesa, Arizona
Local Anesthesia; Dermatologic Procedures

Roger A. Elliott, MPH, PA-C
Associate Professor and Associate Director, University of Oklahoma
Physician Associate Program, University of Oklahoma College of
Medicine, Oklahoma City, Oklahoma
Office Pulmonary Function Testing

Donald R. Frosch, MS, PA-C
Assistant Professor and Research and Assessment Coordinator, Physician
Assistant Program, Butler University/Clarian Health, Indianapolis,
Indiana
Casting and Splinting

F.J. Gianola, PA
Lecturer, MEDEX Northwest Physician Assistant Program, Division of
Physician Assistant Studies, School of Medicine and Center for Health
Sciences Interprofessional Education and Research, University of
Washington, Seattle, Washington
Giving Sad and Bad News

Jonathon W. Gietzen, MS, PA-C
Assistant Professor, Pacific University School of Physician Assistant
Studies, Forest Grove, Oregon
*Trauma-Oriented Ocular Examination, Corneal Abrasion, and Ocular
Foreign Body Removal*

Kenneth R. Harbert, PhD, CHES, PA-C
Dean, South College, Knoxville, Tennesse
  Venipuncture

Theresa E. Hegmann, MPAS, PA-C
Assistant Clinical Professor and Director of Curriculum and Evaluation,
  Physician Assistant Program, University of Iowa Carver College of
  Medicine, Iowa City, Iowa
  Cryosurgery

Paul C. Hendrix, MHS, PA-C
Associate Clinical Professor of Surgery and Director of the Physician
  Assistant Surgical Residency Program, Duke University School of
  Medicine, Durham, North Carolina
  Sterile Technique

Paul F. Jacques, EdM, PA-C
Assistant Professor and Associate Chair for Clinical Research, Department
  of Clinical Services, Medical University of South Carolina, Charleston,
  South Carolina
  Wound Dressing Techniques

P. Eugene Jones, PhD, PA-C
Professor and Chair, Department of Physician Assistant Studies; Editor-in-
  Chief, Journal of Physician Assistant Education, University of Texas
  Southwestern Medical Center, Dallas, Texas
  Cryosurgery

Nikki L. Katalanos, PhD, CDE, PA-C
Professor and Chair, Department of Physician Assistant Studies; Editor-in-
  Chief, Journal of Physician Assistant Education, University of Texas
  Southwestern Medical Center, Dallas, Texas
  Foot Examination of the Patient with Diabetes

Patricia Kelly, EdD, MHS, PA-C
Associate Professor and Chair, Department of Health Science, and Director,
  Doctor of Health Science Program, Nova Southeastern University, Fort
  Lauderdale, Florida
  Clinical Breast Examination

Charles S. King, PA-C
Clinical Coordinator, Physician Assistant Program, University of Utah
  School of Medicine, Salt Lake City, Utah
  Exercise Stress Testing for the Primary Care Provider

Patrick Knott, PhD, PA-C
Associate Professor and Chair, Physician Assistant Department, Rosalind
  Franklin University of Medicine and Science, North Chicago, Illinois
  Casting and Splinting

Daniel L. McNeill, PhD, PA-C
Professor and Director, Physician Associate Program, University of
  Oklahoma College of Medicine, Oklahoma City, Oklahoma
  Office Pulmonary Function Testing

Dawn Morton-Rias, EdD, PA-C
Dean and Assistant Professor, College of Health Related Professions, State
  University of New York, Downstate Medical Center, Brooklyn, New York
  Flexible Sigmoidoscopy

Richard D. Muma, PhD, MPH, PA-C
Chair and Associate Professor, College of Health Professions, Department of
  Physician Assistant, Wichita State University, Wichita, Kansas
  Patient Education Concepts

Karen A. Newell, MMSc, PA-C
Academic Coordinator, Emory University School of Medicine, Physician
  Assistant Program, Atlanta, Georgia
  Wound Closure

Sue M. Nyberg, MHS, PA-C
Assistant Professor, Department of Physician Assistant, College of Health
  Professions, Wichita State University, Wichita, Kansas
  Treating Ingrown Toenails; Anoscopy

Claire Babcock O'Connell, MPH, PA-C
Associate Professor, Physician Assistant Program, University of Medicine
  and Dentistry of New Jersey Robert Wood Johnson Medical School,
  Piscataway, New Jersey
  Arterial Puncture

Daniel L. O'Donoghue, PhD, PA-C
Associate Professor, Physician Associate Program, University of Oklahoma
  College of Medicine, Oklahoma City, Oklahoma
  Office Pulmonary Function Testing

Martha Petersen, MPH, PA-C
Assistant Professor, Department of Physician Assistant, Rangos School of
  Health Sciences, Duquesne University, Pittsburgh, Pennsylvania
  Endometrial Biopsy

Richard R. Rahr, MBA, EdD, PA-C
Professor and Chair, Physician Assistant Studies, School of Allied Health
  Sciences, University of Texas Medical Branch, Galveston, Texas
  Recording an Electrocardiogram

Tammy Dowdell Ream, MPAS, PA-C
Assistant Professor and Coordinator of Clinical Education, Texas Tech
  University Health Sciences Center, School of Allied Health Sciences,
  Physician Assistant Program, Midland, Texas
  Removal of Cerumen and Foreign Bodies from the Ear

Conrad J. Rios, NP, PA, MSN
Clinical Coordinator and Faculty, University of California at Davis Family
  Nurse Practitioner/Physician Assistant Program, Sacramento, California
  Injections

Ted J. Ruback, MS, PA-C
Associate Professor and Head, Division of Physician Assistant Education,
  and Director, Physician Assistant Program, Oregon Health & Science
  University School of Medicine, Portland, Oregon
  Informed Consent

Virginia Fallaw Schneider, PA-C
Assistant Professor, Departments of Pediatrics and Family and Community
  Medicine, Baylor College of Medicine, Houston, Texas
  Lumbar Puncture

Gary R. Sharp, MPH, PA-C
Associate Professor and Clinical Coordinator, Physician Associate Program,
  University of Oklahoma College of Medicine, Oklahoma City, Oklahoma
  Office Pulmonary Function Testing

Shepard B. Stone, MPS, PA
Associate Clinical Professor of Anesthesiology, Yale University School of
  Medicine; Physician Associate Anesthesiologist, Yale–New Haven Hospital,
  New Haven, Connecticut; State Aviation Medicine Officer, Connecticut
  Army National Guard, Niantic, Connecticut
  Endotracheal Intubation

Kirsten Thomsen, PA-C
Adjunct Assistant Professor, The George Washington University School of
  Medicine and Health Sciences, Physician Assistant Program, Washington, DC
  Standard Precautions

Dan Vetrosky, MEd, PA-C
Assistant Professor and Academic Coordinator, Department of Physician
  Assistant Studies, University of South Alabama, Mobile, Alabama
  Nasogastric Tube Placement; Urinary Bladder Catheterization

M.F. Winegardner, MPAS, PA-C
Physician Assistant, Department of Radiation Oncology, Mayo Clinic,
Rochester, Minnesota
Joint and Bursal Aspiration

Preface

In writing this book regarding common clinical procedures for medical practitioners, we hope to fill a unique need for an area of clinical practice that is vital to clinical education and the practice of medicine. Members of both the physician assistant (PA) and nurse practitioner (NP) professions have prided themselves on their ability to function as a part of the health care team that can fill almost any role that is needed, including the performance of clinical procedures. As the professions have evolved, using PAs and NPs in roles that provide greater autonomy and responsibility has served to increase the importance of a curriculum that incorporates common clinical procedures as part of the preparation of competent clinicians.

In attempting to accomplish this goal we have turned to our colleagues who are involved in clinical education, as either core faculty or clinical preceptors, who are very aware of the clinical procedure skills that clinical practice requires. Although we recognize that this textbook does not cover every procedure that a PA or NP may be asked to perform in practice, it does address a majority of the commonly occurring clinical procedures, and most were selected based on data that support the frequency with which PAs perform these procedures in primary care settings.

We are forever indebted to the hundreds of bright, caring, compassionate, and pioneering men and women who founded our profession. They ventured into this career with little assurance that they would have a job or a career, much less a dependable income. They have made it into one of the most rewarding professions in existence today. Their vision, dedication, endurance, ingenuity, and concern for the best interest of their patients continue to be a motivating force for us as PA educators.

We would also like to recognize the hundreds of colleagues with whom we share the role and title of PA educator. These individuals often give up freely the opportunity for the greater income and greater control of their schedule that can often be found in private practice to help prepare the next generation of PAs. We find the dedication and commitment of PA educators to their profession truly inspiring.

We owe a great debt of gratitude to students. Without their eager thirst for information and knowledge, we would find our responsibility to teach them clinical procedures to be simply work. However, their passion and excitement about learning clinical procedures for the purpose of taking care of their patients make this task a true pleasure.

Finally, we would like to acknowledge our publisher for its commitment to making educational materials available to PAs and NPs. Specifically, we would like to thank Shirley Kuhn for pursuing the idea of this book with us and encouraging us to take the leap of faith necessary to publish the first edition. We would also like to thank Rolla Couchman for his help in preparing the second edition.

Contents

Chapter 1

Informed Consent

Ted J. Ruback

Procedure Goals and Objectives

Goal: To provide clinicians with the necessary knowledge and understanding of the principles of informed consent for all clinical procedures.

Objectives: The student will be able to …

- Describe the historical basis of informed consent.
- Describe the philosophical doctrine of informed consent.
- Describe the underlying principles of informed consent.
- List the three essential conditions that must be met to ensure effective informed consent.
- Describe exceptions to the requirement for informed consent.

BACKGROUND AND HISTORY OF THE PATIENT-PROVIDER RELATIONSHIP

Over the last four decades, there has been a dramatic shift in the character of the physician-patient relationship, from one traditionally paternalistic or physician-focused in nature, to one that recognizes patient autonomy and is predominantly patient-centered. This struggle between paternalism and autonomy has been central to the discussions of ethically acceptable medical practice and has formed the basis for the doctrine of informed consent.

Paternalism is based on the principle of beneficence, the desire to do good for the patient. The concept of informed consent asserts that the desire to do good is not a justification for overriding a competent patient's right to personal autonomy and self-determination. Although there is some question about whether consent to medical procedures can ever be truly informed, the process of obtaining informed consent from a patient has been incorporated into American society's expectation of good medical practice.

PURPOSE OF INFORMED CONSENT

In May 2000 (amended May 2004), the House of Delegates of the American Academy of Physician Assistants adopted a policy of comprehensive "Guidelines for Ethical Conduct for the Physician Assistant Profession." The guidelines address the profession's responsibility in protecting a patient's autonomy.

> *Physician assistants have a duty to protect and foster an individual patient's free and informed choices. The doctrine of informed consent means that a PA provides adequate information that is comprehendible to a competent patient or patient surrogate. At a minimum, this should include the nature of the medical condition, the objectives of the proposed treatment, treatment options, possible outcomes, and the risks involved. PAs should be committed to the concept of shared decision making, which involves assisting patients in making decisions that account for medical, situational, and personal factors.*
>
> (American Academy of Physician Assistants, 2004)

Informed consent should be obtained from a patient before all medical interventions that have the potential for harm, including diagnostic and therapeutic procedures. A patient, through the exercise of personal autonomy, may either agree to or refuse a proposed procedure or treatment, but it is the responsibility of the practitioner to make sure that the decision is based on complete and appropriate information.

At the present time, the United States has no federal statute that comprehensively sets national standards of practice regarding patient consent for medical procedures. There is an implied moral obligation on professionals to disclose the necessary information to the patient, but the nature and extent of the legal obligation varies from one jurisdiction to another (Beauchamp, 2001). In most states, health care providers have an "affirmative duty" to disclose information regarding medical treatments, which means that information must be volunteered and not just provided in response to questions posed by the patient. Once the information has been disclosed, the provider's obligation has been met. Weighing the risks and deciding on a course of action then becomes the responsibility of the patient or the patient's surrogate.

Legal actions against health care professionals for failure to obtain informed consent to treatment have been pursued under two separate theories of liability—one based on the concept of battery and the other on the concept of negligence (Applebaum, 1987).

Most early litigation involving informed consent argued that the provision of treatment without consent constituted battery—an intentional, nonconsensual touching of the patient. The concept of battery protects a person's physical integrity against unwanted invasion.

After 1957, most suits alleging lack of informed consent were brought under the legal theory of negligence. Under this theory, an injured patient argues that he or she was harmed by the provider's unintentional failure to satisfy a professional standard of care. When applied in an informed consent case, the alleged negligence results from a failure to disclose sufficient information about the risks or complications of a treatment.

ESSENTIAL COMPONENTS OF INFORMED CONSENT

There are three essential conditions that must be met to ensure effective informed consent. First, the patient must have the capacity, or competence, to make an informed decision. A distinction is sometimes made between the medical judgment of a patient's capacity to consent and the legal judgment of his competence; however, in clinical practice the two are closely linked (Beauchamp, 2001). Second, the patient must be given sufficient information about the procedure or treatment and the alternatives available, to allow him or her to make an informed choice. Third, the patient must give consent to treatment voluntarily, without coercion, manipulation, or duress.

PATIENT CAPACITY

There is no universally accepted test of a patient's capacity to consent to treatment. In general, an adult is presumed to be legally competent unless he or she has been formally and legally declared incompetent. Conversely, a minor is generally presumed to be legally incompetent to make medical decisions, although a number of exceptions to this rule exist and are often state-specific (e.g., emancipation). Additionally, specific legislation sometimes grants minors legal status to make some medical decisions for themselves (e.g., testing for sexually transmitted diseases, reproductive decisions).

Competency is usually established by assessing whether the patient has the capacity to understand the nature of his or her condition and the various options available and whether he or she is capable of making a rational decision. To make a rational choice, patients must be able to understand the treatments available and the likely outcomes in each case. They must also be able to deliberate and consider their options and weigh them against one another to choose the best alternative. To do so effectively, they must assess the options available in relation to a set of values and goals, without which they would have no basis for preferring one outcome to any other (Moskop, 1999). They must also be able to communicate their understanding and their decision in some intelligible way.

ADEQUATE INFORMATION

The second requirement of informed consent is that the patient must be provided with adequate information with which to make a decision. The right to informed consent is embedded in the nature of fiduciary relationships, wherein one party has differential power, and thus that party has the inherent responsibility to share necessary information with the other. General categories of information that must be provided are the diagnosis; the nature of the proposed procedure; the risks, consequences, and benefits of the procedure; an assessment of the likelihood that the procedure(s) will accomplish the desired outcomes; and any reasonable and feasible alternatives to treatment (including the alternative of not having the procedure) and the risks and benefits of each. In clinical practice, the information required to be disclosed is frequently summarized by using the abbreviation PARQ: P (the recommended medical **p**rocedure), A (the reasonable **a**lternatives to the recommended procedure), and R (the **r**isks of the procedure); Q represents the additional step of asking the patient if he or she has any **q**uestions about the proposed procedure not adequately disclosed in the discussion.

States are far from uniform in their views of how much information should be disclosed for meaningful informed consent. Various criteria have been proposed as both legal and moral standards for adequate disclosure. The "reasonable physician" standard bases disclosure of information on the prevailing practice within the profession. What would a typical health care provider in the same specialty and "community" disclose about this procedure? This legal standard, the only judicial standard by which courts judged physicians prior to 1972, allows the practitioner to determine what information is appropriate to disclose. It is often argued that this more paternalistic approach, although still dominant in the courts, is inconsistent with the goals of informed consent and true patient autonomy.

The second standard of disclosure, introduced in 1972, is the "reasonable person" standard. The reasonable person standard requires a health care provider to disclose to a patient any material information that the practitioner recognizes that a reasonable person in the patient's position would consider to be significant to his or her decision making about the recommended medical intervention. Risks that are not serious, or are unlikely, are not considered material. Under this standard, the critical requirement shifts from whether the disclosure met the profession's standard to whether the undisclosed information would have been material to a reasonable patient's decision making.

The great advantage of the reasonable person standard is the focus on the preferences of the patient. A requirement for this standard is that the type and amount of information provided must be at the patient's level of understanding if he or she is truly to be an autonomous decision maker. The disadvantages of this standard include its failure to articulate the nature of the "hypothetical" reasonable person. In addition, the retrospective application of this standard presents a significant problem in that any complication of a procedure is likely to seem material after it has occurred (Nora, 1998).

Although the reasonable person standard does focus more on the patient, it does not require that the disclosure be tailored to each patient's specific informational needs or desires. Instead, it bases the requirements on what a hypothetical reasonable person would want to know. The third standard of disclosure, the "subjective" standard, addresses this limitation by asking the question, What would *this* particular patient need to know and understand in order to make an informed decision? This patient-centered approach allows greater differentiation based on patient preference, relying on the unique nature and abilities of the individual patient to determine the degree of disclosure needed to satisfy the requirements of informed consent. This standard is the most challenging to implement in practice due to its requirement to tailor information specifically to each patient.

In addition to providing information, the clinician has the ethical obligation to make reasonable efforts to ensure comprehension. Communicating highly technical and specialized knowledge to someone who is not conversant in the subject presents a formidable challenge. Patient-centered barriers to informed consent—such as anxiety, language differences, and physical or emotional impairments—can impede the process. Lack of familiarity or sensitivity to the patient's cultural and health care beliefs on the part of the provider can act as a significant barrier to providing effective informed consent. Process-centered barriers, including readability of consent forms, timing of the consent discussion, and amount of time devoted to the process, also may reflect disrespect for the autonomy of the patient.

To optimize information sharing, explanations should be given clearly and simply, and questions should be asked frequently to assess understanding. Whenever possible, a variety of communication techniques should be used, including written forms of educational materials, videotapes, CDs, DVDs, and additional media sources. Computers have taken on a new and ever-expanding role as an effective tool in patient education when integrated into the clinical setting.

VOLUNTARY CHOICE

In a clinical setting, voluntariness may be influenced by the vulnerability of the patient and the inherent imbalance in knowledge and power between the health care professional and the patient. Care needs to be exercised in advising patients carefully so that what professionals construe in good faith as rational persuasion does not unintentionally exert undue influence on a patient's decision making (Messer, 2004). Consent to treatment obtained using manipulation or coercion, or both, is the antithesis of informed consent. Although a health care provider's recommendation regarding treatment typically can have a strong influence on a patient's decision making, a recommendation offered as part of the clinician's responsibility to inform and guide a patient in his or her decision making is not considered coercion.

TYPES OF INFORMED CONSENT

Consent may take many forms, including implied, general, and special. Implied consent is often used when immediate action is required. In the emergency room, consent is presumed when inaction may cause greater injury or would be contrary to good medical practice. General consent is often obtained on hospital admission to provide consent for routine services and routine touching by health care staff. Such "blanket" forms generally do not list specific procedures, risks, benefits, or alternatives that might be encountered by a patient during a hospitalization. Additionally, the risk associated with a procedure may be variable depending upon a patient's condition. Therefore, a consent to "general treatment" upon hospital admission may not be adequate to meet the requirements of informed consent (Manthous, 2003). Finally, special consent is required for specific high-risk procedures and medical treatments.

State laws vary as to which interventions require a signed consent form. Some states require a written consent only for surgical interventions, anesthesia, or other more invasive procedures. Other states require informed consent be documented for a broader range of procedures.

In order to ensure that informed consent is properly obtained, the health care provider should actually discuss with the patient each of the procedures to be performed, including the nature, risks, and alternatives. Consent obtained verbally is as binding as written consent because there is no legal requirement that consent be in written form; however, when disagreements arise, oral consent becomes difficult to prove. The health care provider should always document verbal consent explicitly in the medical record.

Written consent is the preferred form of consent. The consent form provides legal, visible proof of a patient's intentions. A well-drafted informed consent document can provide concrete evidence that some exchange of information was communicated to, and some assent obtained from, the patient. Such a document, supported by an entry in the patient's medical record, is often the key to a successful malpractice defense when the issue of consent to treatment arises.

Some states have laws that specify certain language on consent forms for certain procedures. In cases that do not require specific forms, a general consent form that identifies the patient, the date, and precise time of signature and documents the procedure, the risks associated with it, the indications, and the alternatives can be used. Most states require a consent form to be witnessed. Because of the potential conflict of interest, office personnel (nursing or other staff) should not act as the sole witness to a consent document.

A written informed consent document should be prepared with the patient's needs in mind and should verify that the patient was given the opportunity to ask questions and discuss concerns. Consent forms are often written in great detail and use medical and legal terminology that is far beyond the capacity of many patients. For true autonomy to exist in informed consent, consent forms should be understandable and should include the patient's primary language or languages whenever possible. When appropriate, an interpreter should be made available during the informed consent conference. The issue of comprehension is vital to the process. Health care providers should not make the mistake of equating the written and signed document with informed consent. The provider should always take care to make sure that information-transferring communication did occur.

PATIENT'S RIGHT TO REFUSE TREATMENT

Patients have the right to refuse treatment. In such circumstances, it is essential to document carefully such refusals and, most importantly, the patient's understanding of the potential consequences of refusing treatment. The signature of a witness is helpful in these circumstances.

EXCEPTIONS TO INFORMED CONSENT REQUIREMENTS

Several types of legitimate exceptions to the right of informed consent have been described. In rare instances, courts have recognized limited privileges that potentially can protect health care providers from claims alleging a lack of informed consent. Such exceptions include emergencies, patients unable to consent, a patient waiver of consent, public health requirements, and therapeutic privilege. In all these instances, the provider has the burden of proving that the claimed exception was invoked appropriately.

According to the emergency exception, if treatment is required to prevent death or other serious harm to a patient, that treatment may be provided without informed consent. Courts have upheld that the emergent nature of the situation and the impracticality of conferring with the patient preclude the need for informed consent. This exception is based on the presumption that the patient would consent to treatment to preserve life or health if he or she were able to do so and if there were sufficient time to obtain consent. Despite this exception, a competent patient may refuse interventions even if they are life-saving. For example, courts have repeatedly recognized the rights of Jehovah's Witnesses to refuse blood products.

Care of patients who lack decision-making capacity can be provided without the patient's informed consent. This exception, however, does not imply that no consent is necessary; instead, informed consent is required from a surrogate acting on behalf of the patient. Some surrogate decision makers are clearly identifiable (e.g., the legal guardians assigned to protect the best interests of persons judged to be incompetent and the parents of minor children). In other cases, surrogates are more difficult to determine.

The decision-making authority of surrogates is directed by defined standards. These standards require surrogates to rely first on any treatment preferences specifically indicated by the patient, either written or oral, before he or she lost decision-making capacity. Lacking such direction, surrogates are then empowered to exercise "substituted judgment,"—that is, to use their knowledge of the patient's preferences and values to choose the alternative they believe the patient would choose if he or she were able to do so. In some instances, prior knowledge of a patient's preferences or values is lacking. In such situations, surrogates are directed to rely on their assessment of the patient's best interests and are encouraged to pursue the course of action they deem most likely to foster the patient's overall well-being (Buchanan, 1989).

When a surrogate's treatment choice appears clearly contrary to a patient's previously expressed wishes or best interests, the patient's provider is duty-bound to question that choice. The health care provider does not have the authority to unilaterally override the surrogate's decision but must bring the issue to the attention of an appropriate legal authority for review and adjudication.

In the "Guidelines for Ethical Conduct for the Physician Assistant Profession," the clinician's role with regard to surrogates is clearly delineated.

> *When the person giving consent is a patient's surrogate, a family member, or other legally authorized representative, the PA should take reasonable care to assure that the decisions made are consistent with the patient's best interests and personal preferences, if known. If the PA believes the surrogate's choices do not reflect the patient's wishes or best interests, the PA should work to resolve the conflict. This may require the use of additional resources, such as an ethics committee.*
> (American Academy of Physician Assistants, 2004)

Informed consent, although clearly recognized as a patient's right, is not a patient's duty. Patients can choose to waive their right to receive the relevant information and give informed consent to treatment. The provider may honor the patient's right to choose someone else to make treatment decisions on his or her behalf as long as the request is made competently, voluntarily, and with some understanding that the patient recognizes that he or she is relinquishing a right. Health care providers should not feel obligated to accept the responsibility for making treatment decisions for the patient if they are asked to do so. Instead, they can request that the patient make his or her own choice or designate another person to serve as surrogate.

Sometimes medical interventions have a potential benefit not only to the patient but also to others in the community. In such rare instances, public health statutes may authorize patient detention or treatment without the patient's consent. This exception overrides individual patient autonomy in specific circumstances to protect important public health interests.

The final exception to informed consent is the concept of therapeutic privilege, which allows the health care provider to let considerations about the physical, mental, and emotional state of the patient affect what information is disclosed to the patient. The practitioner should believe that the risk of giving information would pose a serious detriment to the patient. The anticipated harm must result from the disclosure itself and not from the potential influence that the information might have on the patient's choice. The sole justification of concern that the patient might refuse needed therapy is not considered adequate to justify invoking this exception. The therapeutic privilege is extremely controversial and not universally recognized. Thus, the value of therapeutic privilege as an independent exception to informed consent is limited.

CONCLUSIONS

The moral and legal doctrine of informed consent and its counterpart, the refusal of treatment, are products of the last half of the 20th century. During this time, judges sought to protect patient autonomy—that is, the patient's right to self-determination. Informed consent requires the health care practitioner to provide the patient with an adequate disclosure and explanation of the treatment and the various options and consequences.

Informed consent, however, is more than a legal necessity. When conducted properly, the process of communicating appropriate information to patients about treatment alternatives can help establish a reciprocal relationship between health care provider and patient that is based on good and appropriate communication, considered advice, mutual respect, and rational choices. The therapeutic objective of informed consent should be to replace some of the patient's anxiety and unease with a sense of participation as a partner in decision making. Such a sense of participation strengthens the therapeutic alliance between provider and patient. After initial consent to treatment has occurred, a continuing dialogue between patient and practitioner, based on the patient's continuing medical needs, reinforces the original consent. In the event of an unfavorable outcome, the enhanced relationship will prove crucial to maintaining the patient's trust.

In the area of informed consent, as in every other area of risk management, the best recommendation is to practice good medicine. Informed consent is an essential part of good medical practice today and is an ethical and moral responsibility of all health care providers.

REFERENCES

American Academy of Physician Assistants: Guidelines for Ethical Conduct for the Physician Assistant Profession. Alexandria, Va, American Academy of Physician Assistants, 2004.

Applebaum PS, Lidz CW, Meisel A: Informed Consent: Legal Theory and Clinical Practice. New York, Oxford University Press, 1987.

Beauchamp TL, Childress JF: Principles of Biomedical Ethics, 5th ed. New York, Oxford University Press, 2001.

Buchanan AE, Brock DW: Deciding for Others: The Ethics of Surrogate Decision Making. Cambridge, England, Cambridge University Press, 1989.

Manthous CA, DeFirolamo A, Haddad C, Amoateng-Adjepong Y: Informed consent for medical procedures: local and national practices. Chest 124:1978-1984, 2003.

Messer NG: Professional-patient relationships and informed consent. Postgrad Med J 80:277-283, 2004.

Moskop JC: Informed consent in the emergency department. Emerg Clin N Am 17:327-340, 1999.

Nora LM, Benvenuti RJ: Medicolegal aspects of informed consent. Neurol Clin N Am 16:207-215, 1998.

BIBLIOGRAPHY

Jonsen AR, Siegler M, Winslade WJ: Clinical Ethics, 4th ed. New York, McGraw-Hill, 1998.

Mazur DJ: Medical Risk and the Right to an Informed Consent in Clinical Care and Clinical Research. Tampa, Fla, American College of Physician Executives, 1998.

Mazur DJ: Shared Decision Making in the Patient-Physician Relationship. Tampa, Fla, American College of Physician Executives, 2001.

Chapter 2

Standard Precautions

Kirsten Thomsen

PROCEDURE GOALS AND OBJECTIVES

Goal: To use and understand the importance of standard precautions when interacting with a patient.

Objectives: The student will be able to …

- Describe the indications, contraindications, and rationale for adhering to standard precautions.

- Identify and describe common problems associated with adhering to standard precautions.

- Describe the essential infectious disease principles associated with standard precautions.

- Identify the materials necessary for adhering to standard precautions and their proper use.

BACKGROUND AND HISTORY

The concept of isolating patients with infectious diseases in separate facilities, which became known as infectious disease hospitals, was introduced in a published hospital handbook as early as 1877. Although infected and non-infected patients were separated, nosocomial transmission continued, largely because of the lack of minimal aseptic procedures, coupled with the fact that infected patients were not separated from each other by disease. By 1890 to 1900, nursing textbooks discussed recommendations for practicing aseptic procedures and designating separate floors or wards for patients with similar diseases, thereby beginning to solve the problems of nosocomial transmission (Lynch, 1949).

Shortly thereafter, the cubicle system of isolation changed U.S. hospital isolation procedures as patients were placed in multiple-bed wards. "Barrier nursing" practices, consisting of the use of aseptic solutions, hand washing between patient contacts, disinfecting patient-contaminated objects, and separate gown use, were developed to decrease pathogenic organism transmission to other patients and personnel. These practices were used in U.S. infectious disease hospitals. By the 1960s, the designation of specifically designed single- or multiple-patient isolation rooms in general hospitals and outpatient treatment for tuberculosis caused these specialized hospitals (which since the 1950s had housed tuberculosis patients almost exclusively) to close (Garner, 1996).

The lack of consistent infectious patient isolation policies and procedures noted by the Centers for Disease Control (CDC) investigators in the 1960s led to the CDC publication in 1970 of a detailed isolation precautions manual entitled *Isolation Techniques for Use in Hospitals,* designed to assist large metropolitan medical centers as well as small hospitals with limited budgets.

After revision in 1983, the manual was renamed the *CDC Guidelines for Isolation Precautions in Hospitals.* These new guidelines encouraged hospital infection control decision making with respect to developing isolation systems specific to the hospital environment and circumstances or choosing to select between category-specific or disease-specific isolation precautions. Decisions regarding individual patient precautions were to be based on factors such as patient age, mental status, or possible need to prevent sharing of contaminated articles and were to be determined by the individual who placed the patient on isolation status. Decisions regarding the need for decreasing exposure to infected material by wearing masks, gloves, or gown were to be left to the patient caregiver (Garner, 1984; Haley, 1985).

Issues of overisolation of some patients surfaced using the 1983 categories of isolation, which included strict isolation, contact isolation, respiratory isolation, tuberculosis (acid-fast bacilli) isolation, enteric precautions, drainage-secretion precautions, and blood and body fluid precautions. In using the disease-specific isolation precautions, the issue of mistakes in applying the precautions arose if the patient carried a disease not often seen or treated in the hospital (Garner, 1984; Haley, 1985), if the diagnosis was delayed, or if a misdiagnosis occurred. This happened even if additional training of personnel was encouraged. These factors, coupled with increased knowledge of epidemiologic patterns of disease, led to subsequent updates of portions of the CDC reports:

■ Recommendations for the management of patients with suspected hemorrhagic fever published in 1988 (CDC, 1988)

■ Recommendations for respiratory isolation for human parvovirus B19 infection specific to patients who were immunodeficient and had chronic human parvovirus B19 infection or were in transient aplastic crisis (CDC, 1989)

■ Recommendations for the management of tuberculosis, which stemmed from increasing concern for multidrug-resistant tuberculosis, especially in human immunodeficiency virus (HIV)–infected patients in care facilities (CDC, 1990)

■ Recommendations for hantavirus infection risk reduction (CDC, 1994)

■ Expansion of recommendations for the prevention and control of hepatitis C virus (HCV) infection and hepatitis C virus–related chronic disease (CDC, 1998)

■ Occupational exposure recommendations and postexposure management for hepatitis B virus (HBV), HCV, and HIV (CDC, 2001)

■ Recommendations for infection control of avian influenza and management of exposure to severe acute respiratory syndrome–associated coronavirus (SARS-CoV) in the healthcare setting (CDC, 2004; CDC, 2005)

BODY SUBSTANCE ISOLATION

An entirely different approach to isolation, called *body substance isolation* (BSI), was developed in 1984 by Lynch and colleagues (1987, 1990) and required personnel, regardless of patient infection status, to apply clean gloves immediately before all patient contact with mucous membranes or nonintact skin, and to wear gloves if a likelihood existed of contact with any moist body substances. An apron or other barrier was also to be worn to keep the provider's own clothing and skin clean. It was recommended also that personnel be immunized if proof of immunity could not be documented when barriers, such as masks, could not prevent transmission by airborne routes (e.g., rubella, chickenpox). Additionally, when immunity was not possible, as with pulmonary tuberculosis, masks were to be worn during all patient contact. Goggles or glasses, hair covers, and shoe covers were also used as barriers. Careful handling of all used sharps, recapping of needles without using the hands, and the disposal of used items in rigid puncture-resistant containers were stressed. Trash and soiled linen from all patients were bagged and handled in the same manner. This approach sought to protect the patient from contracting nosocomial infections and the provider from bacterial or viral pathogens that might originate with the patient.

UNIVERSAL PRECAUTIONS

In response to increasing concerns by health care workers and others about occupational exposure and the risk of transmission of human immuno-deficiency virus, HBV, and other blood-borne pathogens during provision of health care and first aid, the CDC, in 1987, defined a set of precautions that considered blood and certain body fluids from all patients to be potential sources of infection for human immunodeficiency virus, HBV, and other blood-borne pathogens. These recommendations became known as universal precautions (UP) and have subsequently been integrated into the *Recommendations for Isolation Precautions in Hospitals, 1996,* which includes the current standard precautions (SP) (Table 2-1).

Table 2.1   Recommendations for Isolation Precautions in Hospitals, Hospital Infection Control Practices Advisory Committee, 1996

STANDARD PRECAUTIONS
Use Standard Precautions, or the equivalent, for the care of all patients.

HAND WASHING
Wash hands after touching blood, body fluids, secretions, excretions, and contaminated items, whether or not gloves are worn. Wash hands immediately after gloves are removed, between patient contacts, and when otherwise indicated to avoid transfer of microorganisms to other patients or environments. It may be necessary to wash hands between tasks and procedures on the same patient to prevent cross-contamination of different body sites.
   Use a plain (nonantimicrobial) soap for routine hand washing.
   Use an antimicrobial agent or a waterless antiseptic agent for specific circumstances (e.g., control of outbreaks or hyperendemic infections), as defined by the infection control program. (See "Contact Precautions" for additional recommendations on using antimicrobial and antiseptic agents.)

GLOVES
Wear gloves (clean, nonsterile gloves are adequate) when touching blood, body fluids, secretions, excretions, and contaminated items. Put on clean gloves just before touching mucous membranes and nonintact skin. Change gloves between tasks and procedures on the same patient after contact with material that may contain a high concentration of microorganisms. Remove gloves promptly after use, before touching noncontaminated items and environmental surfaces, and before going to another patient, and wash hands immediately to avoid transfer of microorganisms to other patients or environments.

MASK, EYE PROTECTION, FACE SHIELD
Wear a mask and eye protection or a face shield to protect mucous membranes of the eyes, nose, and mouth during procedures and patient care activities that are likely to generate splashes or sprays of blood, body fluids, secretions, and excretions.

GOWN
Wear a gown (a clean, nonsterile gown is adequate) to protect skin and to prevent soiling of clothing during procedures and patient care activities that are likely to generate splashes or sprays of blood, body fluids, secretions, or excretions. Select a gown that is appropriate for the activity and amount of fluid likely to be encountered. Remove a soiled gown as promptly as possible, and wash hands to avoid transfer of microorganisms to other patients or environments.

PATIENT CARE EQUIPMENT
Handle used patient care equipment soiled with blood, body fluids, secretions, and excretions in a manner that prevents skin and mucous membrane exposures, contamination of clothing,

Table 2.1 Recommendations for Isolation Precautions in Hospitals, Hospital Infection Control Practices Advisory Committee, 1996—cont'd

and transfer of microorganisms to other patients and environments. Ensure that reusable equipment is not used for the care of another patient until it has been cleaned and reprocessed appropriately. Ensure that single-use items are discarded properly.

ENVIRONMENTAL CONTROL
Ensure that the hospital has adequate procedures for the routine care, cleaning, and disinfection of environmental surfaces, beds, bed rails, bedside equipment, and other frequently touched surfaces, and ensure that these procedures are being followed.

LINEN
Handle, transport, and process used linen soiled with blood, body fluids, secretions, and excretions in a manner that prevents skin and mucous membrane exposures and contamination of clothing, and that avoids transfer of microorganisms to other patients and environments.

OCCUPATIONAL HEALTH AND BLOOD-BORNE PATHOGENS
Take care to prevent injuries when using needles, scalpels, and other sharp instruments or devices; when handling sharp instruments after procedures; when cleaning used instruments; and when disposing of used needles. Never recap used needles, or otherwise manipulate them using both hands, or use any other technique that involves directing the point of a needle toward any part of the body; rather, use either a one-handed "scoop" technique or a mechanical device designed for holding the needle sheath. Do not remove used needles from disposable syringes by hand, and do not bend, break, or otherwise manipulate used needles by hand. Place used disposable syringes and needles, scalpel blades, and other sharp items in appropriate puncture-resistant containers, which are located as close as is practical to the area in which the items were used, and place reusable syringes and needles in a puncture-resistant container for transport to the reprocessing area.

Use mouthpieces, resuscitation bags, or other ventilation devices as an alternative to mouth-to-mouth resuscitation methods in areas where the need for resuscitation is predictable.

PATIENT PLACEMENT
Place a patient who contaminates the environment or who does not (or cannot be expected to) assist in maintaining appropriate hygiene or environmental control in a private room. If a private room is not available, consult with infection control professionals regarding patient placement or other alternatives.

AIRBORNE PRECAUTIONS
In addition to standard precautions, use airborne precautions, or the equivalent, for patients known or suspected to be infected with microorganisms transmitted by airborne droplet nuclei (small-particle residue [5 µm or smaller in size] of evaporated droplets containing microorganisms that remain suspended in the air and that can be dispersed widely by air currents within a room or over a long distance).

PATIENT PLACEMENT
Place the patient in a private room that has (1) monitored negative air pressure in relation to the surrounding area, (2) six to twelve air changes per hour, and (3) appropriate discharge of air outdoors or monitored high-efficiency filtration of room air before the air is circulated to other areas in the hospital. Keep the room door closed and the patient in the room. When a private room is not available, place the patient in a room with a patient who has active infection with the same microorganism, unless otherwise recommended, but with no other infection. When a private room is not available and cohorting is not desirable, consultation with infection control professionals is advised before patient placement.

RESPIRATORY PROTECTION
Wear respiratory protection when entering the room of a patient with known or suspected infectious pulmonary tuberculosis. Susceptible persons should not enter the room of patients known or suspected to have measles (rubeola) or varicella (chickenpox) if other, immune caregivers are available. If susceptible persons must enter the room of a patient known or

continued

Table 2.1 Recommendations for Isolation Precautions in Hospitals, Hospital Infection Control Practices Advisory Committee, 1996—cont'd

suspected to have measles (rubeola) or varicella, they should wear respiratory protection. Persons immune to measles (rubeola) or varicella need not wear respiratory protection.

PATIENT TRANSPORT
Limit the movement and transport of the patient from the room to essential purposes only. If transport or movement is necessary, minimize patient dispersal of droplet nuclei by placing a surgical mask on the patient, if possible.

ADDITIONAL PRECAUTIONS FOR PREVENTING TRANSMISSION OF TUBERCULOSIS
Consult CDC *Guidelines for Preventing the Transmission of Tuberculosis in Health Care Facilities* for additional prevention strategies.

DROPLET PRECAUTIONS
In addition to standard precautions, use droplet precautions, or the equivalent, for a patient known or suspected to be infected with microorganisms transmitted by droplets (large-particle droplets [larger than 5 μm in size] that can be generated by the patient during coughing, sneezing, talking, or the performance of procedures).

PATIENT PLACEMENT
Place the patient in a private room. When a private room is not available, place the patient in a room with a patient(s) who has active infection with the same microorganism but with no other infection (cohorting). When a private room is not available and cohorting is not achievable, maintain spatial separation of at least 3 feet between the infected patient and other patients and visitors. Special air handling and ventilation are not necessary, and the door may remain open.

MASK
In addition to standard precautions, wear a mask when working within 3 feet of the patient. (Logistically, some hospitals may want to implement the wearing of a mask to enter the room.)

PATIENT TRANSPORT
Limit the movement and transport of the patient from the room to essential purposes only. If transport or movement is necessary, minimize patient dispersal of droplets by masking the patient, if possible.

CONTACT PRECAUTIONS
In addition to standard precautions, use contact precautions, or the equivalent, for specified patients known or suspected to be infected or colonized with epidemiologically important microorganisms that can be transmitted by direct contact with the patient (hand or skin-to-skin contact that occurs when performing patient care activities that require touching the patient's dry skin) or indirect contact (touching) with environmental surfaces or patient care items in the patient's environment.

PATIENT PLACEMENT
Place the patient in a private room. When a private room is not available, place the patient in a room with a patient(s) who has active infection with the same microorganism but with no other infection (cohorting). When a private room is not available and cohorting is not achievable, consider the epidemiology of the microorganism and the patient population when determining patient placement. Consultation with infection control professionals is advised before patient placement.

GLOVES AND HAND WASHING
In addition to wearing gloves as outlined under "Standard Precautions," wear gloves (clean, nonsterile gloves are adequate) when entering the room. During the course of providing care for a patient, change gloves after having contact with infective material that may contain high concentrations of microorganisms (fecal material and wound drainage). Remove gloves before leaving the patient's environment and wash hands immediately with an antimicrobial agent or

Table 2.1 **Recommendations for Isolation Precautions in Hospitals, Hospital Infection Control Practices Advisory Committee, 1996—cont'd**

a waterless antiseptic agent. After glove removal and hand washing, ensure that hands do not touch potentially contaminated environmental surfaces or items in the patient's room to avoid transfer of microorganisms to other patients or environments.

GOWN
In addition to wearing a gown as outlined under "Standard Precautions," wear a gown (a clean, nonsterile gown is adequate) when entering the room if you anticipate that your clothing will have substantial contact with the patient, environmental surfaces, or items in the patient's room, or if the patient is incontinent or has diarrhea, an ileostomy, a colostomy, or wound drainage not contained by a dressing. Remove the gown before leaving the patient's environment. After gown removal, ensure that clothing does not contact potentially contaminated environmental surfaces to avoid transfer of microorganisms to other patients or environments.

PATIENT TRANSPORT
Limit the movement and transport of the patient from the room to essential purposes only. If the patient is transported out of the room, ensure that precautions are maintained to minimize the risk of transmission of microorganisms to other patients and contamination of environmental surfaces or equipment.

PATIENT CARE EQUIPMENT
When possible, dedicate the use of noncritical patient care equipment to a single patient (or cohort of patients infected or colonized with the pathogen requiring precautions) to avoid sharing between patients. If use of common equipment or items is unavoidable, adequately clean and disinfect them before use for another patient.

ADDITIONAL PRECAUTIONS FOR PREVENTING THE SPREAD OF
VANCOMYCIN RESISTANCE
Consult the HICPAC report on preventing the spread of vancomycin resistance for additional prevention strategies.

HICPAC, Hospital Infection Control Practices Advisory Committee.
From Centers for Disease Control and Prevention: Recommendations for Isolation Precautions in Hospitals, 1996. Available at: *http://www.cdc.gov/ncidod/hip/isolat/isopart1.htm* and *www.cdc.gov./ncidod/hip/isolat/isopart2.htm*

STANDARD PRECAUTIONS

Although universal precautions were designed to address the transmission of blood-borne infections through blood and certain body fluids, they do not address other routes of disease transmission, which were addressed at the time by body substance isolation guidelines. Additionally, confusion developed as to whether one should use universal precautions and body substance isolation guidelines, because both guidelines dealt with similar circumstances but offered conflicting recommendations. The guideline for isolation precautions in hospitals was revised in 1996 by the CDC and the Hospital Infection Control Practices Advisory Committee (HICPAC), which had been established in 1991 to serve in a guiding and advisory capacity to the Secretary of the Department of Health and Human Services (DHHS), the Assistant Secretary of Health of the DHHS, the Director of the CDC, and the Director of the National Center for Infectious Diseases with respect to hospital infection control practices and U.S. hospital surveillance, prevention, and control strategies for nosocomial infections. The CDC guideline revision was designed to include the following objectives:

> *(1) to be epidemiologically sound; (2) to recognize the importance of all body fluids, secretions, and excretions in the transmission of nosocomial pathogens; (3) to contain adequate precautions for infections transmitted by the airborne, droplet, and contact routes of transmission; (4) to be as simple and user friendly as possible; and (5) to use new terms to avoid confusion with existing infection control and isolation systems.*
>
> (Garner, 1996)

The new guidelines were designed to supersede universal precautions and body substance isolation guidelines and in essence combined parts of both these previous guidelines. This synthesis of guidelines allows patients who were previously covered under disease-specific guidelines to now fall under standard precautions, a single set of recommendations. For patients who require additional precautions (defined as *transmission-based precautions,* for use when additional transmission risk exists [e.g., from airborne or droplet contamination]), additional guidelines have been developed to go above and beyond those of standard precautions (Garner, 1996) (see Table 2-1).

GLOVES, GOWNS, MASKS, AND OTHER PROTECTIVE BARRIERS AS PART OF UNIVERSAL PRECAUTIONS

All health care workers should routinely use appropriate barrier precautions to prevent skin and mucous membrane exposure during contact with any patient's blood or body fluids that require universal precautions.

Gloves should be worn as follows:

- For touching blood and body fluids requiring universal precautions, mucous membranes, or nonintact skin of all patients

- For handling items or surfaces soiled with blood or body fluids to which universal precautions apply

Gloves should be changed after contact with each patient. Hands and other skin surfaces should be washed immediately or as soon as patient safety permits if contaminated with blood or body fluids requiring universal precautions. Hands should be washed immediately after gloves are removed. Gloves should reduce the incidence of blood contamination of hands during phlebotomy, but they cannot prevent penetrating injuries caused by needles or other sharp instruments. Institutions that judge routine gloving for all phlebotomies as not necessary should periodically re-evaluate their policy. Gloves should always be available to health care workers who wish to use them for phlebotomy. In addition, the following general guidelines apply:

- Use gloves for performing phlebotomy when the health care worker has cuts, scratches, or other breaks in the skin.

- Use gloves in situations in which the health care worker judges that hand contamination with blood may occur; for example, when performing phlebotomy in an uncooperative patient.

- Use gloves for performing finger or heel sticks, or both, in infants and children.

- Use gloves when persons are receiving training in phlebotomy.

Masks and protective eyewear or face shields should be worn by health care workers to prevent exposure of mucous membranes of the mouth, nose, and eyes during procedures that are likely to generate droplets of blood or body fluids requiring universal precautions. Gowns or aprons should be worn during procedures that are likely to generate splashes of blood or body fluids requiring universal precautions.

All health care workers should take precautions to prevent injuries caused by needles, scalpels, and other sharp instruments or devices during procedures; when cleaning used instruments; during disposal of used needles; and when handling sharp instruments after procedures. To prevent needlestick injuries, needles should not be recapped by hand, purposely bent or broken by hand, removed from disposable syringes, or otherwise manipulated by hand. After they are used, disposable syringes and needles, scalpel blades, and other sharp items should be placed in puncture-resistant containers for disposal. The puncture-resistant containers should be located as close as is practical to the area of use. All reusable needles should be placed in puncture-resistant containers for transport to the reprocessing area.

General infection control practices should further minimize the already minute risk for salivary transmission of human immunodeficiency virus. These infection control practices include the use of gloves for digital examination of mucous membranes and endotracheal suctioning, hand washing after exposure to saliva, and minimizing the need for emergency mouth-to-mouth resuscitation by making mouthpieces and other ventilation devices available for use in areas where the need for resuscitation is predictable.

THE APPLICATION OF STANDARD PRECAUTIONS IN CLINICAL PROCEDURES

Standard precautions should be followed when performing any procedure in which exposure to, or transmission of, infectious agents is possible. These guidelines attempt to minimize exposure to infectious body fluids. Because it is not always possible to determine in advance whether a specific patient is infectious, these precautions should be followed routinely for all patients. The nature of performing clinical procedures often results in exposure to body fluids. Consequently, as practitioners involved in performing clinical procedures, it is imperative that we attempt to anticipate potential exposures and implement preventive guidelines to reduce exposure risks.

Additionally, it is important that the practitioner assess the health status of each patient to determine if additional precautions are warranted and, if so, apply the necessary transmission-based precautions as described in Table 2-1. Standard precautions are the current recommended behaviors designed to prevent the transmission of pathogens from patient to practitioner or practitioner to patient. It is imperative that all providers be knowledgable about standard precautions and transmission-based precautions and how to practice them competently and consistently.

REFERENCES

Centers for Disease Control and Prevention: Interim recommendations for infection control in health-care facillities caring for patients with known or suspected avian influenza. May 21, 2004. Available at http://www.cdc.gov/flu/avian/professional/infect-control.htm, accessed 7/3/06.

Centers for Disease Control and Prevention: Public health guidance for community-level preparedness and response to severe acute respiratory syndrome (SARS) version 2. Supplement I: Infection control in healthcare, home, and community setting. May 3, 2005. Available at http://www.cdc.gov/ncidod/sars/guidance/i/, accessed 7/3/06.

Centers for Disease Control and Prevention: Updated U.S. Public Health Service guidelines for the management of occupational exposures to HBV, HCV, and HIV and recommendations for postexposure prophylaxis. MMWR Morb Mortal Wkly Rep 50:1-42, 2001.

Centers for Disease Control and Prevention: Recommendations for prevention and control of hepatitis C virus (HCV) infection and HCV-related chronic disease. MMWR Morb Mortal Wkly Rep 47:1-39, 1998.

Centers for Disease Control and Prevention: Laboratory management of agents associated with hantavirus pulmonary syndrome: Interim biosafety guidelines. MMWR Morb Mortal Wkly Rep 43:1-7, 1994.

Centers for Disease Control: Guidelines for preventing the transmission of tuberculosis in health-care settings, with special focus on HIV-related issues. MMWR Morb Mortal Wkly Rep 39:1-29, 1990.

Centers for Disease Control: Risks associated with human parvovirus B19 infection. MMWR Morb Mortal Wkly Rep 38:81-88, 93-97, 1989.

Centers for Disease Control: Management of patients with suspected viral hemorrhagic fever. MMWR Morb Mortal Wkly Rep 37:1-16, 1988.

Centers for Disease Control: Update: Universal precautions for prevention of transmission of human immunodeficiency virus, hepatitis B virus, and other blood borne pathogens in health-care settings. MMWR Morb Mortal Wkly Rep 37:377-388, 1988.

Garner JS: Guideline for isolation precautions in hospitals. Part I. Evolution of isolation practices, Hospital Infection Control Practices Advisory Committee. Am J Infect Control 24:24-31, 1996.

Garner JS: Comments on CDC guideline for isolation precautions in hospitals, 1984. Am J Infect Control 12:163-164, 1984.

Haley RW, Garner JS, Simmons BP: A new approach to the isolation of patients with infectious diseases: Alternative systems. J Hosp Infect 6:128-139, 1985.

Lynch P, Cummings MJ, Roberts PL: Implementing and evaluating a system of generic infection precautions: Body substance isolation. Am J Infect Control 18:1-12, 1990.

Lynch P, Jackson MM: Rethinking the role of isolation precautions in the prevention of nosocomial infections. Ann Intern Med 107:243-246, 1987.

Lynch T: Communicable Disease Nursing. St. Louis, CV Mosby, 1949.

BIBLIOGRAPHY

American College of Physicians Task Force on Adult Immunization and Infectious Diseases Society of America: Guide for Adult Immunization, 3rd ed. Philadelphia, American College of Physicians, 1994.

Bell DM, Shapiro CN, Ciesielski CA, Chamberland ME: Preventing blood borne pathogen transmission from health care workers to patients: The CDC perspective. Surg Clin North Am 75:1189-1203, 1995.

Cardo DM, Culver DH, Ciesielski CA, et al: A case-control study of HIV seroconversion in health care workers after percutaneous exposure: Centers for Disease Control and Prevention Needlestick Surveillance Group. N Engl J Med 337:1485-1490, 1997.

Centers for Disease Control and Prevention: Public Health Service (PHS) guidelines for the management of health care worker exposures to HIV and recommendations for postexposure prophylaxis. MMWR Morb Mortal Wkly Rep 47:1-33, 1998.

Centers for Disease Control and Prevention: Immunization of health-care workers: Recommendations of the Advisory Committee on Immunization Practices (ACIP) and the Hospital Infection Control Practices Advisory Committee (HICPAC). MMWR Morb Mortal Wkly Rep 46:1-42, 1997.

Centers for Disease Control and Prevention: Recommendations for follow-up of health-care workers after occupational exposure to hepatitis C virus. MMWR Morb Mortal Wkly Rep 46:603-606, 1997.

Centers for Disease Control and Prevention: Case-control study of HIV seroconversion in health-care workers after percutaneous exposure to HIV infected blood—France, United Kingdom, and United States, January 1988-August 1994. MMWR Morb Mortal Wkly Rep 44:929-933, 1995.

Centers for Disease Control and Prevention: Hospital Infection Control Practices Advisory Committee: Guideline for prevention of nosocomial pneumonia. Infect Control Hosp Epidemiol 15:587-627, 1994.

Centers for Disease Control and Prevention: Guidelines for preventing the transmission of *Mycobacterium tuberculosis* in health-care facilities, 1994. MMWR Morb Mortal Wkly Rep 43:1-132, 1994.

Centers for Disease Control and Prevention: National Institutes for Health: Biosafety in Microbiological and Biomedical Laboratories, 3rd ed. Atlanta, U.S. Department of Health and Human Services, Public Health Service, 1993.

Centers for Disease Control and Prevention: Update on adult immunization: Recommendations of the Immunization Practices Advisory Committee (ACIP). MMWR Morb Mortal Wkly Rep 40:1-94, 1991.

Centers for Disease Control and Prevention: Protection against viral hepatitis: Recommendations of the Advisory Committee on Immunization Practices (ACIP). MMWR Morb Mortal Wkly Rep 39:1-27, 1990.

Chin J (ed): Control of Communicable Diseases Manual, 17th ed. Washington, DC, American Public Health Association, 1999.

Diekema DJ, Alabanese MA, Schuldt SS, Doebbeling BN: Blood and body fluid exposures during clinical training: Relation to knowledge of universal precautions. J Gen Intern Med 11:109-111, 1996.

Garner JS: Hospital Infection Control Practices Advisory Committee: Guidelines for Isolation Precautions in Hospitals. Infect Control Hosp Epidemiol 17:53-80, 1996.

Gerberding JL, Lewis FR Jr, Schecter WP: Are universal precautions realistic? Surg Clin North Am 75:1091-1104, 1995.

Moran G: Emergency department management of blood and fluid exposures. Ann Emerg Med 35:47-62, 2000.

National Committee for Clinical Laboratory Standards: Protection of laboratory workers from infectious disease transmitted by blood, body fluids, and tissue: Tentative guideline. NCCLS Document M29-T2, vol 11. Villanova, Pa, National Committee for Clinical Laboratory Standards, 1991, pp 1-214.

Orenstein R, Reynolds L, Karabaic M, et al: Do protective devices prevent needlestick injuries among health care workers? Am J Infect Control 23:344-351, 1995.

Osborn EH, Papadakis MA, Gerberding JL: Occupational exposures to body fluids among medical students: A seven-year longitudinal study. Ann Intern Med 130:45-51, 1999.

Peter G (ed): Report of the Committee on Infectious Diseases Red Book, 25th ed. Elk Grove Village, Ill, American Academy of Pediatrics, 2000.

U.S. Department of Labor, Occupational Health and Safety Administration: Criteria for recording on OSHA Form 200. OSHA instruction 1993, standard 1904. Washington, DC, U.S. Department of Labor, 1993.

U.S. Department of Labor, Occupational Safety and Health Administration: Occupational exposure to blood borne pathogens, final rule. CFR Part 1910.1030. Fed Reg 56:64004-64182, 1991.

U.S. Department of Labor, Occupational Health and Safety Administration: Record keeping guidelines for occupational injuries and illnesses: The Occupational Safety and Health Act of 1970 and 29 CFR 1904. OMB No. 120-0029. Washington, DC, U.S. Department of Labor, 1986.

Chapter 3

Sterile Technique

Paul C. Hendrix

PROCEDURE GOALS AND OBJECTIVES

Goal: To provide clinicians with the knowledge and skills necessary to perform clinical procedures using accepted sterile technique.

Objectives: The student will be able to …

- Describe the indications and rationale for practicing sterile technique.

- Identify and describe the history and development of the concept of sterile technique.

- List the principles of sterile technique.

- Describe the essential steps performed in the surgical hand scrub.

- Describe the essential steps performed in preparing and draping a sterile field.

- Describe the principles involved in the use of surgical caps, masks, and gowns.

- Describe the principles involved in the use of standard precautions.

BACKGROUND AND HISTORY

The teachings of Hippocrates (460 BC) were instrumental in turning the art of healing away from mystical rites to an approach that everyone could understand and practice. He stressed cleanliness to avoid infection by using boiling water and fire to clean instruments and by irrigating dirty wounds with wine or boiled water (Adams, 1929). Louis Pasteur (1822-1895) developed what would come to be known as the *germ theory of disease.* His experiments revealed that microbes could be found in the air and on the surface of every object (Dubos, 1950). He discovered that the number of microbes could be reduced on surfaces by using heat or appropriate cleansing but that they would still remain in the air. Joseph Lister (1827-1912) is considered the father of sterile technique (Godlee, 1917). When Lister learned of Pasteur's work, he began to experiment with various methods of sterile technique in surgery. He noted a significant decrease in postoperative infections after using carbolic acid to sterilize both surgical wounds and his own hands and by spraying the operative field. His antiseptic methods of performing surgery were refined over the years and eventually incorporated into hospitals worldwide.

PRINCIPLES OF STERILE TECHNIQUE

Sterile technique is the method by which contamination with microorganisms is minimized. Adherence to protocol and strict techniques is required at all times when caring for open wounds and performing invasive procedures. To avoid infection, procedures should be performed within a sterile field from which all living microbes have been excluded. Items entering the sterile field, including instruments, sutures, and fluids, must be sterile. Although it is not possible to sterilize the skin, it is possible to reduce significantly the number of bacteria that is normally present on the skin. Before a procedure, personnel must first perform a surgical hand scrub and then don sterile gloves, sterile gown, and mask. The primary goal is to provide an environment for the patient that promotes healing, prevents infections, and minimizes the length of recovery time. Using the principles of sterile technique will help accomplish that goal. The principles are as follows:

- All items used within a sterile field must be sterile.

- A sterile barrier that has been permeated must be considered contaminated.

- The edges of a sterile container are considered contaminated once the package is opened.

- Gowns are considered sterile in front from shoulder to waist level, and the sleeves are considered sterile to 2 inches above the elbow.

- Tables are sterile at table level only.

- Sterile persons and items touch only sterile areas; unsterile persons and items touch only unsterile areas.

- Movement within or around a sterile field must not contaminate the field.

- All items and areas of doubtful sterility are considered contaminated.

SURGICAL HAND SCRUB

The surgical hand scrub has its own traditions and rituals dating back to the use of chlorinated lime by Semmelweis, who in 1846 recognized the role of contagions on doctors' hands in the spread of puerperal fever, and the use of carbolic acid by Lister to soak his instruments and hands (Lister, 1867). The goal of the surgical hand scrub is to remove dirt and debris and to reduce bacterial flora. An ideal surgical hand scrub should provide the following antimicrobial effects:

- Immediate reduction in the resident bacterial flora

- Sustained effect to maintain a reduced bacterial count under surgical gloves

- Cumulative effect with each additional application of the antiseptic

- Persistent effect providing progressive reduction of bacteria with additional applications

The traditional 10-minute surgical scrub, using a stiff brush and harsh chemicals, does not meet the criteria for satisfactory antimicrobial action (an immediate reduction in microbial count that is sustained, cumulative, and persistent) and is associated with a number of difficulties and problems, chiefly a high incidence of irritation and dermatitis that can paradoxically result in an increased microbial population on the hands (Larson, 1986). Modifications have been made to the traditional surgical hand scrub to increase its beneficial effects and to decrease its harmful effects.

The duration of the recommended scrub time has been decreased so that a 2-minute scrub time is now considered by some to be optimal (Wheelock, 1997). Some authors have recommended eliminating the scrub brush, to decrease abrasion of the hands (Gruendemann, 2001). New antiseptics, emollients, and humectants have been developed to minimize skin dryness and dermatitis resulting from the surgical hand scrub. New procedures and products for hand hygiene and the surgical hand scrub have been consolidated into a publication that was issued by the Centers for Disease Control and Prevention (CDC) in 2002. These guidelines are comprehensive, providing an analysis of the science of hand hygiene and specific recommendations for surgical hand antisepsis (CDC, 2002):

SURGICAL HAND ANTISEPSIS

1. Remove rings, watches, and bracelets before beginning the "surgical hand scrub" (i.e., a process to remove or destroy transient microorganisms and reduce resident flora).
2. Remove debris from underneath fingernails using a nail cleaner under running water.
3. "Surgical hand antisepsis" (i.e., a process for removal or destruction of transient microorganisms) using either an antimicrobial soap or an alcohol-based hand rub with persistent activity is recommended before donning sterile gloves when performing surgical procedures.
4. When performing surgical hand antisepsis using an antimicrobial soap, scrub hands and forearms for the length of time recommended by the manufacturer, usually 2 to 6 minutes. Long scrub times (e.g., 10 minutes) are not necessary.
5. When using an alcohol-based surgical hand scrub product with persistent activity, follow the manufacturer's instructions. Before applying the alcohol solution, prewash hands and forearms with a nonantimicrobial soap and dry hands and forearms completely. After application of the alcohol-based product as recommended, allow hands and forearms to dry thoroughly before donning sterile gloves.

Materials Utilized for Hand Scrub

- Chlorhexidine gluconate or povidone-iodine solutions are rapid-acting, broad-spectrum antimicrobials that are effective against gram-positive and gram-negative microorganisms. Each is prepared in combination with a detergent to give a cleansing action along with the antimicrobial effect.

- Sterile disposable scrub brushes impregnated with chlorhexidine gluconate, povidone-iodine, or other CDC-approved products (CDC, 2002).

Procedures for the Surgical Scrub: Timed (Anatomic) and Counted Stroke Methods

Note: Two methods of surgical scrubbing are typically used: the *timed method* (Fig. 3-1), which is illustrated here, and the *counted stroke method.* Both methods follow a prescribed anatomic pattern of scrubbing beginning with the fingernails, then moving on to the four surfaces of each finger, the palmar and dorsal surfaces of the hands and wrists, and extending up the arms to the elbows. The timed method requires a total of 5 minutes of scrub time. The counted stroke method requires a specific number of bristle strokes for the fingers, hands, and arms. The scrub includes 30 strokes for the fingernails and 20 strokes to each surface of the fingers, hands, wrists, and arms to the elbows.

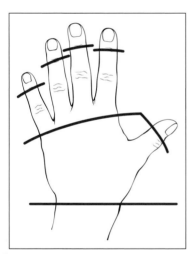

FIGURE 3-1.

1. Organize supplies and adjust water to a comfortable temperature.

2. Wet hands and arms, prewash with soap from a dispenser, rinse.

3. Remove scrub brush from package and use nail cleaner to clean fingernails.

4. Squeeze scrub brush under water to release soap from sponge.

5. With scrub brush perpendicular to fingers, begin to scrub all four sides of each finger with a back-and-forth motion.

6. Scrub dorsal and palmar surfaces of hand and wrist with a circular motion.

7. Starting at the wrist, scrub all four sides of the arm to the elbow.

8. Transfer scrub brush to the other hand and repeat steps 5 to 7.

9. Discard scrub brush and rinse hands and arms, starting with the fingertips and working toward the elbows.

10. Allow contaminated water to drip off the elbows by keeping hands above the waist

Materials Utilized to Prepare the Procedure Site

Note: Preparation trays are commercially available and typically include the listed necessary items.

- Disposable razors to remove hair from the procedure site

- Towels

- Antiseptic soap: There are multiple antiseptic skin scrubs available. The most commonly used are iodine-based soaps and solutions.

- Gauze sponges

- Large clamp or ring forceps to hold the preparation sponge or gauze

Procedure for Preparing the Operative Site

1. Scrub the skin with the antiseptic solution, beginning at the procedure site and working outward in a circular fashion toward the periphery of the field (Fig. 3-2). Make sure the area prepared is much wider than the procedure site.

Note: The scrubbing action must be vigorous, including both mechanical and chemical cleansing of the skin.

2. On reaching the outer boundary, discard the first sponge and repeat the procedure until all prepared sponges are used.

Figure 3-2.

Caution: Do not return to a previously prepared area with a contaminated sponge.

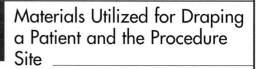

Materials Utilized for Draping a Patient and the Procedure Site

Note: Draping the procedure site and the patient follows preparing the skin.

• Drapes: typically green, blue, or gray to reduce glare and eye fatigue

• Types of drapes: towels, sheets, split sheets, fenestrated sheets, stockinette, and plastic incision drapes

Note: Each type of drape has a specific use; for example, fenestrated sheets have a window that exposes the procedure site, and stockinette is used to cover the extremities circumferentially. Drapes must be lint-free, antistatic, fluid resistant, abrasive-free, and made to fit contours.

Procedure for Draping

Note: Draping is the process of maintaining a sterile field around the procedure site by covering the surrounding areas and the patient with a barrier.

1. Hold the drapes high enough to avoid touching unsterile areas.

2. Always walk around the table to drape the opposite side.

Caution: Never reach over the patient.

3. Handle drapes as little as possible and avoid shaking out wrinkles (contaminants are present in the air).

4. When draping, make a cuff over the gloved hand to protect against touching an unsterile area, and place the folded edge toward the incision to provide a

uniform outline of the surgical site and to prevent instruments or sponges from falling between layers.

Note: Any part of the drape below waist or table level is considered unsterile. Towel clips fastened through the drapes have contaminated points and should be removed only if necessary.

5. If a hole is found in a drape after it is placed, cover it with a second drape.

6. Drapes should not be adjusted after placement. If a drape is placed improperly, either discard it or cover it with another drape.

Procedure for Maintaining a Sterile Field

Note: The sterile field includes the draped patient and any scrubbed personnel.

1. Someone outside the sterile field must hand items needed during the procedure into the sterile field. This is the reason a minimum of two individuals is required to do most procedures—one with unsterile hands to pass instruments and supplies into the sterile field, and one with gloved hands working within the sterile field.

Note: Sterile supplies are uniformly packaged in such a way to allow an unsterile person to open and pass them safely, without contamination, into the sterile field.

2. Contamination of supplies or personnel within the sterile field must be addressed immediately. This includes changing gowns or gloves and removing from the sterile field any instrument or supplies that have become contaminated.

3. Unsterile personnel must avoid contact with the sterile field by remaining at a safe distance (at least 12 inches away) and by always facing the field when passing to avoid accidental contact.

4. Every individual involved with the procedure must immediately call attention to any observed breaks, or suspected breaks, in sterile technique.

5. If the sterility of any item is in doubt, it must be considered contaminated, removed from the sterile field, and replaced with a sterile item.

Caution: There is no compromise with sterility. An item is either sterile or unsterile.

Procedure for Wearing Surgical Masks, Caps, and Gowns

Note: Because of the large number of potentially harmful microbes that reside in the respiratory tract, surgical masks are recommended at all times when there are open sterile items or sterile instruments present.

1. Fit the mask snugly over both the nose and the mouth and tie securely (Fig. 3-3).

2. When wearing a mask, keep conversation to a minimum to prevent moisture buildup.

3. Change surgical masks routinely between procedures or during a procedure if they become moist or wet.

continued

FIGURE 3-3.

FIGURE 3-4.

Note: Surgical caps prevent unsterile material from the hair entering the sterile field. The standard unisex surgical cap is adequate for women and men with short hair, but a more voluminous cap is required for long hair. Both caps and masks generally are made of paper and are disposable.

Note: For lengthy procedures, or when it is necessary to put the forearms into the sterile field, a sterile surgical gown is required (Figs. 3-4 and 3-5). Procedures for which gloves are sufficient include joint aspiration, suturing a minor laceration, and performing a lumbar puncture. A gown is required for repairing a large wound, for cardiac catheterization, or for any procedure that requires it by protocol. Only the front of the gown above the waist level and the lower portion of the sleeves are considered sterile. Even though the entire gown is sterile initially, brushing against an unsterile object with the back, sides, or lower portion of the gown is easy to do.

FIGURE 3-5.

SPECIAL CONSIDERATIONS

Standard Precautions   In 1987, the CDC developed universal precautions, later incorporated into standard precautions, which were designed to protect health care personnel from unknown exposures from the patient and environment. The CDC (1987) stated, "Since medical history and examination cannot identify all patients who are potentially infected with blood-borne pathogens, specific precautions should be used with all patients, thereby reducing the risk of possible exposure to its minimum."

Therefore, all procedures and patients should be considered to be potentially contaminated, and strict protocols should be followed to prevent exposure to blood and body fluids. The CDC advised that health care workers could reduce the risk of exposure and contamination by adhering to the following guidelines:

1. Use appropriate barrier protection to prevent skin and mucous membrane exposure when contact with blood and body fluids of any patient is anticipated. Gloves, masks, and protective eyewear or face shields should be worn during all surgical procedures and when handling soiled supplies or instruments during or after a procedure to prevent exposure of mucous membranes.
2. Wash hands and other skin surfaces immediately and thoroughly if contaminated with blood or other body fluids. Although both sterile and unsterile personnel wear gloves during a surgical procedure, hand washing after the removal of gloves should become a routine practice for all personnel working in a procedure room.
3. Take all necessary precautions to protect against injuries caused by needles, scalpels, and other sharp instruments or devices during procedures; when cleaning used instruments; and when handling sharp instruments after a procedure. Needles should never be recapped or bent after use. Suture needles and sharps should be contained in a puncture-resistant container and sealed for proper disposal according to recommended practices and established protocols. Sharp instruments should be placed in a tray in such a way that their points are not exposed so that injury to persons working with the trays is avoided. During the procedure, care must be taken when handling suture needles to ensure that no one receives an injury by placing the needle on a needle holder and passing it with the point down.
4. Health care workers who have exudative lesions or weeping dermatitis should refrain from all direct patient care and from handling patient care equipment until the condition resolves. Individuals with minor breaks in the skin should restrict scrubbing activities until the breaks have healed. Sterile gloves should be worn if a skin lesion is present, and the lesion covered when working in a procedure room.

The Occupational Safety and Health Administration (OSHA) has adopted these guidelines in its efforts to maintain a safe working environment. In addition, both OSHA and the CDC recommend that aspirated or drainage material never come into contact with health care providers. Thus, the use of an adequate suctioning system is important during procedures, with careful disposal protocols after the procedure is completed. For more information on standard precautions, see Chapter 2.

Disposal of Materials

1. Care should be taken to dispose of contaminated supplies and materials to avoid the transmission of infectious organisms to others.
2. Sharp objects should be disposed in appropriately marked containers.
3. Body fluids, human tissue, disposable gowns, gloves, caps, and drapes should be placed in containers marked with the appropriate biohazard warnings.
4. All receptacles containing biohazardous waste should be properly labeled and identified and processed according to institutional procedures.

REFERENCES

Adams F: The Genuine Works of Hippocrates. New York, W. Wood, 1929.

Centers for Disease Control and Prevention: Guideline for hand hygiene in health-care settings. MMWR Recomm Rep 51(RR-16):1-45, 2002.

Centers for Disease Control and Prevention: Recommendations for prevention of HIV transmission in health-care settings. MMWR Morb Mortal Wkly Rep 36(suppl 2):1S-18S, 1987.

Dubos R: Louis Pasteur: Free Lance of Science. Boston, Little, Brown, 1950.

Godlee RJ: Lord Lister. London, Macmillan, 1917.

Gruendemann BJ: Is it time for brushless scrubbing with an alcohol-based agent? AORN J 74:859-873, 2001.

Larson E: Physiologic and microbiologic changes in skin related to frequent handwashing. Infect Control Hosp Epidemiol 7:59-63, 1986.

Lister J: On a new method of treating compound fractures, abscess, etc. with observations on the conditions of suppuration. Lancet 1:326, 357, 507, 1867.

Wheelock SM: Effect of surgical hand scrub time on subsequent bacterial growth. AORN J 65:1087-1098, 1997.

Chapter 4

Blood Pressure Measurement

Randy Danielsen

PROCEDURE GOALS AND OBJECTIVES

Goal: To accurately measure the systemic arterial blood pressure in any patient in any setting.

Objectives: The student will be able to ...

- Describe the indications, contraindications, and rationale for performing arterial blood pressure measurement.

- Describe the essential anatomy and physiology associated with the performance of blood pressure measurement.

- Identify the necessary materials and their proper use for performing blood pressure measurement.

- Perform the proper steps and techniques for obtaining blood pressure measurement.

- Describe the indications for performing orthostatic blood pressure assessment.

- Perform the proper steps and techniques for obtaining orthostatic blood pressure measurement.

BACKGROUND AND HISTORY

Various theories about circulation and blood pressure (BP) emerged about 400 BC. Hippocrates knew about arteries and veins, but he believed veins carried air. Six hundred years later, Galen demonstrated that both arteries and veins carried blood; however, he also thought that the heart was a warming machine for two separate types of blood. He was convinced that veins and arteries were not connected and that blood flowed both backward and forward from the heart. Subsequently Galen's teachings remained unchallenged for over 1000 years (Stevens, 1978).

It was William Harvey, in 1616, who disagreed with Galen by demonstrating one-way circulation of blood and theorized the existence of capillaries. Thirty years later, Marcello Malpighi was the first to view capillaries microscopically (Stevens, 1978).

The first person to measure BP was Stephen Hales in 1733. An English physiologist, clergyman, and amateur scientist, Hales inserted a brass pipe into the carotid artery of a mare and then attached the pipe to a windpipe taken from a goose. The flexible goose windpipe was then attached to a 12-foot glass tube. Although the experiment had little practical application at the time, it did provide valuable information about BP (Wain, 1970).

Although Ritter von Basch experimented with a device that could measure the BP of a human without breaking the skin, the prototype design of the sphygmomanometer was devised in 1896 by Scipione Riva-Rocci (Lyons, 1987). He introduced a method for indirect measurement of BP based on measuring the external pressure required to compress the brachial artery so that arterial pulsations could no longer be transmitted through the artery. The Riva-Rocci sphygmomanometer was described by Porter (1997) as "an inflatable band that was wrapped around the upper arm; air was pumped in until the pulse disappeared; it then was released from the band until the pulse reappeared, and the reading was taken."

In 1905, a Russian physician named Korotkoff first discovered the auscultatory sounds that are heard while measuring BP. While the artery is occluded during BP measurement, transmitted pulse waves can no longer be heard distal to the point of occlusion. As the pressure in the bladder is reduced by opening a valve on the inflation bulb, pulsatile blood flow reappears through the generally compressed artery, producing repetitive sounds generated by the pulsatile flow. The sounds, named after Korotkoff, change in quality and intensity. The five phases of these changes are characterized in Table 4-1. Around the turn of the 20th century, BP became an accepted clinical measurement. As data increased, physicians and other clinicians were able to establish normal BP ranges and identify abnormalities.

René Laënnec is credited with the invention of the stethoscope in 1816, which became a convenience for physicians who preferred not to place their ears directly on the chest wall of a patient. In 1905, Korotkoff tried using the stethoscope to monitor the pulse while the sphygmomanometer was inflated. He discovered a more accurate BP reading and that the pulse disappeared as the cuff pressure decreased at a point in consonance with the expanding of

Table 4.1	**Korotkoff Sounds***		

PHASE

I	First appearance of clear, repetitive, tapping sounds; this coincides approximately with the reappearance of a palpable pulse
II	Sounds are softer and longer, with the quality of an intermittent murmur
III	Sounds again become crisper and louder
IV	Sounds are muffled, less distinct, and softer
V	Sounds disappear completely

*As the pressure is reduced during deflation of the occluding cuff, the Korotkoff sounds change in quality and intensity.

From Perloff D, Grimm C, Flack J, et al: Human blood pressure determination by sphygmomanometry. Circulation 88:2461, 1993.

the heart. Subsequently, the term *Korotkoff sounds* came to be used (Lyons, 1987).

According to Grim and Grim (2000):

Indirect BP measurement is one of the most frequently performed health care procedures. Because BP measurement is a simple procedure, it is taken for granted that all graduates from medical training programs have the ability to record accurate, precise, and reliable BP readings. However, research since the 1960s has shown this assumption to be false. Most health professionals do not measure BP in a manner known to be accurate and reliable.

The authors describe two factors that contribute to inaccurate BP measurement: (1) lack of depth in the instruction of basic skills in professional education; and (2) relying on nonmercury devices. Subsequently, every clinician who takes BP measurements should know and understand the principles and steps needed to obtain accurate indirect auscultatory BP measurement. The measurement taken is an important tool in screening and diagnosis, which is why it is considered one of the patient's "vital signs."

For the accurate indirect measurement of BP, the American Heart Association (AHA) recommends that the cuff size be based solely on the limb circumference. Manning, Kuchirka, and Kaminski studied prevailing cuffing habits, compared them with AHA guidelines, and reported their findings in *Circulation* in 1983. They found that "miscuffing" occurred in 65 (32%) of 200 BP determinations in 167 unselected adult outpatients, including 61 (72%) of 85 readings taken on "nonstandard-size" arms. Undercuffing large arms was the most frequent error, accounting for 84% of the miscuffings. They concluded that undercuffing elevates the BP readings by an average of 8.5 mm Hg systolic and 4.6 mm Hg diastolic. It is critical, therefore, that the clinician choose the appropriate size cuff based on the circumference of a patient's bare upper arm. The bladder (inside the cuff) length should encircle 80% and the width should cover 33% to 50% of an adult's upper arm. For a child younger than 13 years of age, the bladder should encircle 100% of the child's upper arm. A cuff that is too narrow or too large for an arm may result in an incorrect BP reading. Cuffs that are generally available usually have been classified by the width of the bladder rather than by the length and are labeled *newborn, infant, child, small adult, adult, large adult,* and *thigh.*

Over- and underestimation of BP by using an inappropriate cuff size has been well documented in the literature. Health care settings should have easy access to small, standard, and large cuffs (Graves, 2001).

INDICATIONS

As one of the vital signs, peripheral BP measurement is an indirect method of determining cardiovascular function. Its use is indicated for evaluation of both healthy and unhealthy patients to assess cardiac status. BP measurement is a part of every complete physical or screening examination and is performed to screen for hypertension or hypotension.

CONTRAINDICATIONS

There are no absolute contraindications to measuring BP. Relative contraindications include physical defects and therapeutic interventions, such as indwelling intravenous catheters and renal dialysis shunts.

POTENTIAL COMPLICATIONS

Complications from measurement of BP occur as a result of improper training of the individual performing the assessment. Overinflation or prolonged time of inflation may lead to tissue or vascular damage at the measurement site. Lack of proper care of equipment or flawed equipment may give an inaccurate reading.

REVIEW OF ESSENTIAL ANATOMY AND PHYSIOLOGY

In most clinical settings, BP is measured by the indirect technique of using a sphygmomanometer placed over the brachial artery of the upper extremity. The brachial artery is a continuation of the axillary artery, which lies medial to the humerus proximally and gradually moves anterior to the humerus as it nears the antecubital crease (Fig. 4-1). Placement of the bladder and cuff of the sphygmomanometer circumferentially over the brachial artery allows inflation of the cuff to create adequate pressure so that the artery is fully occluded when the pressure exceeds the systolic pressure within the brachial artery.

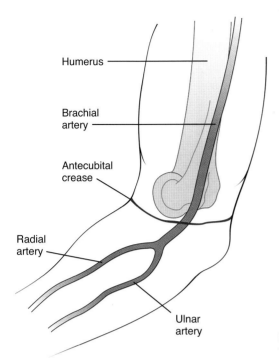

Humerus

Brachial
artery

Antecubital
crease

Radial
artery

Ulnar
artery

FIGURE 4-1. Location of the
brachial artery.

Indirect measurement of the BP involves the auscultatory detection of the initial presence and disappearance of changes and the disappearance of Korotkoff sounds, which are audible with the aid of a stethoscope placed over the brachial artery distal to the BP cuff near the antecubital crease. Korotkoff sounds are low-pitched sounds (best heard with the stethoscope bell) that originate from the turbulence created by the partial occlusion of the artery with the inflated BP cuff.

As long as the pressure within the cuff is so little that it does not produce even partial occlusion (or intermittent occlusion), no sound is produced when auscultating over the brachial artery distal to the cuff. When the cuff pressure becomes great enough to occlude the artery during at least some portion of the arterial pressure cycle, a sound becomes audible over the brachial artery distal to the cuff. This sound is audible with a stethoscope and correlates with each arterial pulsation.

There are five phases of Korotkoff sounds used in determining systolic and diastolic BP (see Table 4-1). Phase I occurs as the occluding pressure of the cuff falls to a point that is the same as the peak systolic pressure within the brachial artery (Fig. 4-2). The tapping sound that is produced is clear and generally increases in intensity as the occluding pressure continues to decrease. Phase II occurs at a point approximately 10 to 15 mm Hg lower than at the onset of phase I, and the sounds become softer and longer with a quality of intermittent murmur. Phase III occurs when the occluding pressure of the cuff falls to a point that allows for large amounts of blood to cross the

FIGURE 4-2. Phase 1 of Korotkoff sounds.

partially occluded brachial artery. The phase III sounds are again crisper and louder than phase II sounds. Phase IV occurs when there is an abrupt muffling and decrease in the intensity of the sounds. This occurs as the pressure is close to that of the diastolic pressure of the brachial artery. Phase V occurs when the blood vessel is no longer occluded by the pressure in the cuff. At this point, the tapping sound disappears completely.

PATIENT PREPARATION

Ideally, the environment should be relaxed and peaceful. BP levels may be affected by emotions, physical activity, or the environment. Subsequently, the examiner should minimize any and all disturbances that may affect the reading. The procedure should be explained to the patient.

The patient is asked to be seated or to lie down with the back supported, making sure that the bare arm is supported horizontally at the level of the heart. According to Mourad and Carney (2004):

> *Choosing the dependent arm is a behavior likely to lead to the overdiagnosis of hypertension and inappropriate treatment of hypertension because the dependent arm falsely elevates both systolic and diastolic blood pressure. These results should encourage national and international organizations to reaffirm the importance of the horizontal arm in the measurement of blood pressure.*

The clinician should avoid an arm that appears injured or has a fistula or an IV or arterial line. If the patient has undergone breast or axilla surgery, avoid the arm on the same side. It is important to note that rolling up the sleeves

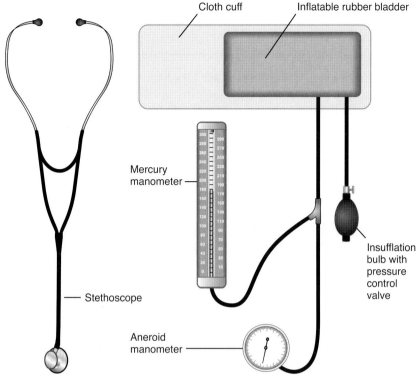

Cloth cuff   Inflatable rubber bladder

Mercury manometer

Insufflation bulb with pressure control valve

Stethoscope

Aneroid manometer

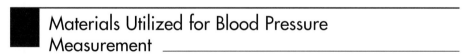

FIGURE 4-3.   Instruments used for recording blood pressure.

has the potential of compressing the brachial artery and may have an even greater effect on the BP than if the shirt is left under the manometer's cuff (Lieb, 2004) The patient should avoid smoking or ingesting caffeine for 30 minutes before the BP is recorded.

Materials Utilized for Blood Pressure Measurement

- Stethoscope

- Calibrated sphygmomanometer (a mercury, aneroid, or hybrid sphygmomanometer with a calibrated scale for measuring pressure; inflatable rubber bladders; tubes; and valves). There continues to be environmental concern over the use of mercury sphygmomanometers because of the hazards of mercury spills and potential exposure (see "Note"). As a result, more automated devices are being used (Valler-Jones, 2005). One of the factors affecting the accuracy of BP measurement is the equipment used. Defects or inaccuracy of aneroid sphygmanometers may be a source of error in BP measurement.

- Recording instruments (Fig. 4-3)

■ Appropriate size cuff: A cuff that has an antimicrobial agent to help prevent bacterial growth is recommended. It has been reported that BP cuffs can carry significant bacterial colonization and actually can be a source of transmission of infection (Base-Smith, 1996).

Note: Modern sphygmomanometers are less likely to spill mercury if dropped. If a spill occurs, however, mercury is fairly simple to clean up unless it is spilled within heated devices or is trapped in upholstery, carpeting, or other surfaces. Unfortunately, mercury in the organic form is extremely toxic via skin contact, inhalation, and ingestion and may require the calling of a hazardous materials team. If mercury manometers are used, a mercury spill kit is recommended.

Procedure for Indirect Blood Pressure Measurement

1. Check to see that the mercury level of the sphygmomanometer is at 0 or, if an aneroid device is used, that the needle rests within the calibration window.

2. Palpate the brachial artery and place the cuff so that the midline of the bladder is over the arterial pulsation. Care should be taken that the cuff is placed at approximately the horizontal level of the heart.

3. Wrap and secure the cuff snugly around the patient's bare upper arm. The lower edge of the cuff should be 1 inch (approximately 2 cm) above the antecubital crease, the point at which the bell of the stethoscope is to be placed (Fig. 4-4). As noted earlier, avoid rolling up the sleeve in such a manner that it may form a tight tourniquet around the upper arm.

4. Place the manometer so that the center of the mercury column or aneroid dial is at eye level and clearly visible to the examiner. Make sure that the tubing from the cuff is unobstructed.

5. Inflate the cuff rapidly to 70 mm Hg and increase by increments of 10 mm Hg while palpating the radial pulse. Note the

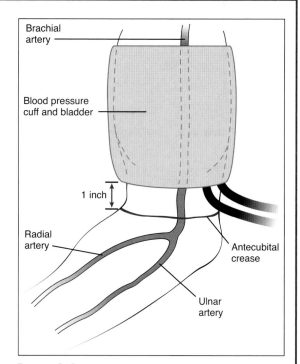

FIGURE 4-4.

level of pressure at which the pulse disappears and subsequently reappears during deflation. This procedure, the palpatory method, provides the necessary preliminary approximation of the systolic pressure to ensure an adequate level of inflation when the actual, auscultatory measurement is accomplished. The palpatory method is particularly useful to avoid underinflation of the cuff in patients with an auscultatory gap and overinflation in those with very low BP. The auscultatory gap occurs at a point between the highest systolic reading and the diastolic reading. The Korotkoff sounds may become absent between the peak systolic measurement and diastole, resulting in underestimation of the peak systolic BP if the cuff is not initially inflated to a high enough pressure.

6. Place the earpieces of the stethoscope into your ear canals, angled forward to fit snugly.

7. Switch the stethoscope head to the low-frequency position (bell).

8. Place the bell of the stethoscope over the brachial artery pulsation just above and medial to the antecubital crease but below the lower edge of the cuff (Fig. 4-5). Hold it firmly in place, making sure the bell makes contact with the skin around the entire circumference. Excessive pressure will result in stretching the underlying skin, causing the bell to function as a diaphragm. This may result in the loss of low-frequency sounds.

9. Inflate the bladder rapidly and steadily to a pressure 20 to 30 mm Hg above the level previously determined by palpation. Partially unscrew the valve and deflate the bladder at 2 mm per second while listening for the appearance of Korotkoff sounds.

Figure 4-5.

10. As the pressure in the bladder falls, note the level of the pressure on the manometer at the first appearance of repetitive sounds, the continuation of the sounds, and when the sounds disappear. During the period of the Korotkoff sounds (see Table 4-1), the rate of deflation should be less than 2 mm per beat, thereby compensating for both rapid and slow heart rates.

11. Record the systolic and diastolic pressure immediately, rounded off upward to the nearest 2 mm Hg. The name of the patient, the date and time of measurement, the arm or site at which the measurement was taken, the cuff size, and the patient's position while taking the measurement should be noted.

12. Neither the patient nor the clinician should talk during the measurement.

SPECIAL CONSIDERATIONS

THE APPREHENSIVE PATIENT OR "WHITE COAT" HYPERTENSION

Ambulatory blood pressure measurement (ABPM) is increasingly being used in clinical practice (O'Brien, 2003). ABPMs correlate better than clinical measurements on patients with end-organ injury (Verdecchia, 2000). Twenty-four-hour ABPM is the most efficient means for assessing white coat hypertension (WCH), particularly in the absence of end-organ disease. WCH has been defined as clinical BP greater than 140 mm Hg systolic and 90 mm Hg diastolic (Al-Hermi, 2004). Ambulatory measurements are also valuable in assessing patients with apparent drug resistance, low BP symptoms, and in patients taking antihypertensive medications. There is now wider acceptance of BP readings taken by patients in their homes. Patients should be encouraged to monitor their BP at home with validated devices followed by appropriate recording and reporting to their clinician.

THE OBESE OR LARGE ARM

It is well known that BP measurement with a standard 12- to 13-inch (27- to 34-cm) wide cuff is inappropriate for large or obese arms. If the arm circumference of the patient exceeds 13 inches (34 cm), use a thigh cuff 17 to 20 inches (18 cm) wide on the patient's upper arm. Table 4-2 gives acceptable bladder dimensions for adult arms of different sizes. In patients with extremely large arms, place the cuff on the patient's forearm and listen over the radial artery. Occasionally, it may be necessary to determine the BP in the leg; this may be required to rule out coarctation of the aorta or if an upper extremity BP determination is contraindicated. To do this, use a wide, long thigh cuff

Table 4.2 **Acceptable Bladder Dimensions for Arms of Different Sizes***			
CUFF	BLADDER WIDTH (CM)	BLADDER LENGTH (CM)	ARM CIRCUMFERENCE RANGE AT MIDPOINT (CM)
Newborn	3	6	<6
Infant	5	15	6-15[†]
Child	8	21	16-21[†]
Small adult	10	24	22-26
Adult	13	30	27-34
Large adult	16	38	35-44
Adult thigh	20	42	45-52

*There is some overlapping of the recommended range for arm circumferences in order to limit the number of cuffs; it is recommended that the larger cuff be used when available.
[†]To approximate the bladder width–to–arm circumference ratio of 0.40 more closely in infants and children, additional cuffs are available.
  From http://www.americanheart.org/presenter.jhtml?identifier=3000861; accessed May 6, 2006.

with a bladder size of 45 to 52 cm and apply it to the mid-thigh. Center the bladder over the posterior surface, wrap it securely, and listen over the popliteal artery (Perloff, 1993).

According to Pickering and colleagues (2005), "wrist monitors may be useful in very obese patients if the monitor is held at heart level. Finger monitors are not recommended." Block and Schulte (1996) discussed ankle BP measurements and found that mean BP readings obtained at the arm and at the ankle were statistically equivalent and concluded that ankle cuff placement provided a reliable alternative to the placement of the cuff on the arm.

INFANTS AND CHILDREN

Measuring BP in infants and children presents special problems to the clinician. The same measuring techniques are used as in adults. As mentioned earlier, pediatric cuff sizes are available to ensure that the bladder completely encircles the upper arm. Various techniques can enforce patient compliance—using relaxation techniques for the child, having the mother inflate the BP cuff, and/or demonstrating BP measurement on a stuffed animal.

ELDERLY PATIENTS

In elderly patients, who may have significant atherosclerosis, it is likely that the systolic pressure is overestimated by the indirect method of BP measurement. BP tends to be more labile in elderly patients, so it is important to obtain several baseline measurements before making any diagnostic or therapeutic decisions (Joint National Committee on Prevention, Detection, Evaluation, and Treatment of High Blood Pressure, 2003). ABPM is very useful in this age group.

ASSESSMENT OF ORTHOSTATIC BLOOD PRESSURE

The measurement of orthostatic BP is an essential clinical tool for the assessment and management of patients suffering from many common medical disorders. The most common causes are volume depletion and autonomic dysfunction. According to Carlson (1999), orthostatic hypotension, which is a decline in BP when standing erect, is the "result of an impaired hemodynamic response to an upright posture or a depletion of intravascular volume. The measurement of orthostatic blood pressure can be done at the bedside and is therefore easily applied to several clinical disorders."

Orthostatic hypotension is detected in 10% to 20% of community-dwelling older individuals (Mader, 1987). This condition is frequently asymptomatic, but disabling symptoms of light-headedness, weakness, unsteadiness, blurred vision, and syncope may occur.

The American Academy of Neurology's consensus statement (1996) defines orthostatic hypotension as a "reduction of systolic blood pressure of at least 20 mm Hg or diastolic blood pressure of at least 10 mm Hg within 3 minutes of standing."

Many clinicians use a combination of a decrease in BP combined with an increase in heart rate to determine the presence of orthostatic hypotension.

Performing these orthostatic measurements requires adequate techniques in BP measurement, appropriate positioning of the patient, and proper timing of the measurements.

Materials Utilized for Measuring Orthostatic Blood Pressure

This technique requires the same equipment as previously mentioned for measuring BP.

Procedure for Measuring Orthostatic Blood Pressure

1. Ask the patient about his or her ability to stand.

2. Make sure the cuffed arm is positioned so that the brachial artery is held at the level of the heart.

3. After 5 to 10 minutes of supine rest, take a baseline BP and pulse.

4. Have the patient sit on the side of the bed with feet dangling for 2 to 3 minutes, then take BP and pulse.

5. Repeat the measurements immediately upon having the patient stand.

6. Repeat the measurements again 1 to 3 minutes after continued standing. When recording the measurements, include the position when you took the readings and any signs or symptoms developed with postural changes.

Throughout the procedure assess the patient for dizziness, light-headedness, pallor, sweating, or syncope. If any of these occur, return the patient to a supine position.

FOLLOW-UP CARE AND INSTRUCTIONS

The results of the BP measurements dictate the follow-up actions and patient instructions. Long-term observations have been made on the contributions of high BP to illness and death. It is important to note that the classification of BP has changed over the years. In 2003, the seventh report of the Joint National Committee (JNC-VII) on prevention, detection, evaluation, and treatment recommended the classification found in Table 4-3.

Table 4.3 **Classification of Blood Pressure (BP) for Adults 18 Years and Older**				
CLASSIFICATION	SYSTOLIC BP (mm Hg)			DIASTOLIC BP (mm Hg)
Normal	<120	*and*		<80
Prehypertension	120-139	*or*		80-89
Stage 1 hypertension	140-159	*or*		90-99
Stage 2 hypertension	≥160	*or*		≥100

Modified from Chobanian AV, Bakris GL, Blach HR, et al: The seventh report of the Joint National Committee on Prevention, Detection, Evaluation, and Treatment of High Blood Pressure: The JNC 7 report. JAMA 289:2560-2572, 2003.

Table 4.4 **Blood Pressure (BP) Record and Follow-up Recommendations**

Date: _____   **Name:** _____   **Age:** _____

BP Measurements   *Right Arm*   *Left Arm*

Sitting:

Lying:

Standing:

Recommendations   *Medications*   *Home BP Readings*

☐ Return in _____ days

☐ Daily BP readings

☐ Salt restriction

Clinicians should explain the meaning of their BP readings to patients and advise them of the appropriate need for periodic follow-up care and re-measurement. Table 4-4 demonstrates a suggested follow-up form to be given to patients after their BP has been taken.

The measurement of orthostatic BP is a simple technique that requires the same equipment as previously mentioned in this chapter for measuring BP. Practical applications include the detection of intravascular volume depletion and autonomic dysfunction and the treatment of hypertension, congestive heart failure, and other clinical disorders.

REFERENCES

Al-Hermi B, Abbas B: The role of ambulatory blood pressure measurements in adolescence and young adults. Transplant Proc 36:1818-1819, 2004.

American Academy of Neurology: Consensus statement on the definition of orthostatic hypotension, pure autonomic failure, and multiple system atrophy. Neurology 46:1470, 1996.

Base-Smith V: Nondisposable sphygmomanometer cuffs harbor frequent bacterial colonization and significant contamination by organic and inorganic matter. AANA 64:141-145, 1996.

Block FE, Schulte GT: Ankle blood pressure measurement: An acceptable alternative to arm measurements. Int J Clin Monit Comput 13:167-171, 1996.

Carlson JE: Assessment of orthostatic blood pressure: Measurement, technique, and clinical applications. South Med J 92:167-173, 1999.

Graves J: Prevalence of blood pressure cuff sizes in a referral practice of 430 consecutive adult hypertensives. Blood Press Monit 6:17-20, 2001.

Grim CM, Grim C: Manual blood pressure measurement—Still the gold standard: Why and how to measure blood pressure the old-fashioned way. Hypertension Medicine October, 131-145, 2000.

Joint National Committee on Prevention, Detection, Evaluation, and Treatment of High Blood Pressure: The seventh report of the Joint National Committee (JNC-VII) on Prevention, Detection, Evaluation and Treatment of High Blood Pressure. JAMA 289:2560-2572, 2003.

Lieb M, Holzgreve H, Schultz M, et al: The effect of clothes on sphygmomanometric and oscillometric blood pressure measurement. Blood Press 13:279-282, 2004.

Lyons SA, Petrucelli RJ: Medicine: An Illustrated History. New York, Abradale Press, 1987.

Mader SL, Josephson KR, Rubenstein LZ: Low prevalence of postural hypotension among community-dwelling elderly. JAMA 258:1511-1514, 1987.

Manning DM, Kuchirka C, Kaminski J: Miscuffing: Inappropriate blood pressure cuff application. Circulation 68:763-766, 1983.

Mourad A, Carney S: Brief communication: Arm position and blood pressure: An audit. Intern Med J 34:290-291, 2004.

O'Brien E: Ambulatory blood pressure monitoring in the management of hypertension. Heart 89:571-576, 2004.

Perloff D, Grim C, Flack J, et al: Human blood pressure by sphygmomanometry. Circulation 88:2460-2470, 1993.

Pickering TG, Hall JE, Appel LJ, et al: Recommendations for blood pressure measurement in humans: An AHA scientific statement from the Council on High Blood Pressure Research Professional and Public Education Subcommittee. J Clin Hypertens (Greenwich) 7:102-109, 2005.

Porter R: The Greatest Benefit to Mankind: A Medical History of Humanity. New York, WW Norton, 1997.

Stevens G: Famous Names in Medicine. East Sussex, England, Wayland Publishers, 1978.

Valler-Jones T, Wedgbury K: Measuring blood pressure using the mercury sphygmomanometer. Br J Nurs 14;145-150, 2005.

Verdecchia P: Prognostic value of ambulatory blood pressure. Hypertension 35:844-851, 2000.

Wain H: A History of Medicine. Springfield, Ill, Charles C Thomas, 1970.

Chapter 5

Venipuncture

Kenneth R. Harbert

PROCEDURE GOALS AND OBJECTIVES

Goal: To obtain a venous sample of blood while observing standard precautions and with the minimal degree of risk to the patient.

Objectives: The student will be able to …

- Describe the indications, contraindications, and rationale for performing venipuncture.
- Identify and describe common complications associated with venipuncture.
- Describe the essential anatomy and physiology associated with the performance of venipuncture.
- Identify the necessary materials and their proper use for performing venipuncture.
- Identify the important aspects of post-procedure care following venipuncture.

BACKGROUND AND HISTORY

Venipuncture evolved from the practice of phlebotomy. The word *phlebotomy* is derived from two Greek words referring to "veins" and "cutting"; thus, phlebotomy can be defined as the incision of a vein for bloodletting or collection. Since early times, humans have appreciated the association between blood and life itself. Many medical principles and procedures have evolved from this belief. Hippocrates (460-377 BC) stated that disease was the result of excess substances such as blood, phlegm, black bile, and yellow bile within the body. It was believed that removal of the excess of these substances would restore balance (McCall, 1998). From this belief arose the practice of bloodletting—the first form of phlebotomy. By the 17th and 18th centuries, phlebotomy was a major therapy for those practicing the healing arts. Lancets were among the primary instruments used by clinicians in the 18th century.

Methods and procedures associated with phlebotomy today are dramatically improved. Only rarely today is phlebotomy used as a therapeutic modality (e.g., for patients with polycythemia). Instead, the primary purpose of phlebotomy is to obtain a sample of blood for diagnostic testing. The development of sophisticated laboratory equipment has reduced the need for venipuncture by requiring smaller quantities of blood for diagnostic assessments, amounts that often can be obtained by simply puncturing the skin without directly accessing the veins. There are many ways to obtain a blood sample using the venipuncture method. The procedures in this chapter describe techniques using Vacutainers, syringes, and infusion sets.

INDICATIONS

There are as many reasons to perform venipuncture as there are different disease entities. This procedure is indicated any time that a sample of venous blood is necessary in quantities larger than those readily available by finger stick methods.

CONTRAINDICATIONS

Once the decision has been made to perform the venipuncture procedure, the next most important decision is the selection of the site from which to draw a sample. Although many suitable sites may exist, some areas should be avoided. Sites to avoid include the following:

■ Obvious areas of skin infection (e.g., cellulitis, skin rashes, newly tattooed areas)

■ Skin sites that have extensive scarring from burns, surgery, injuries, repeated venipuncture, or trauma

- Upper extremity on the ipsilateral side of a mastectomy; use of this site may affect the test results because of the presence of lymphedema, which occurs after dissection and removal of the lymphatic system

- Sites at which a hematoma is present, which might produce erroneous results in certain types of testing; if another site is not available for venipuncture, the sample should be drawn from the distal aspect of the hematoma

- An arm with an intravenous (IV) line for fluids or blood transfusions; it is essential to use the opposite arm as the site of the venipuncture. If this is not possible, satisfactory samples typically can be drawn from a site distal to the IV site. When following this procedure, the IV line should be turned off for at least 2 minutes, if possible. The blood should then be drawn from a vein other than the one in which the IV is placed above the selected site. The first 5 mL of blood should be drawn and discarded before drawing the samples for testing. Blood specimens that are drawn for glucose levels from the same extremity as the IV infusion may be inaccurate, even when obtained from a point distal to the IV site.

- An arm with a fistula or cannula in place without specific directions from your supervising physician; if the extremity is edematous, another site should be chosen

Additionally, patients with diffuse intravascular coagulation, hyperfibrinolysis, thrombocytopenia, or qualitative platelet disorders characteristically bleed for a long time after venipunctures.

POTENTIAL COMPLICATIONS

Several complications may occur when performing venipuncture, including the following:
- Infection of the skin (cellulitis)

- Infection of the vein (phlebitis)

- Thrombosis

- Laceration of the vein

- Hemorrhage or hematoma at the site of the puncture. The risk of complications is increased with repeated puncture at any site. The most common complication is hemorrhage or hematoma at the site of the puncture, which occurs when blood leaks into the tissues after nicking or penetrating the distal wall of the vein when inserting the needle into the vein. Using the right angle of insertion for the needle can minimize the likelihood of this complication. Also, slower insertion of the needle reduces the likelihood of inserting it too deeply. A smaller gauge needle also decreases the risk of hemorrhage or hematoma. If a hematoma does develop, remove the tourniquet, remove the needle, and maintain pressure on the site for at least 10 minutes. Apply pressure for an additional 5 minutes, at least, for patients who take medications that may have an anticoagulant effect.

■ Vasovagal syncope, or fainting, which can occur when performing a venipuncture. Remove the tourniquet, remove the needle, apply pressure to the site, and fix with tape. Carefully lay the patient down and apply appropriate measures to wake up the patient. This potential complication is one of the most compelling reasons why the best position for performing a venipuncture is the supine position, especially with patients who report previous episodes of syncope or present with overwhelming anxiety.

REVIEW OF ESSENTIAL ANATOMY AND PHYSIOLOGY

Blood constitutes 6% to 8% of the total body weight and consists of blood cells suspended in a fluid called *plasma. Serum* refers to the substrate remaining when the fibrinogen has been removed from the plasma. The three main types of blood cells are red blood cells, called *erythrocytes;* white blood cells, called *leukocytes;* and platelets, known as *thrombocytes.* The primary function of blood is the transportation of oxygen via hemoglobin molecules within the erythrocytes. In addition, it serves to transport nutrients, waste products, components of the immune system, hormones, and other specialized materials throughout the body. It also plays a critical role in the constant regulation of body temperature, the regulation of fluids, and acid-base equilibrium. Finally, the platelets are responsible for preventing blood loss from hemorrhage and have their primary influence on the blood vessel walls.

Veins serve as the structures that channel the deoxygenated blood back to the heart and eventually to the lungs. The muscles within the vein walls facilitate the movement of blood within the vein; one-way valves in the vein prevent the backward flow of blood.

The cubital fossa is the triangular hollow area on the anterior aspect of the elbow. The boundaries include an imaginary line connecting the medial and lateral epicondyles superiorly, the pronator teres medially, and the brachio-radialis laterally. In the cubital fossa region, the cephalic and basilic veins are often most prominent.

Because of the prominence and accessibility of these superficial veins, the cubital fossa is the site used most often for venipuncture. Considerable variations can occur in the connection of the basilic and cephalic veins. The median cubital vein crosses the bicipital aponeurosis, which separates it from the underlying brachial artery and median nerve. The median cubital vein often receives the median antebrachial vein and can bifurcate to form a median cephalic vein and a median basilic vein (Fig. 5-1). These veins may be embedded in subcutaneous tissue, making them difficult to visualize, but the

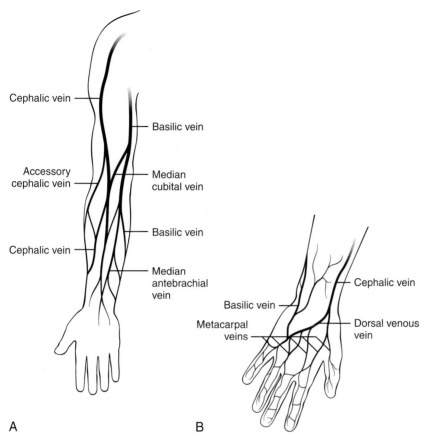

FIGURE 5-1. Superficial veins. **A,** Inner aspect of forearm. **B,** Dorsal aspect of hand and wrist.

use of a tourniquet occludes the veins' return and distends them, making them not only palpable but, in most instances, also visible.

Venipuncture is defined as the collection of a blood specimen or specimens from a vein for the laboratory testing of the blood sample. The tests that are performed on blood offer many important and valuable parameters for aiding in the diagnosis of a variety of different diseases. The integrity of the sample taken is dependent on using good technique, drawing from an appropriate site, and avoiding hemolysis or contamination of a sample.

Standard Precautions   Practitioners should use standard precautions at all times when interacting with patients. Determining the level of precaution necessary requires that the practitioner exercise clinical judgment based on the patient's history and the potential for exposure to body fluids or aerosol-borne pathogens (for further discussion, see Chapter 2).

PATIENT PREPARATION

- Make sure the patient has followed any preparatory instructions before drawing blood (e.g., fasting before a blood glucose or lipid profile, medication withheld or taken prior to procedure, use of medications that may have an anticoagulant effect).

- Discuss with the patient any previous experience with venipuncture to identify any potential difficulties with the procedure (e.g., anxiety, fainting, vomiting). Also ask about previous surgery (mastectomy) or other recent procedures (venous cutdown, dialysis shunt)

- Discuss the need for the procedure with the patient, as well as the potential possibility of an initial stinging pain and possible bruising, while continuing to stress the importance of the patient's cooperation for a successful procedure.

- Instruct the patient to remain as still as possible while the procedure is being carried out.

- Do not say, "This will be only a little uncomfortable." The patient knows that it will hurt. Explain that you will do everything you can to minimize the discomfort, but you will need the patient's cooperation to do so. The practitioner might say, "I want to make this procedure as pain free as I can for you. Follow my directions and we will work together to make that happen."

- Answer any and all questions that the patient may have before you begin the procedure.

Materials Utilized to Perform a Venipuncture

- Gloves: at least two pairs of unsterile gloves (in case one set becomes contaminated; ask patient about latex allergy)

- Needles: 18 gauge to 23 gauge, single and multidraw (Have a needle with a rubber sheath on the part of the needle that inserts into the Vacutainer barrel.)

- Evacuated barrels: Vacutainer barrels are now available with safety release or retract features.

- Evacuated tubes: serum separator tubes, ethylenediaminetetraacetic acid (EDTA), sodium citrate, sodium heparin, plain, and so on (*Always have spare tubes so that if the vacuum is lost or there is a tube with insufficient vacuum you are prepared and do not have to repeat the venipuncture procedure.*) Review color of test tube and test ordered prior to venipuncture procedure.

- Labels for evacuated tubes, ready with patient's name and pertinent information for each tube

- Syringes: 1, 3, 5, and 10 mL, or larger (plastic or glass)

- IV butterfly (useful for children to prevent excessive suction on the vein) infusion sets: 21, 23, or 25 gauge, or all three

- Tourniquets: ¾ inch or 1 inch for adults and ⅛ inch for children. These should be clean, wide strips of latex (check for latex allergies before beginning procedure), or an adult-child blood pressure cuff can be used. Latex-free tourniquets are available. For elderly patients use a blood pressure cuff (maintaining pressure greater than patient's diastolic pressure) instead of a tourniquet, which may be helpful to prevent excessive stress on the vein.

- Gauze pads: 2 inch × 2 inch or 4 inch × 4 inch

- Isopropyl alcohol pads, 70%

- Povidone-iodine (used for cleansing venipuncture sites for blood cultures)

- Adhesive strips (Band-Aids) (again, ask patient if he or she is allergic to adhesive tape before procedure), nylon tape, and paper tape

- Sharps disposal container

- Biohazard waste container

Note: There are many ways to obtain a blood sample using the venipuncture technique. The following procedures describe techniques using Vacutainers, syringes, and infusion sets.

Procedure for Venipuncture Using Vacutainers

Note: When performing a venipuncture, proper planning and preparation are essential to obtaining good results and ensuring a good outcome for your patient. Developing a routine, sequential plan for the venipuncture procedure helps ensure effective and efficient results with the least amount of discomfort for the patient.

1. Know which specific samples you will need to collect for the laboratory studies requested and anticipate the materials and sequence for collecting the needed samples.

2. For each laboratory study to be performed, identify the additive, additive function, volume, and specimen considerations to be followed for each, using the corresponding tubes with color-coded tops. This will save the patient undue distress and will help you in obtaining the best outcome for each sample of blood and corresponding laboratory test that is to be performed. Organize your equipment for procedure before beginning.

continued

3. Wash hands with warm water and bacteriostatic soap. Always observe standard precautions for the prevention of transmission of human immunodeficiency virus (HIV), hepatitis B and C, and other blood-borne infections (Centers for Disease Control and Prevention, 1989).

4. Check patient's identification to ensure that the correct patient is having the procedure.

5. Check the test ordered twice, even if ordered by you.

6. Assemble the equipment, preparing the tubes in the right order and placing the appropriate needle on the Vacutainer barrel.

Note: In some instances, the equipment needed depends on the patient, the medical condition, the site to be used for the procedure, the number of samples required, and the type of setting (hospital, outpatient, pediatric ward, nursery, emergency room) where the procedure will be performed.

7. Talk with the patient and explain what you will be doing. Encourage the patient to take slow, deep breaths as the procedure begins. Position the patient in a manner that is both proper for the procedure and comfortable for the patient. If possible, position the patient in a supine or recumbent position. This assists the patient in relaxing and carries the least likelihood for injury to the patient if he or she experiences vasovagal syncope. If the patient is sitting up, extend his or her arm straight down from shoulder to waist.

8. Observe the patient for any of the contraindications mentioned previously.

9. Inspect the patient's surface anatomy and venous system in the chosen venipuncture site before applying the tourniquet. The cubital fossa is the most common site for sampling and IV injections. Check bilaterally, distally, and proximally to the most common site for venipuncture in the adult, which is the antecubital fossa.

Note: To augment the ability to identify the best site for venipuncture, palpation skills and the sense of touch should be refined by using the palmar aspects of gloved finger pads. Do not rely totally on vision. This can be practiced on oneself or on volunteers until the location of a vein can be identified confidently with eyes closed. Heavily pigmented skin and overlying adipose tissue can make veins difficult to visualize. In particular, difficult venipuncture can occur in patients who have had a number of venipunctures, or in patients who are using IV drugs. In these instances, selecting an adequate site may be difficult. Patients who are frequently subjected to venipuncture may be able to direct you to sites with the highest likelihood of success. A warm compress applied lightly before the procedure can facilitate vein dilation and thus assist with the identification of an adequate vein. The selection of a good site should include a vein that is easily palpated, is large and well anchored, and does not roll when palpated.

Note: The best veins for venipuncture in the right order of choice are as follows:

- Median cubital vein, which is easily palpated, well anchored, least painful, least likely to bruise, and usually the largest vein in the antecubital space

- Cephalic vein, which is a large vein that is easily palpated but poorly anchored; venipuncture here can be painful to the patient

- Basilic vein, which is easy to palpate, not well anchored, and very close to the brachial artery and the median nerve

Note: For finding difficult veins:

- Have the patient keep the extremity below the level of the heart for a few minutes.

- Apply a warm towel to the extremity to promote vasodilation from the heat—the towel should be less than 42° C and should be left on no longer than 2 minutes.

- Use a blood pressure cuff inflated to a point between the systolic and diastolic pressures as a tourniquet to allow for greater control and less discomfort to the patient.

- Carefully rub or tap the vein over the potential puncture site to increase the vein's vasodilation (should be done before the site is prepared).

10. Firmly place the tourniquet about 3 to 4 inches above the venipuncture site, not too tight, and use a wide tube band tied with easily removable bow ties pointing up and away from the site (Fig. 5-2).

Note: Be sure the patient has no contraindications against the use of a latex

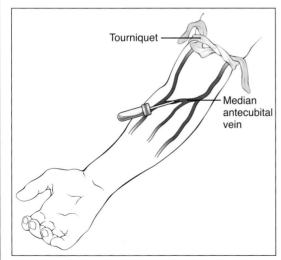

Figure 5-2.

tourniquet. Apply the tourniquet in a manner in which it can be easily removed. Or use a blood pressure cuff.

Caution: Never leave the tourniquet on for more than 2 minutes. The vein may collapse if the tourniquet is too close to the puncture site.

11. After applying the tourniquet, begin palpation of the identified site to locate a desirable vein.

Note: The vein can also be tapped to cause it to dilate and become more prominent. Allow gravity to help the vein become engorged and thus enlarged. If the vein being palpated feels very tight and has no flexibility, it may be a tendon or may overlie a tendon. If it has a palpable pulse, it is an artery. Be certain of the underlying anatomy before performing the procedure.

12. Put on latex gloves. Make sure that all tubes and equipment are within easy reach in the order that they will be used.

13. Before cleansing the area, secure the site by anchoring the vein distal to the venipuncture site, using a finger to apply pressure over the top of the vein (useful with large veins) and thus serving to hold the vein still.

14. Open several alcohol or povidone-iodine pads. Clean the procedure area, beginning at the vein site and circling outward to a 2-inch diameter. Allow the area to air dry thoroughly. This is especially true when using povidone-iodine.

Note: Alcohol lyses red blood cells and can cause intense stinging. Be sure the site is dry.

15. Visualize what you are going to do and begin by stretching the skin downward below the anticipated venipuncture site with the opposite hand to anchor the vein and limit vein movement.

continued

Bevel of needle 15 degrees

Vein

Figure 5-3.

16. Maintaining needle sterility, insert needle into the straightest section of the vein, puncture the skin with the bevel facing up directly over and parallel to the vein, and enter the vein or a point immediately adjacent to the vein. Insert the needle with the bevel up at about a 15- to 30-degree angle so that the needle penetrates halfway into the vessel (Fig. 5-3). When the needle has entered the skin, lower the needle until it is almost parallel with the skin.

Note: Use caution when using Vacutainers because they can exert excessive vacuum, causing the vein to collapse. When using a syringe, watch for a backflow of blood. If backflow is not present with a syringe, carefully advance the needle slightly further into vein.

17. Remove the protective covering from the threaded hub and screw the needle into the holder.

18. Place the Vacutainer tube inside the barrel without puncturing the top of the tube with the needle. Be sure to have extra tubes close at hand in the right order of draw.

Note: Determine the correct order of drawing the samples in the tube or slide, depending on the laboratory or the tests required, or both. This prevents interference by carryover of additives between tubes. Usually the order is as follows:

   1. Blood cultures, usually performed with a syringe using *only iodine as the skin preparation*

   2. Red top (chemistry, immunology, and serology panels; blood bank)

   3. Gold top (chemistry, immunology, and serology panels)

   4. Light blue top (requires a full draw of sample; uses include coagulation tests, such as thrombin and prothrombin times)

   5. Green or lavender top (requires a full draw and inverting slowly at least eight times to prevent clotting and platelet clumping; uses include hematology, blood bank)

   6. Gray top (requires a full draw to prevent hemolysis; uses include lithium, sodium heparin, and glucose levels)

This order changes when using a syringe for drawing blood (see "Procedure for Syringe Venipuncture").

Note: Inserting the needle at less than a 15- to 30-degree angle may allow the needle to puncture through the far wall of the vein.

19. Hold the needle steady. You may want to prop your hand against the patient's arm, so if he or she moves, you move, then engage the Vacutainer tube. Avoid rotating the needle because this may result in excessive damage to the vessel wall.

20. Keeping the needle very steady and still, move the Vacutainer tube down into the barrel so that the tube is punctured. A drop of blood will be visible at the top of the inside needle when it is in the vein. Let the tube fill three-fourths full. After blood finishes flowing into the last Vacutainer tube, release the tourniquet and ask the patient to relax his or her hand.

21. When removing the filled tube and inserting the next tube, grasp the barrel holder securely in the nondominant

hand and anchor it by holding it against the extremity to avoid inadvertently removing the needle from the lumen of the vein.

Note: The existing vacuum gently draws blood into the tubes. Most Vacutainer tubes are unsterile and have additives. The tube will cease drawing blood when its vacuum is expired (i.e., when the tube is appropriately filled).

22. Have the next tube ready for insertion into the Vacutainer. Remove the Vacutainer tube from the holder before removing the needle.

Note: Remember that multiple tubes of blood can be drawn at this one venipuncture site without resticking the patient.

23. If multiple tubes are drawn, carefully invert tubes and mix as required for each specific tube. Do not shake the tubes vigorously because disruption of the cell membranes may result, thus altering the concentrations of intracellular and extracellular components.

24. Have sterile gauze ready. Carefully remove the needle from the skin. Cover with alcohol pad or sterile gauze.

25. Once the needle is removed completely, apply firm pressure for hemostasis by holding a sterile 2 inch × 2 inch covering over the site while the arm is outstretched or raised. Avoid bending the arm. Apply firm pressure to the site until the bleeding stops, for at least 3 to 4 minutes, or for 5 minutes or more if the patient has been taking anticoagulant medications.

26. Dress the site with gauze using multicolored sponge tape or adhesive

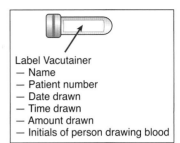

Label Vacutainer
— Name
— Patient number
— Date drawn
— Time drawn
— Amount drawn
— Initials of person drawing blood

Figure 5-4.

strip (ask about allergies before applying dressing).

Note: If the procedure was unsuccessful, do not attempt to repeat it at the same site until healing has occurred. After three unsuccessful attempts, stop and ask for help.

27. Discard the needle in a puncture resistant sharps container.

28. Clean any blood spillage with appropriate cleaning agent.

29. Label all Vacutainer tubes according to facility procedure (Fig. 5-4).

30. Properly dispose of all contaminated materials in the appropriate biohazardous waste container.

31. Talk with the patient, recheck the venipuncture site, and assess the site dressing.

32. Make sure the patient is feeling fine and shows no signs of vertigo, lightheadedness, or discomfort before leaving.

33. Remove gloves and wash your hands.

Procedure for Syringe Venipuncture

Note: Syringes may be used for venipuncture when the patient's veins are small or fragile and Vacutainer tubes may cause the veins to collapse. Using a syringe with a 20- or 21-gauge needle or butterfly allows for greater control. The procedure for using a syringe follows the same steps as those for using the Vacutainer tubes except it differs in the order of samples drawn, the aspiration of blood into the syringe, and the transfer of blood into the vacuum tubes. Self-capping needles are extremely useful when using a syringe.

The order of draw is as follows:

- Blood cultures, using only iodine as a skin preparation

- Light blue top (requires a full draw of sample; uses include coagulation tests such as thrombin and prothrombin times)

- Lavender top (requires a full draw and inverting at least eight times slowly to prevent clotting and platelet clumping; uses include hematology, blood bank)

- Green top

- Gray top (requires a full draw to prevent hemolysis; uses include lithium, sodium heparin, and glucose levels).

- Red top (chemistry, immunology, and serology panels; blood bank)

1. Wash your hands. Cleanse the area, select the venipuncture site, and palpate the vein in the same manner as when using a Vacutainer system. The steps associated with the entry into the vein are the same as well.

2. Once the needle is in the vein, keep the needle steady and still, and then pull back gently on the syringe plunger while holding the syringe securely to keep the needle in the vein.

3. Using the syringe to brace against you, pull back on the plunger and fill the syringe with the desired amount of blood (usually three quarters full) needed for the tubes to be filled.

4. Release the tourniquet and complete the dressing procedure using the same technique as described for the Vacutainer system.

5. When transferring from the syringe to the tubes, remove the 20- or 21-gauge needle from the syringe and replace it with an 18- or 19-gauge needle.

6. Take extreme care to puncture the tubes in the right order and allow the tubes to fill by using the pressure of the vacuum tube.

7. Do not use the plunger to fill the tubes.

Note: Use caution with a syringe, because the temptation is to push the blood sample into the vacuum tube using the syringe plunger, which will affect the sample. Vacuum tubes draw blood into the tubes using their own vacuum. The Vacutainer system consists of vacuum tubes, a needle holder (Vacutainer barrel), and a disposable multi-sample or single-sample needle (Fig. 5-5). New multi-sample needles have guard sheaths.

8. Continue with the same labeling procedure and ensure the status of the patient before allowing him or her to leave.

Needle

Vacutainer barrel (hub)

Vacutainer tube

Vacutainer System

FIGURE 5-5.

Procedure for an Infusion Set Venipuncture

Note: An IV infusion set or butterfly can be used for venipuncture when you are drawing from a hand or a foot or from a very small or difficult vein. The procedure for cleansing the area and site selection are the same as for the syringe and Vacutainer procedures; however, with the infusion set the hand and the foot may be included as new sites.

1. Insert the needle at a lesser angle than for either of the other methods.

Caution: It is important to take great care with the needle so as not to miss the vein.

Note: Infusion sets come in different sizes of needles, and the appropriate one for the adult, child, or difficult vein should be selected carefully.

2. Attach a syringe to the set and be careful not to use excessive suction from the syringe; the blood is drawn slowly and carefully.

Note: The infusion set has plastic "wings" that are attached to a short length of flexible plastic tubing, which is then attached to either a syringe or IV tubing.

Note: As soon as the needle is in the vein, blood will be visible in the tubing, and this will allow for easy access by the syringe.

3. Fill the tube with the appropriate amount of blood, release the tourniquet, and attach a needle. Transfer to the appropriate tubes using the same order as for a syringe.

4. When using a safety infusion set, slide the safety cover over the needle and discard the set.

5. In order to prevent an accidental restick with the infusion set needle, hold the base of the needle or the wings as you remove the needle, and do not let go of the needle base until it is being placed in the biohazard sharps container.

SPECIAL CONSIDERATIONS

- If no blood is obtained, change the position of the needle carefully. Move it forward or backward. Watch for formation of a hematoma. If this occurs, stop the procedure. Also consider adjusting the angle of the needle.

- If blood stops flowing into the vacuum tube, the vein may have collapsed. Resecure the tourniquet to increase venous filling. If this is not successful, remove the needle, take care of the puncture site, and redraw.

- Never draw from a thrombosed or scarred vein. Thrombosed veins lack resilience, feel cordlike, and roll easily.

- Never attempt venipuncture in an artery. Arteries pulsate, are very elastic, and have a thick wall. If you see bright red blood, be cautious: Remove the tourniquet, carefully remove the needle, and apply a firm steady pressure for at least 10 minutes.

- Never draw above an IV site. The fluid may dilute the specimen; collect from the opposite arm. Do not use alcohol when drawing a blood alcohol sample.

- Never draw over scars or new tattoo sites. It is difficult to puncture the scar tissue, and the needle and the tourniquet should not come in contact with the inflamed tattoo site. Edematous extremities with swollen tissue alter the test results.

- Avoid leaving a tourniquet on for more than 2 minutes. This can cause hemoconcentration of nonfilterable elements. The hydrostatic pressure causes some water and filterable elements to leave the extracellular space.

- Make sure the venipuncture site is dry.

- When using a syringe, avoid drawing the plunger back too forcefully.

FOLLOW-UP CARE AND INSTRUCTIONS

- Advise the patient that he or she may experience some minor discomfort and discoloration at the site of the venipuncture for the following 48 to 72 hours.

- Instruct the patient to keep the site clean and dry to reduce the likelihood of infection.

- Educate the patient about signs of infection and phlebitis and advise him or her to call or return to the office if such signs are seen.

REFERENCES

Centers for Disease Control and Prevention: Guidelines for the prevention of transmission of human immunodeficiency virus and hepatitis B virus to health-care and public-safety workers. MMWR Morb Mortal Wkly Rep 38(suppl 6):1-37, 1989.

McCall RE, Tankersley CM: Phlebotomy Essentials. Philadelphia, JB Lippincott, 1998, pp 2-4.

BIBLIOGRAPHY

Bardes CL: Essential Skills in Clinical Medicine. Philadelphia, FA Davis, 1996, pp 104-106.

Chesnutt MS, Dewar TN, Locksley RM, Turee JH: Office and Bedside Procedures. Norwalk, Conn, Lange, 1992, pp 27-29.

Fischbach F: A Manual of Laboratory and Diagnostic Tests, 5th ed. Philadelphia, JB Lippincott, 1996, pp 25-27.

Greene HL, Fincher RM, Johnson WP, et al: Clinical Medicine, 2nd ed. St. Louis, CV Mosby, 1996, pp 874-878.

Jacobs DS, DeMott WR, Grady HJ, Horvat RT: Laboratory Test Handbook. Lexicomp, 1996, pp 197-200.

Jandl JH: Blood: Textbook of Hematology. Boston, Little, Brown, 1997, pp 53-55.

McClatchey KD: Clinical Laboratory Medicine. Baltimore, Md, Williams & Wilkins, 1996, pp 84-90.

Sacher RA, McPherson RA: Wildmann's Clinical Interpretation of Laboratory Tests, 11th ed. Philadelphia, FA Davis, 2000, p 31.

Wallach J: Interpretation of Diagnostic Tests, 7th ed. Philadelphia, Lippincott Williams & Wilkins, 2000, pp 3-17.

Chapter 6

Obtaining Blood Cultures

Darwin Brown

Procedure Goals and Objectives

Goal: To obtain a blood culture sample successfully while observing standard precautions and with the minimal degree of risk to the patient.

Objectives: The student will be able to ...

- Describe the indications, contraindications, and rationale for obtaining a blood culture sample.

- Identify and describe common complications associated with obtaining a blood culture sample.

- Describe the essential anatomy and physiology associated with obtaining a blood culture sample.

- Identify the materials necessary for obtaining a blood culture sample and their proper use.

- Identify the important aspects of patient care after a blood culture sample is obtained.

BACKGROUND AND HISTORY

A blood culture is performed when an infection of the blood (bacteremia or septicemia) is suspected in the presence of fever, chills, low blood pressure, or other symptoms. The blood culture helps identify the infection's origin and provides a basis for determining appropriate antimicrobial therapy.

Bacteremia is a microbial infection of the bloodstream. Identification of pathogens within the bloodstream is accomplished primarily by blood culture. Culturing blood is one of the most important procedures that can be performed in individuals who are severely ill and febrile as well as those in whom an intravascular infection is suspected. Isolation and identification of an infectious agent from the blood have obvious diagnostic significance and provide an invaluable guide for selecting the most appropriate antimicrobial agent for therapy (Hoeprich, 1994).

Sources of bacteremia include focal sites of infection most often associated with the respiratory tract, the genitourinary tract, the abdomen, and the skin and soft tissues. The infecting organism results from organisms indigenous to the site.

Until approximately 1985, broth culture was the most conventional blood culture method. Conventional broth culture methods call for inoculating blood to liquid media contained in bottles or tubes. Today there is a wide variety of media from which to choose. The obtained cultures are incubated either aerobically or anaerobically for 7 to 14 days at 35° C. They are then examined visually every day for evidence of growth; in addition, blind subcultures and smears are prepared at scheduled intervals.

INDICATIONS

Blood cultures are a useful diagnostic tool for the evaluation of patients with a history and clinical physical examination findings that are indicative of bacteremia or septicemia.

- Blood cultures should be obtained only if there is reasonable suspicion of a bloodstream infection (bacteremia). A thorough history and physical examination can provide important information for determining the potential of an infectious state.

- Documentation should be made of the specific infecting organism in bacteremia or focal infection sites.

- Blood cultures are useful for monitoring the efficacy of pharmacologic treatments of blood-borne infections.

- Other specific indications for obtaining blood cultures include severely ill and febrile patients, suspected infective endocarditis, intravascular catheter site infection, meningitis, osteomyelitis, septic arthritis, bacterial pneumonia, and fever of unknown origin.

CONTRAINDICATIONS

There are few true contraindications to obtaining blood cultures.

■ Patients currently being treated with warfarin (Coumadin) should be assessed carefully to determine if the benefit of performing the procedure outweighs the potential risk.

■ Obtaining blood cultures should be avoided at the site of an active skin infection because of the probability of introducing bacteria into the blood circulation and the increased possibility of contamination of the culture by organisms originating from the infected structures.

■ If multiple previous blood cultures have failed to identify an infecting agent, the likelihood of obtaining a useful result is diminished and must be considered in view of all the available clinical evidence.

POTENTIAL COMPLICATIONS

Complications resulting from the collection of a blood culture are limited.

■ The development of a hematoma at the site of the venipuncture is not uncommon.

■ Continued bleeding from the puncture site also may occur.

■ Other possible complications include the development of a localized skin infection or phlebitis.

■ Contaminated blood samples may result in the inappropriate use of antibiotics, which, in turn, may enhance selection for multidrug-resistant organisms. This may increase the rate of nosocomial infections and antibiotic-related complications, possibly raising health care costs (Chien, 1998).

In general, contamination should be suspected if:

■ A common component of the skin flora is recovered and the patient's history does not warrant consideration of a "nonpathogen" as being significant.

■ A mixture of several kinds of bacteria is recovered.

■ Growth is found in only one of several specimens from separate venipunctures (Hoeprich, 1994).

REVIEW OF ESSENTIAL ANATOMY AND PHYSIOLOGY

It is important to know the specific anatomy of each area from which blood cultures will be obtained. It is generally accepted that for each septic episode,

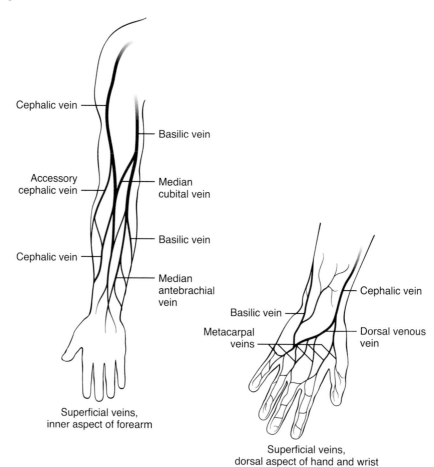

FIGURE 6-1. Venous anatomy of the arm and hand.

at least two sets of blood culture specimens should be collected. This results in two separate venipunctures at different sites. The median cubital vein usually is the easiest to locate. Other acceptable locations include the cephalic and basilic veins and veins in the back of the hand (Fig. 6-1). For more information regarding the anatomy and physiology of veins, see Chapter 5.

Standard Precautions   Practitioners should use standard precautions at all times when interacting with patients. Determining the level of precaution necessary requires the practitioner to exercise clinical judgment based on the patient's history and the potential for exposure to body fluids or aerosol-borne pathogens (for further discussion, see Chapter 2).

PATIENT PREPARATION

Instruct the patient about the need for the procedure and the potential benefits and risks associated with having the procedure performed.
- Explain that the procedure includes skin preparation and the potential need to use two separate venipuncture sites.

- If the patient notes an allergy to iodine, use chlorhexidine or 70% isopropyl alcohol for site cleansing.

Materials Utilized for Obtaining Blood Cultures

- 20-mL syringe with 21-gauge needle or vacuum tube adapter and needle

- 70% isopropyl alcohol swabs or wipes

- 1% to 2% tincture of iodine, povidone-iodine, or chlorhexidine gluconate swabs or wipes

- Alcohol swabs for cleaning blood culture bottle tops

- Aerobic and anaerobic vacuum blood culture bottles with properly identified patient labels

- Tourniquet

- Gloves

- 2-inch × 2-inch gauze pads

- Bandages

Procedure for Obtaining a Blood Culture

1. Identify the patient. Ask the patient to state his or her name and then check and confirm other identification information.

2. Initial setup: Assemble and lay out equipment for collecting the blood culture specimen. Wash your hands before putting on gloves.

3. Position the patient. Make sure patient is in a comfortable position and that the arm is supported appropriately.

4. Apply tourniquet 3 inches above intended site. Locate an appropriate vein and then release tourniquet.

5. Clean the site using sterile 70% isopropyl alcohol wipes; starting at the intended site, move outward in concentric circles (Fig. 6-2). Repeat this two or three times, being sure to use a new, clean wipe each time.

continued

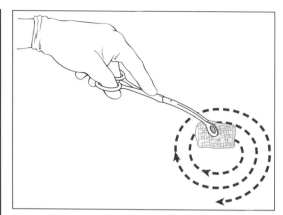

FIGURE 6-2.

6. Next apply povidone-iodine in the same manner two or three times and allow site to air dry. Once dry, the site should not be touched again. Sterile gloves must be worn if the site is to be repalpated.

7. Replace the tourniquet and remove the iodine with 70% isopropyl alcohol just before venipuncture.

8. Perform the venipuncture using a syringe or vacuum tube system.

9. Draw blood in the correct order. If specimens for multiple laboratory tests are to be obtained, always collect the blood culture specimens first, and then fill the other tubes as needed. Swab the top of the blood culture bottle with an alcohol wipe before blood insertion. Inoculate anaerobic bottle, followed by aerobic bottle.

10. Release the tourniquet after the first tube has been filled. The tourniquet should not be left on for more than 1 minute.

11. After the specimen has been collected, remove the needle and apply pressure until bleeding has stopped.

12. Immediately dispose of the needle in the proper container. Do not attempt to recap needles.

13. After the specimen has been collected, label all cultures with appropriate patient information, which should include patient's full name, identification number, culture site location, time, date, and your initials.

14. Clean the patient's arm of iodine before placing an adhesive bandage. Check to make sure the site is not bleeding before covering with bandage.

15. Pick up and account for all materials before leaving the patient's room. Remove your gloves and wash your hands. Thank the patient for his or her cooperation.

SPECIAL CONSIDERATIONS

The issue of using indwelling central catheters for obtaining blood cultures is somewhat controversial, and studies are conflicting (DesJardin, 1999). If a blood sample for culture is to be obtained during the placement of a central venous catheter, the catheter must be one that is placed in a completely sterile manner above the chest. If an indwelling central venous or arterial catheter is already in place, samples must be taken from both the catheter port and peripheral venipuncture sites to rule out line sepsis (Chien, 1998).

For infants, collect 1 to 5 mL of blood per 100-mL blood culture bottle (Hall, 1995).

FOLLOW-UP CARE AND INSTRUCTIONS

■ Advise the patient that he or she may experience some minor discomfort and discoloration at the site of the venipuncture for the following 48 to 72 hours.

■ Instruct the patient to keep the site clean and dry to reduce the likelihood of infection.

■ Explain to the patient the signs of hematoma, infection, and phlebitis and instruct him or her to call or return to the office or clinic if any of these occurs.

■ Advise the patient to report any adverse events associated with the venipuncture. These may include development of a hematoma or continued bleeding from the venipuncture site.

REFERENCES

Chien JW: Making the most of blood cultures. Postgrad Med 104:120, 1998.
DesJardin JA, Falagas ME, Ruthazer R, et al: Clinical utility of blood cultures drawn from indwelling central venous catheters in hospitalized patients with cancer. Ann Intern Med 131:641-647, 1999.
Hall G: Microbiology. In Tietz NW (ed): Clinical Guide to Laboratory Tests, 3rd ed. Philadelphia, WB Saunders, 1995, p 904.
Hoeprich PD, Rinaldi MG: Diagnostic methods for bacterial, rickettsial, mycoplasmal, and fungal infections. In Hoeprich PD, Jordan MC, Ronald AR (eds): Infectious Diseases: A Treatise of Infectious Processes, 5th ed. Philadelphia, JB Lippincott, 1994, pp 169-171.

BIBLIOGRAPHY

Flynn JC: Procedures in Phlebotomy, 2nd ed. Philadelphia, WB Saunders, 2005.
Garza D, Becan-McBride K: Phlebotomy Handbook: Blood Collection Essentials. Upper Saddle River, NJ, Pearson Prentice Hall, 2005.
Gill VJ, Fedorko DP, Witebsky FG: The clinician and the microbiology laboratory. In Mandell GL, Bennett JE, Dolin R (eds): Mandell, Douglas, and Bennett's Principles and Practice of Infectious Diseases, 6th ed, vol I. Philadelphia, Elsevier/Churchill Livingstone, 2005, pp 209-210.
Lehmann CA (ed): Saunders Manual of Clinical Laboratory Science. Philadelphia, WB Saunders, 1998.

Chapter 7

Inserting Intravenous Catheters

Ellen Davis-Hall

PROCEDURE GOALS AND OBJECTIVES

Goal: To insert an intravenous (IV) line successfully while observing standard precautions and with the minimal degree of risk to the patient.

Objectives: The student will be able to …

- Describe the indications, contraindications, and rationale for insertion of an IV line.
- Identify and describe common complications associated with IV line insertion.
- Describe the essential anatomy and physiology associated with the insertion of an IV line.
- Identify the necessary materials for insertion of an IV line and their proper use.
- Identify the important aspects of patient care after insertion of an IV line.

BACKGROUND AND HISTORY

Once William Harvey described the circulation of blood in 1628, experimentation with this system was inevitable. It was in 1656, however, that Sir Christopher Wren used a quill and bladder to inject opium intravenously into a dog, and IV therapy was begun (Gardner, 1982). Because of the sepsis accompanying such endeavors, IV therapy did not come into general use until the 1920s (Weinstein, 1997).

Little controversy exists over the value of IV therapy, and its use is widespread. Performance of this activity is highly technical and demands careful instruction and supervised experience. Various professionals and technicians can initiate IV therapy. This is regulated by state law and may vary.

INDICATIONS

Indications for IV therapy include the following:
- The administration of fluids (e.g., in clinical situations such as volume depletion, burn injury, blood loss, heat illness, shock, electrolyte imbalance)

- The provision of rapid and efficient delivery of medications (e.g., in various medical and surgical states and emergencies)

- The administration of blood or blood products

CONTRAINDICATIONS

There are few contraindications to IV therapy.
- Venipuncture should be avoided at the site of an active skin infection, because of the probability of introducing bacteria into the blood circulation.

- IV lines should not be inserted distal to any area of preexisting thrombophlebitis.

- Lower extremity venipunctures should be avoided in elderly patients and those with peripheral vascular disease and venous insufficiency. These compromised veins will not be effective vessels for fluid or medication administration, and the veins may suffer further injury.

POTENTIAL COMPLICATIONS

LOCAL

- Thrombosis or thrombophlebitis is the result of mechanical trauma to the vein at the time of insertion and the subsequent indwelling nature of the IV cannula. To prevent or minimize these complications, avoid trauma at time of insertion, tape the cannula securely to prevent movement, and avoid inserting IV lines in close proximity to joints. Infiltration of an IV line may cause the patient discomfort and increase the risk of infection and local tissue damage. Close observation and early detection will prevent or minimize this complication.

■ Local infection may also develop but can usually be avoided by adherence to sterile technique and regular dressing changes at the puncture site.

SYSTEMIC

■ Catheter embolization is a rare occurrence that results from shearing off of a distal portion of the catheter end by the beveled needle tip. This may occur when either an over-the-needle or a through-the-needle catheter is advanced into the vein and is then pulled back over or through the needle. This serious complication is avoidable by strict adherence to proper technique.

■ Septicemia can usually be avoided by adherence to sterile technique and established institutional IV line care protocols.

■ Pulmonary embolism may occur when a small blood clot that may form near the IV site dislodges and travels through the circulation until it lodges in the small capillary bed of the lungs. Avoidance of lower extremity veins helps prevent this occurrence.

■ Air embolism occurs when air, inadvertently left in or allowed into the IV tubing, travels into the bloodstream. This can be avoided by careful attention to flushing all lines before connection.

REVIEW OF ESSENTIAL ANATOMY AND PHYSIOLOGY

The anatomy of the veins that are most commonly considered for IV line placement is presented in Figure 7-1. Use of veins in the arm is recommended because they are most accessible, most comfortable for the patient, and the easiest to secure for long-term therapy. Often the easiest access is available on the dorsal aspect of the hand and the lower aspects of the arm; the metacarpal and cephalic veins are used most frequently. Valves may be palpable as knotlike lumps in a vein. These valves, as well as bifurcations, should be evaluated to ascertain adequate length and straightness for threading of the IV needle and catheter.

The choice of a vein for IV line insertion is based on the prescribed therapy, the duration of therapy, the condition of the extremity and the patient in general, and the condition, size, and location of the veins.

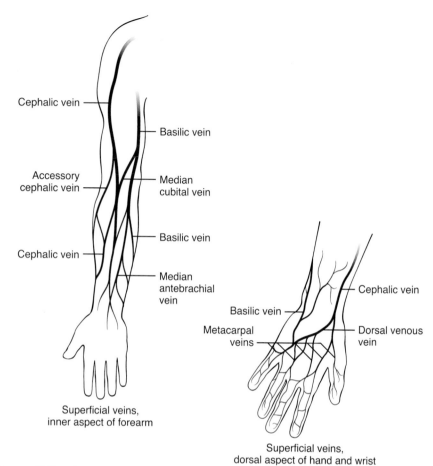

FIGURE 7-1. Anatomy of the veins most commonly considered for intravenous (IV) line placement.

Standard Precautions   Practitioners should use standard precautions at all times when interacting with patients. Determining the level of precaution necessary requires the practitioner to exercise clinical judgment based on the patient's history and the potential for exposure to body fluids or aerosol-borne pathogens (for further discussion, see Chapter 2).

PATIENT PREPARATION

- The patient should be informed of the indications for the IV line, the benefits and risks associated with the procedure, and the steps involved in the procedure. The patient may be anxious or afraid of the IV line itself or the anticipated pain, and explaining the procedure may help alleviate some of the anxiety.

- Inquire about iodine, latex, and tape allergies.

- The patient should also be advised of the need to limit movement of the extremity once the IV line is in place.

- Occasionally, in pain-sensitive individuals, an injection of 0.5% to 1.0% lidocaine (Xylocaine), to raise a wheal at the puncture site, may help minimize discomfort. This can be accomplished with a needle as small as 27 gauge. This may be helpful especially when a larger gauge butterfly or catheter is required. The patient should be warned, however, of the "bee sting and burn" nature of the lidocaine injection. The patient must be carefully screened for the possibility of previous allergic reactions to lidocaine before using this technique.

Materials Utilized for Inserting Intravenous Lines

- Intravenous catheter or butterfly

Note: There are a large number of catheters available for IV cannulation. The most common choice is the over-the-needle catheter. An alternative to this is the butterfly or winged small vein needle. The use of these two types of infusion devices is the focus of this section. They are presented in Figure 7-2. Beginning in 2001, IV catheters with safety mechanisms were required. These retract the steel needle into a closed device to minimize the chance of a needle stick. The gauge of the catheter or butterfly needle is chosen based on the vein used and the purpose of the infusion. A plan to administer blood, for example, demands a larger gauge, such as 16 gauge,

Butterfly

Over-the-needle catheter with safety retraction device

FIGURE 7-2. Butterfly and over-the-needle catheters.

whereas IV fluids alone can be administered with a needle having a gauge as small as 23. While closed infusion systems have been in use for some time, recently this concept has also been applied to the IV catheter system. Such a closed system combines the over-the-needle catheter, short extension set or needleless access connector, or both. This system reduces the chance of blood spills, and decreases the potential for contamination.

- Gloves and eye protection

- A topical antimicrobial to cleanse the skin

- Intravenous fluid

- Administration set (tubing with a drip chamber, a roller clamp flow regulator, and a standard connector that fits into the hub of the cannula or butterfly needle)

- Tourniquet

- ½-inch tape

- Arm board (if necessary to prevent flexion of a joint near the IV insertion point)

- Scissors to trim hair (if necessary)

- 2-inch × 2-inch or 4-inch × 4-inch gauze bandages or other occlusive dressing

- IV catheter pole

- Biohazardous waste and needle containers

- Antibiotic ointment (optional)

Procedure for Inserting an Intravenous Catheter

1. Apply the tourniquet above the elbow to ensure adequate filling of the veins, first to one arm and then to the other, to identify the best vein for IV catheter insertion.

Note: The most distal vein that is large enough to accommodate the size of the required butterfly needle or catheter should be chosen.

2. Palpate the veins for firmness and stability.

Note: Selection of the vein should be determined more by how the vein feels than by how it looks. Choose a vein that is straight and void of palpable valves for at least 1 inch proximal to your intended insertion site.

3. Release the tourniquet and recheck all supplies. Make certain that all necessary materials are within easy reach, the fluids are hung, and the tubing is flushed with the IV solution.

4. Reapply the tourniquet above the elbow. Use low tourniquet pressure to avoid damaging the vein in a geriatric patient. A blood pressure cuff will be gentler to sensitive tissue than a tourniquet.

5. If tourniquet pressure does not distend the vein adequately, ask the patient to open and close the hand several times, tap or pat the vein lightly, apply a warm moist towel, or have the patient place the extremity lower than the heart to facilitate vein dilation.

6. Apply gloves and eye protection.

7. Cleanse the puncture site with an approved antimicrobial solution such as chlorhexidine gluconate (O'Grady, 2002). This particular topical should be applied using a back and forth motion, with friction, and allowed to dry for 30 seconds.

8. With the nondominant hand, hold the patient's hand or arm and retract the skin distal to the insertion site toward the fingers.

Note: This serves to make the skin taut and anchors the vein to help prevent it from "rolling" (Fig. 7-3).

9. Puncture the vein using direct or indirect entry:

Note: Direct entry (one step) is useful for larger veins.

- Warn the patient of the "stick."

- With the dominant hand, insert the butterfly or catheter needle (bevel up) through the skin at a 15- to 30-degree angle at the site of anticipated vein entry.

- As soon as the skin is punctured, and with one continuous motion, drop the hub down close to the skin, if needed, and enter the vein from the top (see Fig. 7-3).

Note: Indirect entry (two steps) is useful for smaller veins.

- Warn the patient of the "stick."

- With the dominant hand, insert the butterfly or catheter needle (bevel up) through the skin and tissue at a 15- to 30-degree angle slightly distal to the anticipated point of vein entry.

- Relocate the vein and while maintaining the distal anchor, enter the vein either from the top or the side. A "pop" may be felt with vein puncture.

Over-the-needle catheter

Vein

15 degrees

FIGURE 7-3.

continued

Note: If the vein is successfully entered, there will be a flashback of blood into the butterfly or catheter hub tubing.

10. In the case of the catheter, after the initial appearance of the flash, advance the device 2 to 3 mm further to help ensure that the catheter is not inadvertently removed from the vein when the stylette is removed.

11. If the IV line insertion attempt is unsuccessful (no flashback), pull the butterfly and intact catheter back slightly, but not out of the skin.

12. Reassess the location and anchoring of the vein and advance the butterfly or catheter again in the direction of the vein. If the attempt is unsuccessful, the tourniquet should be released and the butterfly or catheter removed (Heckman, 1993).

13. Apply pressure for 1 minute and then attempt insertion at a more proximal site or in the other extremity.

14. Once removed from the skin puncture, properly discard the butterfly or catheter.

Caution: Never reuse a catheter.

15. Once the flashback is achieved, the vein can be cannulated with the butterfly needle or catheter.

Over-the-Needle Catheter Cannulation

- Hold the needle base firmly in place with the nondominant hand while advancing the catheter with the dominant hand over the needle and threading into the vein all the way to the catheter hub (Fig. 7-4).

- Hold the catheter flange in place with the nondominant hand.

- Apply light pressure to the vein proximal to the indwelling catheter tip with the little or long finger of the nondominant hand, release the tourniquet, and activate the needle retraction safety device (Fig. 7-5).

- If you do not have a closed unit system, attach the administration set and release proximal pressure on the vein (Fig. 7-6). The infusion may begin.

Needle

Over-the-needle catheter

FIGURE 7-4.

FIGURE 7-5.

FIGURE 7-6.

Caution: Once the stylette has been separated or withdrawn from the catheter (even partially), it should never be reinserted. Attempting to do so can result in the shearing off of a small portion of the distal catheter, which then floats free in the circulatory system. This small piece of catheter floats until it lodges in a smaller vessel and potentially creates a site for embolism and infarction.

Butterfly Needle Cannulation

- Once the flashback is noted, thread the needle in gently up the distended vein to its hub with the dominant hand (Fig. 7-7). Be careful not to puncture the vein's posterior wall.

- Hold the plastic butterfly portion of the IV line in place against the skin with the

continued

FIGURE 7-7.

FIGURE 7-8.

nondominant hand and apply light pressure to the vein proximal to the indwelling needle tip with the little finger of this hand.

- Release the tourniquet and, if you do not have a closed unit system, attach the administration set.

- Last, release the proximal pressure on the vein and begin the infusion.

16. Inspect the site for any signs of swelling. If swelling is observed, turn off the infusion of fluids and remove the IV line. Apply pressure to the site for at least 3 to 5 minutes. Insertion of the IV line should next be attempted at a more proximal site or in the other extremity.

17. Secure the butterfly or catheter with chevron taping. Slip a 4- to 5-inch-long piece of ½-inch tape under the base of the IV line, adhesive side up, and then cross over the hub to adhere it to the skin proximal to the insertion site.

18. Tape the distal end of the administration set tubing to the skin. Avoid taping over the insertion site (Fig. 7-8).

Note: Some institutions recommend the use of an antibiotic ointment at the IV insertion site.

19. Apply either a gauze bandage or an occlusive dressing over the site.

20. Loop and secure the tubing separate from the butterfly or catheter (Fig. 7-9).

FIGURE 7-9.

SPECIAL CONSIDERATIONS

- Butterfly IV line equipment is especially useful in the pediatric population. It has also been termed a *scalp vein IV line* because of this historically useful site for infants (Weinstein, 1997). However, scalp veins are no longer the first choice for IV access in babies. With small IV catheters available, the sites currently recommended are the hand, forearm, upper arm, foot, and antecubital fossa. Proper securing of the IV line in children is paramount.

- In the geriatric population, the smallest catheter possible (based on infusion indication) should be used. Skin care is an important consideration, with careful securing of the catheter onto the often fragile skin. A tourniquet may not be necessary. Although the site selection process is the same as the one for adults presented earlier, in geriatric patients, the smaller vessels may be fragile and rupture easily. At the other extreme, the larger, hardened, distended veins may represent sclerotic vessel walls, which may make puncture and threading difficult. It is important to avoid lower extremity IV lines in this population.

FOLLOW-UP CARE AND INSTRUCTIONS

■ Instruct the patient receiving IV therapy or the caregiver to notify the IV therapist if there is burning, stinging, redness, bleeding, or swelling at the insertion site. These may be initial signs of infection. The IV solution should be discontinued immediately if these symptoms occur.

■ The rare patient on home IV therapy will require additional education in regard to fluid management, dressings, and possible complications. The most common complication of any IV therapy is phlebitis, which is often a result of movement of the needle or catheter within the vein. This vein may appear indurated, tender, erythematous, hardened, and very warm to the touch. The IV line should be removed immediately (Way, 1994). If the patient experiences significant discomfort, oral analgesics and warm, moist soaks to the area may be administered (Sager, 1980).

REFERENCES

Gardner C: United States House of Representatives honors the National Intravenous Therapy Association, Inc. J Natl Intravenous Ther Assoc 5:14, 1982.

Heckman J: Emergency Care and Transportation of the Sick and Injured. Rosemont, Ill, American Academy of Orthopaedic Surgeons, 1993.

O'Grady NP, Alexander M, Dellinger EP, et al: Guidelines for the prevention of intervascular catheter-related infections. MMWR Recomm Rep 51(RR-10):1-29, 2002.

Sager D, Bomar S: Intravenous Medications. Philadelphia, JB Lippincott, 1980.

Way L: Current Surgical Diagnosis and Treatment. Norwalk, Conn, Appleton & Lange, 1994 .

Weinstein S: Plummer's Principles and Practices of Intravenous Therapy. New York, Lippincott-Raven, 1997.

Chapter 8

Arterial Puncture

Claire Babcock O'Connell

Procedure Goals and Objectives

Goal: To obtain a high-quality sample of arterial blood while observing standard precautions and with a minimal degree of risk to the patient.

Objectives: The student will be able to …

- Describe the indications, contraindications, and rationale for performing an arterial puncture.

- Identify and describe common complications associated with arterial punctures.

- Describe how to perform an Allen test.

- Describe the essential anatomy and physiology associated with the performance of an arterial puncture.

- Identify the materials necessary for performing an arterial puncture and their proper use.

- Properly perform the actions necessary to collect an arterial sample of blood.

- Identify the important aspects of post-procedure care after an arterial puncture.

BACKGROUND AND HISTORY

Gaining intentional access to the circulatory system has been practiced for centuries. As discussed in Chapter 5, at approximately 400 BC, Hippocrates expressed the view that disease was a result of excess substances such as blood, phlegm, black bile, and yellow bile within the body. Resulting from this view, it was believed that the removal of the excess could restore balance. Bloodletting, which involved cutting into a vein with a sharp instrument to release blood from the circulatory system, was commonplace.

Accessing the arterial system specifically is a relatively recent procedure. The first recorded arterial puncture was performed in 1912, and the first arterial sample used for blood gas analysis was obtained in 1919. However, routine blood gas analysis was not practiced until after 1953, with the introduction of technology designed to measure oxygen pressure (McCall, 1998).

INDICATIONS

Arterial puncture is indicated whenever a sample of arterial blood is required. Unlike in venous blood, the level of dissolved gases in an arterial sample is constant throughout the arterial system. Therefore, a sample obtained from any arterial site represents the true level of gases dissolved in the blood within the arterial system and provides a more accurate assessment of ventilation and oxygenation. Arterial blood is preferred whenever an assessment of the level of dissolved gases is needed for diagnostic or therapeutic purposes. The following is a list of conditions that may necessitate arterial sampling:

- Diagnosis of an acute dysfunction in CO_2/O_2 exchange or acid-base balance: Conditions include severe exacerbations of asthma, suspected pulmonary thromboembolism, coma of unknown cause, suspected drug overdose, shock states and cardiac arrhythmias that are refractory to medical intervention.

- Monitoring the severity and progression of a documented disease process in patients with a chronic condition that affects CO_2/O_2 exchange or acid-base balance: Progressive chronic obstructive pulmonary disease (COPD) may be monitored through changes from baseline arterial blood gas values. Patients receiving long-term oxygen therapy should be monitored when changes in status occur and periodically to document status.

- After therapeutic hyperventilation therapy or cardiopulmonary resuscitation, arterial blood gas determinations assist with the need to quantify the patient's response to therapeutic interventions, thus monitoring a return to baseline or the need for further intervention.

Procurement of an arterial sample may be preferred for a specific laboratory test that offers the most accurate assessment when performed on arterial blood. An arterial blood sample is preferable to venous blood samples when

FIGURE 8-1. Modified Allen test. (Redrawn from Pfenninger JL, Fowler GC [eds]: Procedures for Primary Care Physicians. St. Louis, Mosby–Year Book, 1994, p 343.)

assessing ammonia levels, carbon monoxide levels, and lactate levels. Other laboratory tests can be performed using an arterial sample when venous access cannot be readily obtained, such as emergency situations of severe hypovolemia.

CONTRAINDICATIONS

■ Arterial puncture for blood sampling is absolutely contraindicated whenever the arterial pulse is not palpable.

■ For the radial artery, negative results of a modified Allen test (collateral circulation test) suggest an inadequate collateral blood supply to the hand, and an alternate arterial site should be selected. To perform the Allen test (Fig. 8-1), have the patient make a tight fist and elevate the hand; occlude both the radial and ulnar arteries using firm pressure for approximately 1 minute until the hand appears blanched. Lower the hand while maintaining pressure and instruct the patient to open the fist. Release only the ulnar compression while maintaining the radial artery pressure. Color should return to the entire hand within 15 seconds (positive test). Failure of color to return to normal indicates occlusion of the collateral circulation (negative test); radial artery puncture in this setting may result in ischemia and gangrene distal to the site and should not be attempted.

■ Attempting an arterial puncture when surface landmarks are not visible is not recommended.

■ Arterial puncture is inadvisable in the presence of arterial disease, including atherosclerosis, arterial inflammatory conditions, or known or suspected aneurysm.

■ The higher pressure inherent to the arterial system makes arterial puncture a considerably higher risk in a patient with a coagulopathy, severe thrombocytopenia, or in a patient undergoing anticoagulant therapy; a possible future need for such therapy should also be considered.

- Arterial puncture should also be avoided in a patient undergoing therapy for end-stage renal disease who has an arteriovenous shunt or may need placement in the near future.

- Local skin irritations, including infections (such as cellulitis), chronic skin rashes, and burned areas should be avoided. If these conditions are present in the site desired for arterial puncture, an alternative site should be selected.

POTENTIAL COMPLICATIONS

Arterial puncture is an invasive procedure with the potential for significant complications and must be performed with priority given to the safety of the patient. Any break from the proper safety technique can cause injury to the patient, which may result in loss of form and function to the body distal to the arterial puncture site. The risk of complications is increased any time repeated punctures are attempted at the same site.

- The most common complication is hemorrhage or hematoma formation at the puncture site. This occurs more often in brachial and femoral punctures than in radial punctures. Using the smallest gauge needle acceptable for the task helps decrease the risk of hemorrhage or hematoma formation. Hematoma development can best be minimized by prompt pressure placed on the puncture site continuously for 10 minutes after the procedure is complete.

- Thrombosis is more common at the radial artery than at the brachial or femoral artery. It is more likely if the arterial puncture is performed on a vessel with occlusive disease. Thrombosis may lead to ischemia and gangrene distal to the puncture. Thrombosis may also lead to distal embolization of a clot or plaque with resultant arterial occlusion. The potential for loss of function of the hand or fingers is considerable if arterial embolism occurs and is not quickly recognized and treated. The likelihood of thrombosis can be reduced by varying the site of repeated puncture and by using the smallest gauge needle possible. It is imperative to check for collateral circulation (Allen test) before a radial puncture.

- A transient arterial spasm may occur during or after arterial puncture. If this occurs, continue to monitor and assess the collateral circulation. If the circulation remains impaired, vascular consultation should be obtained. If the collateral circulation is compromised, immediate surgical intervention is warranted.

- Nerve damage may result from the inadvertent direct needle insertion into the nerve bundle or by excessive nerve compression secondary to a large hematoma in the adjacent area. If the patient has a coagulopathy that delays clotting, the risk is increased.

■ Infection is rare when proper technique is followed. Proper sterile technique and avoidance of broken or damaged skin when choosing the site for arterial puncture minimizes this risk.

REVIEW OF ESSENTIAL ANATOMY AND PHYSIOLOGY

RADIAL ARTERY

The radial artery is the site most frequently used for arterial puncture. It is close to the skin surface and readily accessible. It also carries the lowest risk of complications. The radial artery runs along the lateral aspect of the anterior forearm and can be easily palpated between the styloid process of the radius and the flexor carpi radialis tendon. The point of maximal pulsation is just proximal (1 to 2 cm) to the transverse wrist crease.

Before attempting radial artery puncture, check for collateral circulation by performing the Allen test. The distal forearm and wrist should be slightly hyperextended and placed on a firm surface. A small, rolled towel placed under the wrist helps achieve hyperextension. The forearm, wrist, and towel can be secured to an arm board with tape for greater stability if necessary.

BRACHIAL ARTERY

The brachial artery can be accessed if the radial artery has recently been punctured or is otherwise not available (Fig. 8-2). It carries a greater risk of complication, including trauma to the basilic vein or median nerve. If occlusive complications occur, there is greater potential for tissue loss distal to the artery because the collateral circulation is less extensive. The brachial artery courses along the medial surface of the antecubital fossa and should be accessed above the antecubital crease. The arm should be fully extended and secured to a firm surface, ulnar side up.

Puncture site

FIGURE 8-2. The right brachial artery, its branches, and the anatomic site for brachial artery puncture. (Redrawn from Pfenninger JL, Fowler GC [eds]: Procedures for Primary Care Physicians. St. Louis, Mosby–Year Book, 1994, p 345.)

Puncture site

FIGURE 8-3. The right femoral artery and branches. (Redrawn from Pfenninger JL, Fowler GC: Procedures for Primary Care Physicians. St. Louis, Mosby–Year Book, 1994, p 345.)

FEMORAL ARTERY

The femoral artery should be punctured only if radial or brachial artery access is not possible or advisable (Fig. 8-3). If the patient is severely volume depleted or is in shock, the femoral artery may be the only pulse with enough pressure to obtain arterial blood. The femoral artery can be located using the mnemonic NAVEL (*n*erve, *a*rtery, *v*ein, *e*mpty space, *l*ymphatics) from lateral to medial in the inguinal crease. The patient should be supine on a firm surface with hip extended and rotated externally.

Standard Precautions   Practitioners should use standard precautions at all times when interacting with patients. Determining the level of precaution necessary requires the practitioner to exercise clinical judgment based on the patient's history and the potential for exposure to body fluids or aerosol-borne pathogens (for further discussion, see Chapter 2).

PATIENT PREPARATION

- The patient should be educated concerning the purpose of the test and advised of the potential level of discomfort and complications associated with performing the procedure.

- If consent forms are available, consent should be obtained.

- It is important that the patient remain as still as possible during the procedure; a supine position is recommended.

- If oxygen therapy is adjusted or the patient has been suctioned, wait at least 15 minutes before sampling to allow gas levels to stabilize.

Materials Utilized for Arterial Puncture

- 3- to 5-mL glass or special heparinized syringe made for arterial blood gas collection.

Note: If not available, use plastic syringe and heparinize (see later).

- 21- to 25-gauge, ½- to ⅝-inch needle

- Bag or cup of ice for transport

- Iodine-containing skin preparation pads

- Cork board or rubber for needle safety

- Rubber stopper or plug for syringe

- Sterile gloves (two pairs)

- Sterile gauze, 2 inch × 2 inch or 4 inch × 4 inch

- Arm board

- Tape (½ to 1 inch)

- Goggles

- 1:1000 lidocaine without epinephrine (1 to 2 mL)

- Syringe and needle for local anesthesia

Procedure for Arterial Puncture

1. Secure and stabilize the site by placing the patient's supinated arm on the arm board and securing with tape. Prepare a sterile field and gather all equipment.

2. Put on sterile gloves.

3. Cleanse skin with an iodine solution (e.g., povidone-iodine [Betadine], iodophor).

Note: Some practitioners prefer to follow this with an alcohol cleansing. Allow the area to air dry.

4. Coat the syringe and needle with heparin; use a plain plastic syringe if a preheparinized syringe is not available. Heparinize by aspirating 0.5 mL heparin, 10,000 U/mL, and pulling the plunger to

continued

the end of the syringe while holding the syringe and needle vertically. Slowly push back on the plunger to evacuate the heparin. The syringe and needle are now adequately coated with heparin.

Note: Heparinization of the syringe is necessary to prevent coagulation of the sample.

Local Anesthesia

Note: Traditionally, arterial puncture has been performed without the use of local anesthesia. Several studies have proved that there is a significant decrease in pain when local anesthesia is administered before arterial puncture. Concerns that local anesthesia inhibits proper placement by obliterating landmarks have been unfounded. The use of local anesthesia does make arterial puncture a "two-stick" procedure rather than a "one-stick" procedure. However, the intensity of the pain associated with arterial puncture may support the use of the less painful stick required with local anesthesia.

    Note: Use a small amount (1 to 2 mL) of lidocaine without epinephrine to anesthetize the local area. Overzealous anesthesia may obscure landmarks or dull the pulse.

5. Anesthize the area. Advance the needle to just above the periosteum on each side of the artery without entering or making direct contact with the artery. Aspiration should be attempted before injecting the anesthetic to ensure that the anesthetic is injected into the surrounding tissues and not a blood vessel.

Note: Allow several minutes for the anesthetic to take effect before performing the arterial puncture. (For more information regarding local anesthesia techniques, refer to Chapter 22.)

40- to 60-degree angle

Figure 8-4. Needle insertion. (Redrawn from Pfenninger JL, Fowler GC [eds]: Procedures for Primary Care Physicians. St. Louis, Mosby–Year Book, 1994, p 345.)

6. Palpate the artery with the nondominant hand and locate the point of maximal pulsation.

7. Face the patient. Hold the syringe like a dart or a pencil with the bevel facing proximally.

8. Insert the needle at a 40- to 60-degree angle (60- to 90-degree angle for femoral puncture) (Fig. 8-4).

9. Advance the needle until blood is seen entering the hub.

10. If no blood is seen, pull back until the needle is just below the skin and redirect the point 1 mm to either side. If the patient complains of sharp pain radiating up the arm withdraw slightly and reposition. Do not exit completely.

11. Once blood enters the hub of the needle, the arterial pressure should cause blood to fill the syringe spontaneously.

12. In severely hypotensive patients, slight aspiration may be required, but this is rarely necessary.

13. Collect 3 to 5 mL of blood and then remove the needle with a swift, smooth motion.

FIGURE 8-5. Application of pressure. (Redrawn from Potter P: Fundamentals of Nursing, 4th ed. St. Louis, Mosby–Year Book, 1997.)

14. Immediately apply firm, continuous pressure to the area for a minimum of 10 minutes, longer if the patient is hypertensive or is receiving anticoagulant therapy. Pressure should be applied even if no sample is obtained (Fig. 8-5). Apply a pressure dressing and leave intact for the next several hours.

Note: It is not advisable to have the patient apply the pressure; an assistant is recommended.

15. Hold the syringe and needle upright and allow any air bubbles to rise; tapping gently on the side of the syringe may help. Expel any air from the syringe.

16. Insert the needle into a cork or rubber piece for safety; remove the needle from the syringe, dispose of it properly, and close the syringe with a rubber stopper.

17. Gently roll the syringe between your palms to ensure uniform mixing of the sample with the heparin.

18. Label the syringe and place it on ice for immediate transport to the laboratory.

19. Check the arterial puncture site for hematoma formation and adequate distal perfusion.

20. Return to the patient for a repeat check in 5 minutes and again in 15 minutes. Monitor for any changes in color, temperature, vascular incompetency, or function. Inquire if the patient has experienced any numbness, increased pain, or coldness.

21. Record date and time of sampling, patient temperature, and whether the patient is on oxygen therapy at the time of sampling.

SPECIAL CONSIDERATIONS

- Prompt analysis of the sample is imperative. Delay in analysis or improper chilling causes the blood to dissociate from the hemoglobin, thus affecting oxygen levels.
- If air is trapped in the syringe, an open system exists, which may cause O_2 to be dissolved into the sample, causing a relative decrease in Pco_2 and an increase in Po_2. The use of a Vacutainer system also allows O_2 to enter the sample. A plain plastic syringe may lose O_2 through diffusion.
- In the presence of leukocytosis ($>100,000/mm^3$) or thrombocytosis ($>10^6/mm^3$), consumption of O_2 may be great because of the breakdown of the excess cells. This is accompanied by a release of CO_2, causing a pseudoacidosis. A delay in analysis or improper chilling enhances this effect. The Pco_2 rises approximately 3 to 10 mm Hg per hour in an un-iced specimen, but it is stable for approximately 1 to 2 hours in a properly iced specimen.
- Excess heparin in the syringe causes a decrease in pH. This is due to the low pH of heparin and the dilutional effects on the bicarbonate present in the sample.

FOLLOW-UP CARE AND INSTRUCTIONS

- Patients who have undergone this procedure must be monitored to ensure that hemostasis has been achieved.

- Advise the patient that a small amount of tenderness and ecchymosis may result from the procedure.

- Advise the patient to seek evaluation if he or she experiences increasing pain, redness, or coolness of the extremity distal to the arterial puncture site.

- Patients should avoid rigorous activity for at least 24 hours.

REFERENCE

McCall RT, Tankersley CM: Phlebotomy Essentials, 2nd ed. Philadelphia, JB Lippincott, 1998.

BIBLIOGRAPHY

Bhardwaj D, Norris A, Won DT: Is skin puncture beneficial prior to arterial catheter insertion? Can J Anaesth 46:129-132, 1999.

Chestnutt MS, Dewar TN, Locksley RM, Chestnutt M: Office and Bedside Procedures. New York, McGraw-Hill, 1996, pp 116-127.

Fowler GC: Arterial puncture. In Pfenninger JL, Fowler GC (eds): Procedures for Primary Care Physicians. St. Louis, Mosby–Year Book, 2003, Ch 79.

Giner J, Casan P, Belda J, et al: Pain during arterial puncture. Chest 110:1443-1445, 1996.

Gomella LG: Clinician's Pocket Reference, 10th ed. New York, McGraw-Hill, 2004, pp 249-251.

Lightowler JV, Elliot MW: Local anesthetic infiltration prior to arterial puncture for blood gas analysis: A survey of current practice and a randomised double blind placebo controlled trial. J R Coll Phys Lond 31:645-646, 1997.

Macklis RM, Mendelsohn ME, Mudge GH: Introduction to Clinical Medicine, 3rd ed. Philadelphia, Lippincott-Raven, 1994, pp 123-129.

Marini JJ, Wheeler AP: Critical Care Medicine: The Essentials. Philadelphia, Lippincott Williams & Wilkins, 1997, pp 105-107.

Okeson GC, Wulbrecht PH: The safety of brachial artery puncture for arterial blood sampling. Chest 114:748-751, 1998.

Chapter 9

Injections

Conrad J. Rios

This chapter was adapted from the 1st edition chapter written by Robert J. McNellis, MPH, PA-C. Mr. McNellis is the Director of Clinical Affairs and Education for the American Academy of Physician Assistants in Alexandria, Virginia.

PROCEDURE GOALS AND OBJECTIVES

Goal: To perform an injection successfully while observing standard precautions and with the minimal degree of risk to the patient.

Objectives: The student will be able to ...

- Describe the indications, contraindications, and rationale for administering an injection.

- Identify and describe common complications associated with administering injections.

- Describe the essential anatomy and physiology associated with performing an injection.

- Identify the materials necessary for performing an injection and their proper use.

- Identify the important aspects of patient care after an injection.

BACKGROUND AND HISTORY

This chapter covers the most common procedures for parenteral administration of medications. Although *parenteral* means any route other than enteral (gastrointestinal), it ordinarily refers to methods of giving drugs by injection. The most common routes of parenteral medication administration are intradermal, subcutaneous, intramuscular, and intravenous. Intravenous procedures are covered in Chapter 7.

Injections are part of the armamentarium of most medical disciplines. In addition to this common ground, each specialty has its own particular applications (Brokensha, 1999).

The first experiments with intravenous injections were carried out in 1642 by a gentleman's hunting servant in eastern Germany. Similar experiments were performed in 1656 by Christopher Wren (an astronomer, mathematician, and architect in Oxford, England) and by a group of scientists associated with the physicist Robert Boyle. These experiments were prompted by new knowledge about blood circulation provided by William Harvey in 1628. The first books on the applications of intravenous infusions in humans were published in 1664 and 1667. Bladders of animals or enema syringes were used as instruments. Because of lethal accidents, the infusions soon fell out of favor (Feldmann, 2000).

Reinier de Graaf has been credited with the invention of the injection syringe in the late 1660s. De Graaf studied under anatomist Johannes van Horne at the newly established University of Leyden in Holland. As a young student, De Graaf helped Van Horne prepare anatomic specimens, and he used the injection syringe to introduce liquids and wax into the prepared blood vessels as a coloring and preservation medium.

In 1853, Charles Pravaz, a French surgeon in Lyon, invented a small syringe, the piston of which could be driven by a screw, allowing exact doses. A sharp needle with a pointed trocar could be introduced into a vessel, making dissection unnecessary. Pravaz used his syringe for obliteration of arterial aneurysms by injection of ferric sesquichlorate. Pravaz's syringe initiated the invention of a great number of various calibrated syringes made of glass or metal combined with glass. The calibrated syringes were commonly used in the treatment of syphilis by mercurialization.

Also in 1853, in a paper entitled "A New Method of Treating Neuralgia by Direct Application of Opioids to the Painful Point," Alexander Wood introduced his hollow needle in London, England. Within 5 years, injections of morphine had become enormously popular; thriving practices developed in response to what was seen as a potent, benign, and beneficial treatment. Patients were treated with hundreds of injections. Their doctors seemed blissfully unaware of the systemic effects of the drug they were injecting and the nature of the demand for the new treatment.

Charles Hunter, another English physician, was discouraged from using the new technique when his first two patients developed local abscesses. In 1858, he discovered that patients gained just as much benefit from injections distant from the painful site. Hunter coined the term hypodermic and claimed that his treatment was superior to that of Wood. Physicians debated the merits of the two physicians' claims and decided in Hunter's favor. During the debate, physicians continued with both treatments, apparently blind to the addiction underlying the huge and increasingly lucrative demand (Howard-Jones, 1971).

Since the 19th century, there have been great advances in understanding the mechanisms of action of parenteral medications and improvements in the technology of injections. However, the basic principles remain the same. Today, injections can be given in any space or potential space; they can be administered hypodermically under direct vision or guided by ultrasonography or radiography, as well as through the use of endoscopic techniques. The widespread use of needleless (jet) injection systems is just on the horizon. Delivery systems that are less invasive, such as nasal sprays, transdermal patches, and continuous infusion devices, may make injections less and less common.

INDICATIONS

Indications include an illness or injury that requires parenteral medication to improve, treat, or maintain the patient's condition, as well as administration of vaccines for disease prevention.

Caution: As with other medical therapies, the patient has the right to refuse an invasive procedure such as an injection.

CONTRAINDICATIONS

Potential contraindications to injections include the following conditions:
- Allergy to the intended medication
- Lack of a suitable site for injection
- Coagulopathy
- Occlusive peripheral vascular disease
- Shock
- Impairment of peripheral absorption

POTENTIAL COMPLICATIONS

- Anaphylactic or toxic reaction to the medication: Treatment is supportive for anaphylaxis and may vary depending on the severity of the reaction. Medication to reverse the toxic effect of the drug should be readily available. Risk of anaphylaxis can be minimized by asking the patient about allergies or checking medical alert bracelets before injection.

- Medication error: Errors often can be avoided by using the "five rights" as guidelines for the administration of medication. These guidelines ensure that the right drug is given to the right patient in the right dose by the right route at the right time:
  - Right drug: The medication label should be checked three times: when the drug is taken from storage, when the amount of drug is removed, and when the container is returned to storage.
  - Right patient: Always check the patient's identification bracelet or ask the patient to state his or her name.
  - Right dose: Errors in dose are minimized when the unit system is used and a pharmacist prepares drugs. If a drug dose for an infant or child must be calculated, have a second person check the arithmetic, because even a small error can lead to a serious overdose. It is good practice to have a second person double check doses of heparin, insulin, and epinephrine.
  - Right route: Only give injections of substances prepared for parenteral use; it should say "injectable" on the label. Avoid giving an inadvertent intravenous injection by drawing back before pushing the drug.
  - Right time: It is important to know why a drug is ordered for a certain time. Be sure to document when drugs were given.
- The practitioner is responsible for the medications that are administered. Administer only the drugs prepared personally or those that were prepared by the pharmacist, unless there is an emergency situation.
- Infection or abscess at the site: Infection typically occurs as the result of improper aseptic technique. Sterile abscesses can occur after injecting concentrated or irritating solutions. Rotating injection sites can minimize this complication. Injections should be avoided at sites that are inflamed, edematous, or irritated and at sites with moles, birthmarks, scar tissue, or other lesions.
- Lipodystrophy or atrophy of subcutaneous fat, which is caused by repeated injections at the same site: Rotating injection sites can minimize this complication.
- Injection pain: Minimize the use of irritating solutions given subcutaneously to reduce pain. Techniques to reduce the pain of intramuscular injections include having the patient relax the muscle, avoiding extrasensitive areas, waiting until the antiseptic is dry before injecting the medication, using a new needle for injection, inserting and withdrawing the needle rapidly, massaging the muscle after injection to distribute the medication better and increase its absorption, and using ice or topical spray to numb the area before injection.

Figure 9-1. Sites for subcutaneous injection.

REVIEW OF ESSENTIAL ANATOMY AND PHYSIOLOGY

Intradermal injections are given in the outer layers of the skin. There is little systemic absorption of intradermally injected agents, so this type of injection is given primarily to produce a local effect. The ventral forearm is the most commonly used site because of its easy accessibility and lack of hair. In extensive allergy testing, the outer aspect of the upper arms and the area of the back between the scapulae are used.

Subcutaneous injections are given into the adipose tissue beneath the skin. The most common sites are the outer aspects of the upper arm, anterior thigh, loose tissue of the lower abdomen, upper buttocks, and upper back (Fig. 9-1).

Intramuscular injections deposit medication deep into muscle tissue, where it can be readily absorbed. The rate of drug absorption is faster than with the subcutaneous route but slower than with the intravenous route.

Intramuscular sites (Fig. 9-2) include the following:

■ Deltoid muscle: The deltoid muscle is located on the lateral side of the humerus. Place four fingers across the deltoid muscle, with the top finger along the acromion process. The injection site is two to three fingerbreadths below the acromion process (Fig. 9-3). Injecting lower or more posterior in the muscle can result in injury to the radial and ulnar nerves or brachial artery.

■ Dorsogluteal (gluteus medius): Locate the posterior superior iliac spine and the greater trochanter of the femur. Draw an imaginary line between the two landmarks. The injection site is above and lateral to the line. A less accurate method is dividing the buttocks into quadrants. The

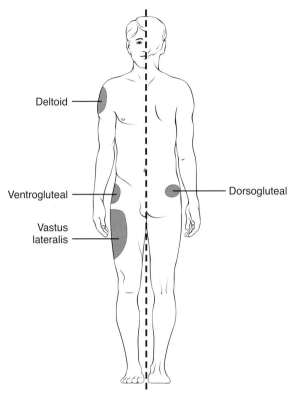

FIGURE 9-2.   Sites for intramuscular injection.

FIGURE 9-3.   Deltoid muscle.

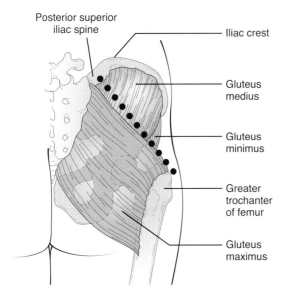

Posterior superior
iliac spine

Iliac crest

Gluteus
medius

Gluteus
minimus

Greater
trochanter
of femur

Gluteus
maximus

FIGURE 9-4. Inject above and lateral to dotted line.

vertical dividing line extends from the gluteal fold up to the iliac crest. The injecting horizontal line extends from the medial fold to the lateral aspect of the buttock. The injection site is the upper outer quadrant, about 2 to 3 inches below the iliac crest. The risk of injury to the sciatic nerve can be great at this site; injury can cause paralysis of the affected leg (Fig. 9-4).

■ Ventrogluteal (gluteus medius and gluteus minimus): Place the heel of your hand over the greater trochanter. Point the thumb toward the groin and fingers toward the head. Place the index finger over the anterosuperior iliac spine and extend the middle finger along the iliac crest. The index finger and middle finger form a V. Inject into the center of the V. The muscles of this site are deep and away from major nerves and blood vessels (Fig. 9-5).

■ Vastus lateralis muscle: This muscle is located at the anterolateral aspect of the thigh and extends from a handbreadth above the knee to a handbreadth below the greater trochanter of the femur. The middle third of the muscle is the best site for injection. This site is a well-developed muscle that lacks major nerves and blood vessels. The branches of the lateral femoral cutaneous nerve are located superficially, and a few cases of damage to these branches have been reported. It is the preferred site for infants, children, and adults (Fig. 9-6).

Parenteral medication administration provides longer action and avoids the first-pass metabolic effects of the liver. Each route of administration has advantages and disadvantages:

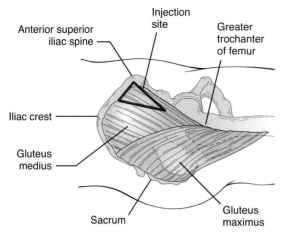

Anterior superior iliac spine

Injection site

Greater trochanter of femur

Iliac crest

Gluteus medius

Sacrum

Gluteus maximus

FIGURE 9-5. Ventrogluteal site.

Gluteus maximus

Biceps femoris

Rectus femoris

Vastus lateralis

Injection site

Knee

FIGURE 9-6. Vastus lateral site.

- Intradermal injections have slow absorption, which is an advantage when testing for allergies.

- The disadvantages of intradermal injections are that only small amounts of drug may be administered and they require an aseptic technique.

- Subcutaneous injections have the advantage of faster onset of drug action than the oral route.

- Disadvantages of subcutaneous injections include the need for aseptic technique, their greater expense when compared with oral medication, the small volume that can be administered, and the potential to produce anxiety; some drugs can irritate tissues and cause pain.

- Intramuscular injections minimize pain from irritating drugs, have larger volumes of drug that can be administered compared with the subcutaneous route, and provide rapidly absorbed medication.

- Disadvantages of intramuscular injections include the need for aseptic technique, the possibility of blood vessel and nerve damage, and the potential to produce anxiety.

Standard Precautions   Every practitioner should use standard precautions at all times when interacting with patients, especially when performing procedures. Determining the level of precaution necessary requires the practitioner to exercise clinical judgment based on the patient's history and the potential for exposure to body fluids or aerosol-borne pathogens (for further discussion, see Chapter 2).

PATIENT PREPARATION

- Explain to the patient why it is necessary to administer the injection.

- Obtain verbal consent to give an injection.

- Ask the patient if he or she is allergic to any medications and the type of reaction that occurs.

- Inform the patient of the benefits and risks in understandable language.

- Inform the patient which site will be used for administering the injection.

- Tell the patient that there will be a sting or pricking sensation felt when the needle is inserted.

- Warn the patient of potential side effects, and advise the patient of signs and symptoms to watch for.

- Ask again about allergies.

Materials Utilized for Administering an Injection

- Appropriate medication
- Syringe and needle
- Materials for cleansing the skin: alcohol pad, most commonly saturated with 70% isopropyl alcohol
- Sterile or unsterile gloves
- Needle disposal box
- Bandage strips and gauze pads

Note: Medication comes in many forms:

- Ampule containing a single drug dose

- Vial containing single or multiple drug doses

- Vial containing powder to which a sterile diluent or solvent must be added with some drugs

- Prefilled cartridge package

- Syringe

Note: Syringes range in size from a capacity of 1 mL to 50 mL, but syringes larger than 5 mL are rarely used for injections. A 2- or 3-mL syringe is adequate for most subcutaneous and intramuscular injections. Most institutions use plastic syringes, although some medications in prefilled cartridges require cartridge syringes (e.g., Tubex).

Insulin syringes have a capacity of 1 mL and are calibrated in units. There is a syringe designed for use with each strength of insulin. For example, a syringe marked U100 is coded to match the label of a vial of insulin that contains 100 units/mL. Tuberculin syringes also have a capacity of 1 mL, but they are long, slender, and calibrated in 0.01-mL units. This fine calibration makes it possible to administer very small amounts of potent drugs, such as those used for intradermal skin testing.

- Barrel of the syringe, handle of the plunger, and hub of the needle

Note: These parts must, out of necessity, be handled during the preparation and administration of an injection, but the inside and tip of the barrel and the shaft of the plunger must be kept sterile, as must the entire length of the needle (Fig. 9-7).

- Needle

Note: Needles that are commonly used for injections vary in length from $\frac{1}{2}$ to $1\frac{1}{2}$ inches; they vary in diameter from 14 to 26 gauge (the larger the gauge, the smaller the diameter). A common size for a subcutaneous injection is 25 gauge, $\frac{5}{8}$ inch; the needle for an intramuscular injection is larger and longer: 18 to 22 gauge, $1\frac{1}{2}$ inches. Typically, needles for intradermal injections are 26 or 27 gauge and $\frac{1}{2}$ to $\frac{5}{8}$ inch long. Needles are packaged individually to permit greater flexibility in selecting the right needle for a specific patient. A syringe and needle may be packaged

FIGURE 9-7. Parts of a syringe and needle.

together if the size of the needle is relatively standard, such as an insulin or tuberculin syringe and needle.

Note: The length of the needle is determined by the size and weight of the patient and whether the drug will be injected subcutaneously or intramuscularly. The gauge depends on the viscosity of the fluid to be injected. A thin, watery, nonsticky solution can be injected easily through a fine-gauge needle (25 or 26), but a thicker, sticky solution requires a larger gauge needle (20 to 22).

Note: Many institutions are beginning to move toward needleless or safety needle systems for injections. In these systems, medication can often be drawn through vials without needles, and, after the injection, needles retract into the plunger, or a sheath covers the needles. Follow the manufacturer's instructions for proper use of these systems.

Procedure for Aspirating from an Ampule

1. Identify the patient.

2. Wash your hands and put on gloves.

3. Select and assemble the appropriately sized needle and syringe (use filter needle with glass ampule if the medication requires it).

4. Remove the liquid from the neck of the ampule by flicking it or swinging it

   quickly in a downward, spiraling motion while holding it by the top (Fig. 9-8A).

5. Tap around the neck of the ampule.

6. Protect your fingers with gauze if the ampule is made of glass.

7. Carefully break off the top of the ampule (for a plastic ampule twist the top) (see Fig. 9-8B).

A   B   C

Figure 9-8.

continued

8. Aspirate fluid from the ampule (see Fig. 9-8C).

9. Remove any air from the syringe as needed.

10. Clean up and dispose of working needle and ampule in accordance with your institution's policy for disposing of contaminated materials and sharp objects (see Chapter 2).

Procedure for Aspirating from a Vial

1. Identify the patient.

2. Wash hands and put on gloves.

3. Disinfect the top of the vial with an alcohol pad.

4. Select a syringe with a volume twice the required amount of drug or solution and add the needle.

5. Draw up as much air as the amount of solution that will be aspirated.

6. Insert the needle into the top of the vial and turn upside down (Fig. 9-9A).

7. Push air out of the syringe into the vial (see Fig. 9-9B).

8. Aspirate the required amount of solution.

Note: Make sure the tip of the needle is below the fluid surface.

9. Pull the needle out of the vial.

10. Remove air from the syringe as needed (see Fig. 9-9C).

11. Clean up and dispose of materials in accordance with your institution's policy for disposing of contaminated materials and sharp objects (see Chapter 2).

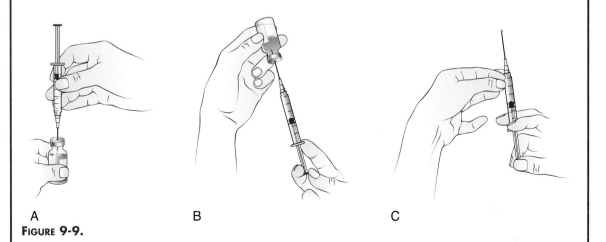

A   B   C

FIGURE 9-9.

Procedure for Administering an Intradermal Injection

1. Identify the patient.

2. Wash hands and put on gloves.

3. Select a tuberculin syringe with a 26- or 27-gauge needle: ½ to ⅝ inch long is generally used.

4. Using aseptic technique, withdraw the appropriate amount of medication from the vial or ampule.

5. With the patient sitting up, have him or her extend the forearm and lay it on a flat surface with the ventral side exposed.

6. Cleanse the surface of the ventral forearm about two to three fingerbreadths distal to the antecubital space using an alcohol pad.

Note: Be sure the test site is free of hair and lesions. Allow the skin to dry completely before administering the injection.

7. While holding the patient's forearm in your hand, stretch the skin taut with your thumb.

8. With your free hand, hold the needle at a 15-degree angle to the patient's arm, with its bevel facing up.

9. Insert the needle about ⅛ inch below the epidermis (Fig. 9-10). Stop when the needle bevel is beneath the skin, and inject the antigen slowly. You should feel some resistance as you do this, and a wheal or bleb should form as you inject the antigen. If no wheal forms, you have injected the antigen too deeply; withdraw the needle and administer

Figure 9-10.

another test dose at least 2 inches from the first site.

10. Withdraw the needle at the same angle at which it was inserted.

11. Do not rub the site. This could cause irritation of the underlying tissue and may affect the test results.

12. Dispose of the syringe and needle according to your institution's policy regarding disposal of contaminated items and sharp objects (see Chapter 2).

13. Document which agents were given, including the lot number and expiration date; where, how (which specific injection method), and when they were given; and by whom.

14. Assess the patient's response in 24 to 48 hours.

Note: In patients hypersensitive to the test antigen, a severe anaphylactic response can result. This requires immediate epinephrine injection and other emergency resuscitation procedures. Be especially alert after giving a test dose of penicillin or tetanus antitoxin.

Procedure for Administering a Subcutaneous Injection

1. Identify the patient.

2. Wash hands and put on gloves.

3. Select a 2- to 3-mL syringe with a 24- to 26-gauge needle that is ⅜ to 1 inch long, depending on the amount of subcutaneous fat.

Note: A longer needle is needed for an obese adult, a shorter needle for a thin child.

4. Using aseptic technique, withdraw the appropriate amount of medication from the vial or ampule.

5. Select an appropriate site.

6. Rotate sites according to a planned schedule for patients who require repeated injections. Use different areas of the body unless contraindicated by the specific drug.

7. Position and drape the patient.

8. Cleanse the injection site with a sterile alcohol pad, beginning at the center of the site and moving outward in a circular motion.

Note: Allow the skin to dry so that alcohol is not introduced into subcutaneous tissues as the needle is inserted.

9. With the nondominant hand, pinch the skin around the injection site.

10. Insert the needle with the bevel facing up at a 45-degree angle (Fig. 9-11). If a fat fold is more than 1 inch, the needle may be injected at a 90-degree angle.

11. Release the patient's skin to avoid injecting into compressed tissue and irritating nerve fibers.

12. Pull back on the plunger slightly. If no blood is aspirated, begin injecting the

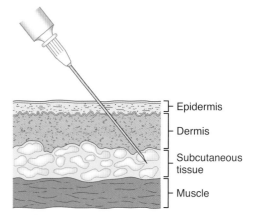

Epidermis

Dermis

Subcutaneous tissue

Muscle

FIGURE 9-11.

drug slowly. If blood appears on aspiration, withdraw the needle, prepare another syringe, and repeat the procedure.

13. After injection, remove the needle gently but quickly at the same angle used for insertion.

14. Cover the site with an alcohol sponge or sterile gauze pad and massage the site gently (unless contraindicated [e.g., heparin]) to distribute the drug and facilitate absorption.

15. Remove the sponge and check the injection site for bleeding.

16. Dispose of the syringe and needle according to your institution's policy regarding disposal of contaminated items and sharp objects (see Chapter 2).

17. Document the medication given, including the lot number and expiration date; where, how (specific injection method), and when it was given; and by whom.

SPECIAL CONSIDERATIONS

ADMINISTERING INSULIN

Note: To establish more consistent blood levels, rotate insulin injection sites within anatomic regions. Absorption varies from one region to another. Preferred insulin injection sites are the arms, abdomen, thighs, and buttocks.

1. Make sure the type of insulin, dose, and syringe are correct.
2. When combining different types of insulin in a syringe, make sure they are compatible. Regular insulin can be mixed with all types.
3. Before drawing up insulin suspension, gently roll and invert the bottle to ensure even particle distribution. Do not shake the bottle, because this can cause foam or bubbles to develop, changing the potency and altering the dose.

ADMINISTERING HEPARIN

Note:
■ The preferred site for heparin injections is the lower abdominal fat pad, 2 inches beneath the umbilicus, between the iliac crests. Injecting heparin into this area, which is not involved in muscular activity, reduces the risk of local capillary bleeding. Always rotate the sites from one side to the other.

■ Do not administer any injections within 2 inches of a scar, bruise, or the umbilicus.

■ Do not aspirate to check for blood return because this may cause bleeding into the tissues at the site.

■ Do not rub or massage the site after the injection. Rubbing can cause localized minute hemorrhages or bruises.

■ If the patient bruises easily, apply ice to the site for the first 5 minutes after the injection to minimize local hemorrhage.

Procedure for Administering an Intramuscular Injection

1. Identify the patient.

2. Wash hands and put on gloves.

3. Select a 2- to 5-mL syringe with an 18- to 22-gauge needle 1 to 2 inches in length, depending on the injection site and the amount of muscle mass of the patient.

4. Using aseptic technique, withdraw the appropriate amount of medication from the vial or ampule and then draw about 0.2 mL of air into the syringe.

5. Select an appropriate intramuscular site.

6. Position and drape the patient.

continued

7. Cleanse the injection site with a sterile alcohol sponge, beginning at the center of the site and moving outward in a circular motion. Allow the skin to dry so that alcohol is not introduced into subcutaneous tissues as the needle is inserted.

8. With the thumb and index finger of your nondominant hand, press down and stretch the skin of the injection site.

Note: This reduces the thickness of subcutaneous tissue that must be pierced to reach the muscle. This is required in an obese patient. If the patient is emaciated, raise the underlying muscle mass by pinching the tissue between the thumb and index finger.

9. Position the syringe at a 90-degree angle to the skin surface, with the needle a couple of inches from the skin. Quickly and firmly thrust the needle through the skin and subcutaneous tissue deep into the muscle (Fig. 9-12).

10. Hold the syringe with your nondominant hand, if desired. Pull back slightly on the plunger with your dominant hand. If no blood is aspirated, place your thumb on

FIGURE 9-13.

the plunger rod and slowly inject the medication into the muscle.

Note: A slow, steady injection rate allows the muscle to distend gradually and accept the medication under minimal pressure. There should be little or no resistance against the force of injection. The air bubble added to the syringe when it was prepared should follow the medication into the injection site to create an air block and prevent tracking of the medication back into the subcutaneous tissue (Fig. 9-13).

11. If blood appears in the syringe on aspiration, the needle is in a blood vessel. If this occurs, withdraw the needle, prepare another injection with new equipment, and inject another site. Do not inject the bloody solution. (Follow your institution's policy for disposal of contaminated items and sharp objects.)

12. After the injection, gently but rapidly remove the needle at a 90-degree angle.

13. Cover the injection site immediately with an alcohol sponge or sterile gauze pad, apply gentle pressure and, unless contraindicated, massage the muscle to

Epidermis

Dermis

Subcutaneous tissue

Muscle

FIGURE 9-12.

help distribute the drug and promote absorption.

14. Remove the alcohol sponge and inspect the injection site for signs of active bleeding. If bleeding continues, apply pressure to the site.

15. Dispose of the syringe and needle according to your institution's policy

regarding disposal of contaminated items and sharp objects. (see Chapter 2).

16. Document the medication given, including the lot number and expiration date; where, how (specific injection method), and when it was given; and by whom.

Procedure for Administering a Z-track Intramuscular Injection

Note: The Z-track method of intramuscular injection prevents leakage of medication back into subcutaneous tissue after the injection is given. It is used with certain drugs—primarily iron preparations—that irritate or discolor subcutaneous tissue. Lateral displacement of the skin before injection helps seal the drug in the muscle after the skin is released. This procedure requires careful attention to technique, because leakage into subcutaneous tissue can cause patient discomfort or may permanently stain tissue if an iron preparation is being given. This type of injection is given only in the outer upper quadrant of the buttocks.

1. Identify the patient.

2. Wash hands and put on gloves.

3. Select a 3- to 5-mL syringe with two 20-gauge needles at least 2 inches long.

4. Using aseptic technique, withdraw the appropriate amount of medication from the vial or ampule and then draw about 0.2 to 0.5 mL of air into the syringe. Remove the first needle and attach the second needle to prevent introduction of medication from the outside of the first needle into the subcutaneous tissue.

Note: For this type of injection, be sure to provide privacy for the patient.

5. Select an appropriate site in an upper outer buttock.

6. Position and drape the patient in the prone or lateral position.

7. Cleanse the area with a sterile alcohol pad.

8. Displace the skin laterally by pulling it about ½ inch away from the injection site (Fig. 9-14A and B).

Air lock
Medication

During injection

A

Injection tract seals
as skin is released

Skin

Subcutaneous
tissue

Air lock

Muscle

Medication

After release

B

FIGURE 9-14.

continued

9. Insert the needle into the muscle at a 90-degree angle.

10. Pull back on the plunger slightly. If no blood is aspirated, inject the drug slowly, followed by the air, which helps clear the needle and prevents tracking of the medication through the subcutaneous tissue.

11. Encourage the patient to walk or move around in bed to facilitate absorption from the injection site.

12. Dispose of the syringe and needle according to your institution's policy regarding disposal of contaminated items (see Chapter 2).

13. Document the medication given, including the lot number and expiration date; where, how (specific injection method), and when it was given; and by whom.

Caution: Never inject more than 5 mL into a single site using the Z-track method.

Note: Alternate gluteal sites to avoid repeated injections in the same site. If the patient is on bed rest, encourage active range of motion exercises or perform passive range of motion exercises to facilitate absorption from the injection site.

Note: If you must inject more than 5 mL of solution, divide the solution and inject it at two separate sites unless the gluteal muscles and vastus lateralis are well developed. Intramuscular injections can traumatize local muscle cells, causing elevated serum levels of enzymes (creatine phosphokinase [CPK]) that can be confused with the elevated enzyme levels resulting from damage to cardiac muscle, as in myocardial infarction. Oral or intravenous routes are preferred for administration of drugs that are poorly absorbed by muscle tissue, such as phenytoin, digoxin, chlordiazepoxide, diazepam, and haloperidol.

SPECIAL CONSIDERATIONS

PEDIATRIC PATIENTS

- Subcutaneous injections are usually administered into the thigh of infants and into the deltoid area of older children.

- The preferred sites for intramuscular injections are the anterolateral aspect of the upper thigh and the deltoid muscle of the upper arm.

- Among most infants, the anterolateral thigh provides the largest muscle mass and is therefore the recommended site.

- The deltoid can also be used with the thigh when multiple injections (such as vaccinations) are needed.

- In toddlers and older children, the deltoid may be used if the muscle mass is adequate.

- Never use the gluteal muscles, which develop from walking, as the injection site for children younger than age 3 or for those who have been walking less than a year.

■ The buttock should not be used routinely in children because of the risk of sciatic nerve injury (Bergeson, 1982).

FOLLOW-UP CARE AND INSTRUCTIONS

■ Immediately dispose of needle and syringe properly in an appropriate needle disposal (sharps) container.

Caution: Never recap needles. It is important to follow this advice diligently to help prevent the 600,000 to 800,000 needlesticks and other percutaneous injuries reported in the United States each year among the 8 million health care workers. (Henry, 1995; EPINet, 1999).

■ Monitor the patient's response, especially after injections of large doses of antibiotic. Patient should be monitored for approximately 30 minutes for signs of anaphylaxis.

■ Instruct the patient to report a new onset of fever, joint pain, shortness of breath, or rash. Also, tenderness, erythema, or ecchymosis at the injection site should be reported to the health care provider.

REFERENCES

Bergeson PS, Singer SA, Kaplan AM: Intramuscular injections in children. Pediatrics 70:944-948, 1982.

Brokensha G: The hollow needle: Inappropriate injection in practice. Aust Prescr 22:145-147, 1999.

EPINet: Exposure prevention information network data reports. University of Virginia, International Health Care Worker Safety Center, 1999.

Feldmann H: History of injections. Laryngorhinootologie 79:239-246, 2000.

Henry K, Campbell S: Needlestick/sharps injuries and HIV exposures among health care workers: national estimates based on a survey of U.S. hospitals. Minn Med 78:1765-1768, 1995.

Howard-Jones N: The origins of the hypodermic medications. Sci Am 224:96-102, 1971.

BIBLIOGRAPHY

American Diabetes Association: Insulin administration. Diabetes Care 23(suppl 1):S86, 2000.

Centers for Disease Control and Prevention: General recommendations on immunization recommendations of the Advisory Committee on Immunization Practices (ACIP). MMWR Recomm Rep 43(RR-01):1-38, 1994.

D'Angelo HH, Welsh NP (eds): Medication Administration and IV Therapy Manual, 2nd ed. Springhouse, Pa, Springhouse, 1993.

De Vries PG, Henning RH, Hogerzeil HV: WHO Guide to Good
Prescribing: The Use of Injections. World Health Organization, 1995.
Available at: http:// www.med.rug.nl/pharma/ggp.htm

Elkin MK, Perry AG, Potter PA: Nursing Interventions and Clinical Skills,
2nd ed. St. Louis, CV Mosby, 1999.

Gilles FH, French JH: Postinjection sciatic nerve palsies in infants and
children. J Pediatr 58:195-204, 1961.

Newton M, Newton D, Fudin J: Reviewing the "big three" injection
routes. Nursing 22:34-42, 1992.

Smith SF, Duell DJ, Martin BC: Clinical Nursing Skills: Basic to Advanced
Skills. Upper Saddle River, NJ, Prentice Hall Health, 2000.

Chapter 10

Recording an Electrocardiogram

Richard R. Rahr and Salah Ayachi

PROCEDURE GOALS AND OBJECTIVES

Goal: To perform an electrocardiogram (ECG) safely and accurately.

Objectives: The student will be able to ...

- Describe the indications, contraindications, and rationale for performing an ECG.
- Identify and describe potential complications associated with performing an ECG.
- Describe the essential anatomy and physiology associated with performing an ECG.
- Identify the materials necessary for performing an ECG and their proper use.
- Identify the proper steps for performing an ECG.

FIGURE 10-1. Electrocardiographic methodology in 1911. (Redrawn from Rawlings CA: Electrocardiography. Redmond, Wash, SpaceLabs, 1991, p 26.)

BACKGROUND AND HISTORY

In 1790 Salvori demonstrated that stimulation of a charged glass rod attached to a frog's leg muscle causes contraction of the muscle, as if the frog willed it to do so. In 1855 Kollickes and Mueller dissected a frog's heart and attached it to the leg muscle; they noted the frog's leg twitched with each heartbeat. In 1880 Ludig and Waller developed a crude capillary electrometer and recorded the electrical activity of the heartbeat from the skin surface. It was not until 1901 that Einthoven developed a machine that passed light over a moving wire and recorded the PQRSTU waveform (Fig. 10-1). He was the first to develop the first three leads (I, II, and III) that make up the equilateral triangle that today bears his name.

INDICATIONS

Numerous technologic advances (cardiac catheterization, echocardiography, nuclear medicine imaging, and magnetic resonance imaging [MRI]) in the study of heart function notwithstanding, the 12-lead ECG continues to be an effective and inexpensive method to screen for heart disease and monitor patients with acute and chronic heart conditions. Some of these conditions include the following:

- Ischemic heart disease, including myocardial infarction

- Heart block

- Dysrhythmias (including wide ventricular tachycardia)

- Electrolyte disturbances

- Abnormality in chamber size or myocardial hypertrophy

The use of the 12-lead ECG is essential in the following scenarios:
- At sites of accidents or emergency calls, it enables the paramedic to identify heart disease with 62% to 90% specificity and 71% to 90% sensitivity in the presence of chest pain (Taylor, 1998).

- It gives hospital personnel warning signs of a patient's condition during transport to the hospital for treatment with thrombolytics or for control of advanced arrhythmias. In some instances, paramedics are allowed to administer thrombolytics prior to arrival at the hospital.

The 12-lead ECG plays a critical role in reducing morbidity and mortality in patients with coronary artery disease, because it enables the practitioner to detect early danger signs and administer reperfusion medications.

CONTRAINDICATIONS

The only relative contraindications to performing an ECG are as follows:
- Concern that the equipment may be malfunctioning

- Hypersensitivity to the electrode adhesive

POTENTIAL COMPLICATIONS

- The most common complication is misinterpretation of the 12-lead ECG. A tracing can be misinterpreted as being "normal" when it is not (i.e., false negative), leading to acquiescence and lowering of the practitioner's index of suspicion, thus failure to intervene, and possibly to patient demise. The lesson is that a "normal ECG" does *not* preclude underlying pathology.

- Errors in interpretation could actually be due to errors in lead placement. It is incumbent on the practitioner to repeat the ECG should unusual waveform patterns for a set of leads appear.

- Because electrodes are attached to the patient's skin, either by adhesives or suction, skin damage may result, especially in elderly or diabetic patients, potentially leading to infections.

- Although extremely unlikely, it is possible that a patient could receive an electrical shock if there is a short in the wiring. Electrocardiographs today are protected by a third ground wire to prevent such events.

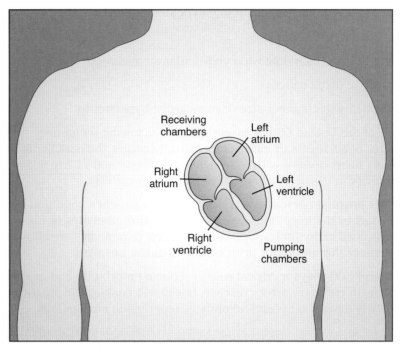

FIGURE 10-2. Anatomy of the heart.

REVIEW OF ESSENTIAL ANATOMY AND PHYSIOLOGY

A review of the anatomy and physiology of the heart is necessary for proper understanding of the 12-lead ECG. The heart is a complex organ whose primary function is to pump blood through the pulmonic and systemic circulations. Four muscular chambers—right and left atria (collecting chambers) and right and left ventricles (pumping chambers)—compose the heart (Fig. 10-2). An intricate network of specialized muscle cells coordinates the sequential contractions of the chambers to make it an effective pump.

The pulmonary artery arises from the right ventricle, whereas the aorta originates from the left ventricle. Each of these large vessels has a valve (pulmonic and aortic, respectively) that opens to accommodate ejection of blood during systole and closes to prevent backward flow during diastole. Atria and ventricles are separated by a valve—the tricuspid between the right atrium and ventricle, and the mitral between the left atrium and ventricle. As in the case of the pulmonic and aortic valves, the tricuspid and mitral valves open to accommodate forward flow and close to prevent retrograde flow. Unlike the pulmonic and aortic valves, the tricuspid and mitral valves open during diastole and close during systole. The left main and right coronary arteries arise from the root of the aorta. The coronary sinus drains venous blood into the right atrium.

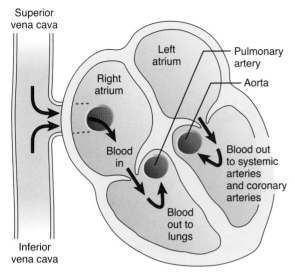

Superior
vena cava

Inferior
vena cava

Right
atrium

Left
atrium

Pulmonary
artery

Aorta

Blood
in

Blood out
to systemic
arteries
and coronary
arteries

Blood
out to
lungs

FIGURE 10-3. The heart box.

Poorly oxygenated blood returning from the systemic circulation, through the superior and inferior venae cavae, to the right atrium enters the right ventricle in large part (70%) by gravity; atrial contraction contributes only 30% to ventricular filling during diastole. The right ventricle pumps blood into the pulmonary artery and the lungs where it is oxygenated and then returned to the left atrium by the pulmonary veins. As in the case of the right side of the heart, atrial contraction contributes only 30% of the blood that enters the left ventricle during diastole.

The left ventricle pumps blood into the aorta and the systemic circulation, including the coronary arteries, which originate from the base of the aorta and supply the myocardium with oxygen-rich blood mostly during diastole (Fig. 10-3). The larger and thicker walled left ventricle maintains the pressure necessary to effect forward flow to the systemic circulation. Deoxygenated blood from the myocardium returns to the right atrium via the coronary sinus.

The electrical pathways (or conduction system) (Fig. 10-4) are essential to the coordinated activity of the heart. The sinoatrial (SA) node, located near the junction of the superior vena cava and the right atrium, has an intrinsic (spontaneous) electrical discharge of 60 to 100 cycles per minute, whereas the atrioventricular (AV) node, located between the right atrium and the right ventricle, spontaneously discharges at 40 to 60 cycles per minute. Adjacent to the AV node and traveling through the ventricular septum are specialized fibers—His bundle, bundle branches, and Purkinje fibers—that conduct electrical impulses at a high rate of speed.

Normally, the SA node initiates the electrical impulse, which rapidly spreads through internodal tracts and depolarizes the left and right atria, ultimately reaching the AV node. At this node, conduction velocity slows considerably to allow atrial activity to complete before ventricular activity begins. Following

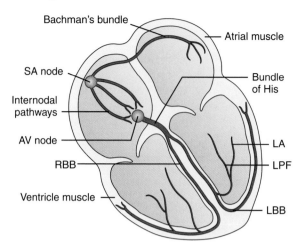

FIGURE 10-4. Electrical pattern of the heart. AV, atrioventricular; LA, left atrium; LBB, left bundle branch; LPF, left posterior fascicle; RBB, right bundle branch; SA, sinoatrial.

this delay, the impulse moves very rapidly through the bundle of His and its branches (the left has two fascicles) and the Purkinje fibers, resulting in the nearly simultaneous depolarization of the right and left ventricles (Fig. 10-5). The atria and ventricles are separated by a fibrous ring that serves to insulate the chambers from their respective activities and permit spread of electrical activity from atria to ventricles only through the AV node area. The system allows the atria and ventricles to beat synchronously, resulting in effective and efficient pumping activity.

The electrical activity of the heart can be measured on the surface of the body using an electrocardiograph, thereby producing ECG tracings that consist of repeating waveforms (PQRST) in which the P wave represents depolarization of atrial tissues, the QRS complex represents depolarization of the ventricles, and the T wave represents repolarization of the ventricles; no waveform is noted that represents atrial repolarization (Fig. 10-6).

PATIENT PREPARATION

Patient preparation is important. Time should be taken to explain to the patient what the procedure entails and what the patient should expect as well as to answer any questions the patient may have. Preparing the patient's skin helps ensure optimal conditions for recording the ECG. The following steps should be taken to prepare the patient:

■ Introduce yourself to the patient.

■ Explain the 12-lead electrocardiography procedure, and proceed by draping the patient's chest.

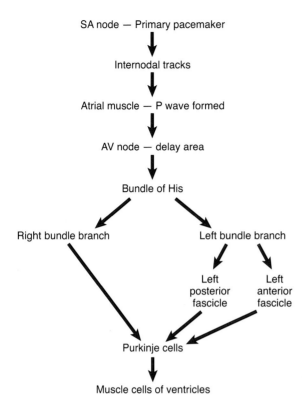

FIGURE 10-5. Electrical sequence of the normal heart. AV, atrioventricular; SA, sinoatrial.

FIGURE 10-6. Electrocardiographic 12-lead tracing.

■ Identify the six precordial leads (you may choose to mark them with a felt-tipped pen).

■ If necessary, shave the areas where the electrodes are to be placed.

■ Use alcohol pads to cleanse the skin and, if necessary, rub with a mild abrasive pad.

■ Use alcohol pads again to remove any residue.

■ Attach the adhesive pads and connect the electrodes.

Materials Utilized for Electrocardiography

■ The machine used to do routine 12-lead ECGs is a standard electrocardiograph mounted on a cart that can be easily wheeled from one location to another. Modern systems have a resting electrocardiographic analysis system with quick reference readout.

■ Electrodes for the six precordial sites

■ Razor to shave hair from a male patient's chest, if necessary.

■ Alcohol to clean skin surface

■ Felt pen to mark site (optional)

■ Abrasive pad to remove epidermal skin layer at electrode sites; pads are used to gently remove felt-pen marks.

Procedure for Performing the Electrocardiogram

Note: The following steps are for performing a routine 12-lead ECG at the bedside.

1. Assemble supplies (leads, alcohol, abrasive pads, etc.).

2. Verify the order on the patient's chart.

3. Verify the patient's identity.

4. Wash hands.

5. Plug in power cord and turn on electrocardiograph.

6. Position the patient in a comfortable supine position and provide a drape or gown to maintain the patient's modesty yet afford adequate access to the patient's chest for lead placement.

7. Cleanse skin at the six precordial sites.

8. Attach limb and precordial leads (refer to Figures 10-7 and 10-8 for correct lead placement).

9. Confirm that all leads are connected.

10. Enter patient's information.

11. Ask the patient to lie quietly for 30 seconds.

12. Press the 12-lead (or the record ECG) button to record the tracing.

Right   Left

R.A.   L.A.

R.L.   L.L.
(ground)

V1   V2   V3   V4   V5   V6
                  (mid-   (mid-
                  clavicular) axillary)

V1 - Fourth intercostal space at right
     border of sternum.

V2 - Fourth intercostal space at left
     border of sternum.

V4 - At the mid-clavicular line and the
     inter-space in which the apex is
     located (the 5th intercostal space
     is used if the apex is not palpable).

V3 - Midway between positions 2 and 4.

V5 - At the anterior axillary line on a
     horizontal level with V4.

V6 - At the mid-axillary line on the same
     horizontal level as V4 and V5.

Spine   Heart

R.V.   L.V.   V6

                V5

Chest   V1   V2   V3   V4
wall   Sternum

FIGURE 10-7.

FIGURE 10-8.

continued

13. "Acquired data" message will appear; wait for "ECG acquisition complete" message to appear.

14. Enter number of extra copies desired.

15. Print report to attach to chart and for cardiology reading station.

16. Press "Store" and "Data in store" to store data for comparison with future tracings.

17. Enter your name, date, and identification number.

18. Remove electrodes and adhesive pads

19. Assist patient with cleaning up and redressing, as necessary.

20. Dispose of used supplies.

SPECIAL CONSIDERATIONS

In case the patient is unable to remain in one position for 30 seconds because of pain, shortness of breath, or confusion, the operator may need assistance to complete the procedure. Similarly, assistance may be required if the patient is a child who is anxious about or fearful of the equipment or procedure.

FOLLOW-UP CARE AND INSTRUCTIONS

■ No follow-up care is necessary provided the skin has not been damaged by the adhesive pads.

■ Patients should be given an estimate of the time it takes before they are given the results and interpretation of the ECG.

REFERENCE

Taylor RV, Key CB, Trach M: Advanced Cardiac Care in the Streets. Philadelphia, Lippincott, 1998.

BIBLIOGRAPHY

Constant J: Essentials of Learning Electrocardiography: A Complete Course for the Non-Cardiologist. New York, Parthenon, 1997.
Dubin D: Rapid Interpretation of EKGs. Tampa, Fla, Cover, 1996.
Goldschlager N, Goldman MJ: Electrocardiography: Essentials of Interpretation. Los Altos, Calif, Lange Medical, 1984.
Lewis KM, Handal KA: Sensible ECG Analysis. Albany, NY, Delmar, 2000.
Lipman BC: ECG Pocket Guide. Chicago, Ill, Year Book Medical, 1987.
Murphy KR, Pelton JJ: ECG Essentials. Chicago, Ill, Quintessence, 1991.
Rawlings CA: Electrocardiography. Redmond, Wash, SpaceLabs, 1991.
Schamroth L: An Introduction to Electrocardiography. Oxford, England, Blackwell Scientific, 1976.

Chapter 11

Exercise Stress Testing for the Primary Care Provider

Charles S. King

PROCEDURE GOALS AND OBJECTIVES

Goal: To identify appropriate candidates for exercise stress testing and to administer the test safely.

Objectives: The student will be able to …

- Describe the indications, contraindications, and rationale for performing exercise stress testing.

- Identify and describe common complications associated with exercise stress testing.

- Describe the essential anatomy and physiology associated with the effective and safe performance of exercise stress testing.

- Identify the necessary materials and their proper use for performing an exercise stress test.

- Identify the important aspects of patient care after an exercise stress test.

BACKGROUND AND HISTORY

Despite advances in disease prevention, coronary artery disease (CAD) remains a major cause of death and disability in the United States. There are considerable costs associated with treating this disease, which are compounded by expenses related to time lost from work and lost wages. Since the 1950s, electrocardiographic analysis during patient exercise has been employed in the pursuit of objective evidence for the presence or progression of CAD. More recently, and perhaps more importantly, the role of exercise testing has taken on the goal of predicting patient outcomes. The *prognostic* value of the Duke treadmill scoring system has added considerable dimension to cardiac stress testing. Although not perfectly applicable to all patients under consideration for stress testing, its usefulness in estimating prognosis in a large segment of patients has been well established. The physiologic stress of exercise can elicit cardiovascular abnormalities not present at rest. Although exercise testing was initially used as a diagnostic tool, it is also a powerful predictor of subsequent cardiac events. Exercise stress testing provides a controlled environment for observing the effects of increased myocardial oxygen demand and can be used to determine the adequacy of cardiac perfusion.

The exercise stress test is a valuable tool for detecting CAD and for evaluating medical therapy, percutaneous or surgical revascularization, and cardiac rehabilitation after myocardial infarction.

Electrocardiographic changes during exercise can provide evidence of ischemia if significant stenosis from CAD is present. Healthy persons who are asymptomatic may be considered candidates for exercise testing if they intend to engage in strenuous or high-risk occupations. The American College of Sports Medicine (ACSM) recommends an exercise test for all women 50 years of age and older and all men 40 years of age and older who plan to engage in vigorous exercise. The ACSM does not recommend exercise testing for asymptomatic, healthy persons who are not planning vigorous exercise, regardless of the person's age (Pate, 1991).

In addition to the standard exercise stress test, other methods of cardiovascular stress testing include scintigraphy and echocardiography. Exercise stress scintigraphy uses a radioactive tracer to enhance abnormal areas of myocardial blood flow and can be performed with pharmacologic agents instead of exercise if a patient's condition warrants. Echocardiography has been used in combination with exercise or pharmacologic stress testing as another form of noninvasive cardiac evaluation.

INDICATIONS

By exposing the cardiopulmonary system to increased metabolic demands using standardized methods and protocols of stress, the clinician is provided a useful tool for detecting the initial presence of cardiopulmonary pathology and for assessing the efficacy of various therapies and rehabilitation programs.

Employing electrocardiographic monitoring and patient vital signs alone or in concert with established and developing imaging modalities, stress testing adds a valuable adjunct to the well-thought-out history and physical examination. Cardiac stress testing is indicated as follows:

- To establish the initial diagnosis of obstructive CAD

- To stratify risk and monitor treatment of patients with previously diagnosed or treated CAD

- To screen asymptomatic individuals (CAD risks or occupations that place the public at risk)

- To assess exercise capacity in patients with valvular, congenital abnormalities or congestive heart failure (CHF)

- To document and monitor therapy in those with exercise-related heart dysrhythmia

As with all laboratory testing, exercise stress testing should be used to augment an already high clinical suspicion of disease that is based on a quality history and physical examination. Accordingly, the rationale for using exercise stress testing in the primary care setting should be based on the "predictive value" of the given test. Attention should be paid to the prevalence of the disease in the patient population under consideration (i.e., the pretest probability of detecting pathology in a given patient).

The sensitivity and specificity of exercise stress testing with electrocardiographic monitoring alone have been validated for its use in detecting CAD by comparison of ST segment changes (depression or elevation) with the gold standard of coronary angiography (Gianrossi, 1989). True positives—that is, the percentage of patients with disease who have electrocardiographic changes indicative of ischemia—are the measures of sensitivity in exercise stress testing, which in the general patient population varies from 40% to 90% (Fletcher, 1992). The sensitivity of exercise stress testing in detecting cardiac pathology other than CAD is less clear.

The occurrence of false negatives—that is, tests in which there is an absence of diagnostic electrocardiographic changes in the presence of true CAD—can be minimized by sound test candidate selection and practicing good testing technique (e.g., achieving target heart rate, getting quality data). The specificity of exercise stress testing with electrocardiographic monitoring alone, described as the percentage of normal patients (i.e., those without CAD) who manifest no electrocardiographic changes indicative of CAD, is reported to be 84% (Fletcher, 1992). False-positive results—that is, tests in which electrocardiographic changes suggest CAD that cannot be substantiated by subsequent coronary angiography—are often associated with patient selection (gender), electrocardiographic abnormality (left ventricular hypertrophy), Q waves at baseline, and associated drug therapy (digoxin).

Both sensitivity and specificity are improved when the pretest probability of detecting the target pathology in a group of patients is high at the onset. Prevalence tables for a variety of illnesses are published and usually broken

Table 11.1 **Pretest Probability of Coronary Artery Disease by Age, Gender, and Symptoms**					
AGE (yr)	GENDER	TYPICAL—DEFINITE ANGINA PECTORIS	ATYPICAL—PROBABLE ANGINA PECTORIS	NONANGINAL CHEST PAIN	ASYMPTOMATIC
30-39	Men	Intermediate	Intermediate	Low	Very low
	Women	Intermediate	Very low	Very low	Very low
40-49	Men	High	Intermediate	Intermediate	Low
	Women	Intermediate	Low	Very low	Very low
50-59	Men	High	Intermediate	Intermediate	Very low
	Women	Intermediate	Intermediate	Low	Very low
60-69	Men	High	Intermediate	Intermediate	Low
	Women	High	Intermediate	Intermediate	Low

High, >90%; intermediate, 10%-90%; low, <10%; very low, <5%.

Adapted from Pate RR, Blair SN, Durstine JL, et al: Guidelines for Exercise Testing and Prescription. American College of Sports Medicine, 4th ed. Philadelphia, Lea & Febiger, 1991, p 87.

down by gender, age, and clinical presentation (Gibbons, 1997). An example of the prevalence of CAD in Western society is detailed in Table 11-1.

Designing a strategy for determining the appropriateness of testing in a given population is often as much an art as a science. An incremental testing strategy for detecting CAD in individuals with a normal resting electrocardiogram (ECG) and those with an abnormal resting ECG is detailed in Figure 11-1.

When considering the predictive value of exercise treadmill testing with electrocardiographic monitoring, it may be the clinical history alone that provides the best guidance. It has been reported that the highest predictor of positive stress testing in either gender is the presentation of "typical" angina pectoris as opposed to atypical or non-anginal symptoms (Weiner, 1979). Enhancement of predicted value may be appreciated with the use of newer, more sophisticated computer analysis of exercise electrocardiographic ST-segment changes, although many of these methods require further validation. The appropriate addition of imaging by radionuclide or, most recently, echocardiography can improve both specificity and sensitivity of exercise stress testing.

Stress testing with electrocardiographic monitoring (with or without an imaging modality) is most commonly used in patients in whom the suspicion for cardiac ischemia is high based on clinical history and physical examination.

The American College of Cardiology guidelines for exercise stress testing consider symptomatic adult patients with at least an intermediate pretest probability of CAD (including those with right bundle branch block or less than 1 mm resting ST depression, or both) candidates for exercise treadmill testing with electrocardiographic monitoring alone (Gibbons, 1997). Patients with suspected CAD (high pretest probability as dictated by age, symptoms, and gender, less than 1 mm of ST depression) who have abnormal ECGs that are at least in part attributed to glycoside therapy (digitalis), left ventricular

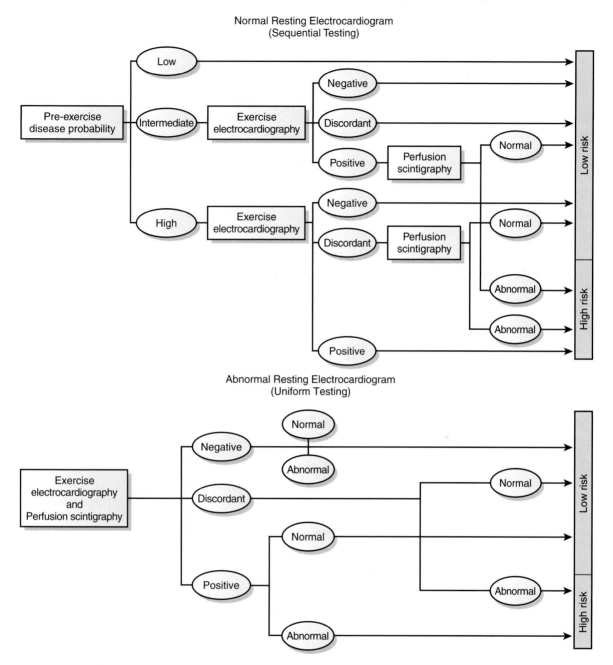

FIGURE 11-1. Incremental testing strategy for coronary artery disease (CAD) risk using serial results of pretest clinical risk (high, intermediate, low), exercise electrocardiography, and radionuclide perfusion scintigraphy. *Top panel* shows sequential testing in patients with a normal baseline electrocardiogram (ECG). *Bottom panel* uses combined electrocardiographic and perfusion scintigraphy (uniform) testing in patients with an abnormal baseline ECG. Results of these tests define low- and high-risk groups. (Negative exercise test [≤ET], <1 mm ST[1], >85% maximal heart rate; discordant ET, ≤1 mm ST[1], <85% maximal heart rate; positive ET, ≥1 mm ST[1], <85% maximal heart rate). (Adapted from Ladenheim ML, Kotler TS, Pollack BH, et al: Incremental prognostic power of clinical history, exercise electrocardiography and myocardial perfusion scintigraphy in suspected coronary artery disease. Am J Cardiol 59:270-277, 1987.)

hypertrophy, left bundle branch block, or other baseline electrocardiographic abnormalities are candidates for exercise stress testing; however, an imaging modality also should be used to improve test sensitivity and specificity.

In addition to its purely "diagnostic" applications, exercise stress testing may be used to assess previous therapy. After infarction, patients are often "risk-stratified" before hospital discharge through the use of exercise stress testing in a "sub-maximal" protocol. Typically, patients without recurrence of angina symptoms are stressed to 70% of their age-predicted maximal heart rate while symptoms and the ECG are assessed. This testing alerts the provider to patients who are likely to have recurrent symptoms with activities of daily living and provides reassurance to the patient and family about the safety of leaving the hospital.

Patients receiving antianginal agents or who have undergone or are being considered for revascularization procedures (percutaneous transluminal coronary angioplasty [PTCA], coronary artery bypass graft [CABG], or both), may benefit from a functional assessment of areas of myocardium treated. After initiation of antiarrhythmic therapy (pharmacologic or a device), especially in patients with a history of exercise-related abnormalities, exercise stress testing in a controlled environment can evaluate management and provide reassurance to the patient. Functional testing using exercise is often directed toward assessing cardiovascular capacity or response in healthy individuals as well as a variety of those with known pathology.

Functional testing often can be offered to those who have undergone congenital heart defect repair, valvular replacement or repair, or cardiac transplantation in an effort to provide a baseline or document improvement in those who were previously physically restricted. Patients who suffer from stable but chronic heart failure, diabetes, chronic renal insufficiency, or pulmonary pathology fall into the group that benefits from functional exercise testing. With the exception of asymptomatic patients with multiple cardiac risk factors and patients with occupations that place the public at risk, exercise treadmill testing with electrocardiographic monitoring should not be considered a screening tool. The indiscriminate use of exercise stress testing in an effort to expose silent ischemia leads to misleading false-positive results that are financially burdensome and lead to undue patient worry (Sox, 1989).

CONTRAINDICATIONS

As with any testing modality, the anticipated benefits of information provided to the clinician by a test should outweigh the potential risks associated with obtaining the information. There are few absolute contraindications to performing exercise treadmill testing, but the test administrator must always weigh the anticipated benefits carefully against the perceived risks of the test.

- Generally, exercise stress testing is likely to worsen myocardial ischemia in patients already suffering from myocardial infarction or unstable angina. Testing should be delayed until rest pain is absent and the infarction has stabilized and been appropriately treated.

■ Patients with symptoms of congestive heart failure should be stabilized to the point at which they are likely to be able to perform the planned test protocol and are not having pulmonary edema.

■ Patients with symptomatic conduction abnormalities, such as high-degree atrioventricular block and symptomatic supraventricular tachycardia, and most ventricular tachycardia, and patients with demonstrated "chronotropic incompetence" should not be stressed until an adequate ventricular rate in response to increased metabolic demand can be anticipated or controlled.

■ Pacemaker therapy is not a contraindication to exercise stress testing, but reprogramming the rate and response settings may be necessary and an imaging modality used if evidence of ischemia is being sought. Persistent ventricular or supraventricular tachycardia should be corrected before testing. Some antiarrhythmic agents may prevent patients from reaching target heart rate during testing, and the addition of an imaging modality may improve the value of the test.

■ Severe systemic arterial hypertension defined as a pretest systolic pressure of 200 mm Hg or greater or pretest diastolic pressure of 110 mm Hg or greater is generally considered an absolute contraindication. Excessive myocardial wall stress imparted by this degree of hypertension exerts a significant increase in myocardial oxygen demand at baseline. These patients are better candidates for testing when their hypertension is controlled.

■ Exercise stress testing in patients with severe aortic stenosis is prohibited because the myocardial oxygen demand at baseline is already significantly elevated. Although testing is used in determining the timing of surgery, it is reserved for patients who have not yet manifested the associated triad of angina, syncope, or congestive heart failure.

Other clinical conditions that should be controlled before exercise stress testing follow:

■ Recent pulmonary embolism or infarct and severe peripheral vascular disease (deep venous thrombosis, phlebitis, claudication)

■ Limitations to ambulation (cerebrovascular accident, orthopedic disability, severe vertigo or dizziness)

■ Inability of the patient to follow instructions (mental disability, catatonia, psychosis)

■ Concomitant illnesses, especially when associated with fever.

RELATIVE CONTRAINDICATIONS

In some patients, the anticipated benefits of exercise testing outweigh the higher than average risks or impediments. These "relative contraindications" are usually more minor versions of the previously mentioned "absolute contraindications" and, as such, are not prohibitive. Common examples follow:

■ Presence of preexisting electrocardiographic abnormalities when the examiner is focusing on non-electrocardiographic criteria (e.g., conditions such as new left ventricular segmental wall motion abnormality seen on echocardiography or perfusion defects and redistribution abnormalities in the setting of radionuclide studies)

■ The patient who cannot mount an adequate heart rate response to exercise stress testing (β-blocker pharmacologic therapy) has an inability to exercise because of ambulation difficulties, or is not otherwise willing to work physically

■ Patients using agents such as dobutamine, dipyridamole, or adenosine, which cause pharmacologic stress and may increase myocardial oxygen demand or myocardial perfusion during which the ECG, blood pressure, heart rate, and imaging can be observed for changes suggesting ischemia

POTENTIAL COMPLICATIONS

■ The risks of cardiac stress testing via a treadmill, cycle ergometer (use of a stationary bike with varying degrees of resistance), or arm exercise testing (use of an exercise wheel analogous to the pedals of a bicycle with varying degrees of resistance) are small when attention is paid to appropriate patient selection. Pooled data suggest that approximately 0.5 deaths per 10,000 tests in large heterogeneous populations can be expected (Gordon, 1993).

■ Most sudden death episodes during stress testing occur in middle-aged and older individuals with advanced atherosclerotic CAD. A detailed medical history and physical examination often identify individuals at higher risk for complication associated with stress testing. Ironically, these individuals are the very group for which stress testing is most often indicated. Specifically, they are individuals with diabetes mellitus, multiple organ system failure, ambulatory impairment associated with orthopedic disorders, and electrolyte imbalance. Proper patient monitoring provided by well-trained individuals who can administer emergent care is essential to reduce known complications.

■ Complications related to the mechanics of walking on an exercise treadmill include, but are not limited to, injury sustained from a fall; prolonged episodes of myocardial oxygen demand in excess of supply, resulting in prolonged myocardial ischemia or infarct, or both; hemodynamically significant tachycardia or bradycardia; and sudden cardiac death.

■ Aggressive efforts at screening patients for contraindications before performing stress testing may significantly reduce the incidence of complications. Continuous patient monitoring for rhythm disturbances, ST segment changes, and other electrocardiographic manifestations of myocardial ischemia, as well as disruptions in the patient's cognitive and psychomotor function, can minimize the incidence of complications associated with exercise stress testing.

REVIEW OF ESSENTIAL ANATOMY AND PHYSIOLOGY

Dynamic or isotonic exercise (muscular contraction resulting in movement) is preferred for testing because it puts a volume stress rather than a pressure load on the heart. It also can be performed in increments. According to the American Heart Association statement on exercise standards, when dynamic exercise is begun or enhanced, oxygen uptake by the lungs quickly increases. After the second minute, oxygen uptake usually remains relatively stable (steady state) despite progressive levels of intensity of exercise. During steady state, heart rate, cardiac output, blood pressure, and pulmonary ventilation are maintained at reasonably constant levels.

Maximal oxygen consumption ($\dot{V}o_2$max) is the highest level of oxygen consumption a subject can achieve during maximal exercise. During exercise, a physically fit subject progressively increases his or her oxygen consumption, cardiac output, and pulmonary ventilation as the circulatory system provides blood and oxygen to the exercising tissues. The definition of a unit of metabolic equivalent (1 MET) is the total oxygen consumption measured in milliliters of oxygen per kilogram of body weight per minute for an adult sitting quietly at rest. 1 MET has been measured at approximately 3.5 mL/kg per minute. MET can and should be used as a work equivalent when comparing the level of physical work during different activities or different exercise protocols (Cintron, 1996).

Heart rate is one of the determinants of myocardial oxygen consumption, and thus peak heart rate is used as an indirect index of the workload imposed on the heart during exercise. Tables and formulas have been developed that provide the expected peak heart rate that should be attained during an exercise test carried out to maximal effort. The maximal achieved heart rate is usually expressed as a percentage of maximal predicted heart rate for a given age. A test that is limited by noncardiac factors at an attained heart rate less than 85% of maximal heart rate (MHR) may not have challenged the circulatory cardiac reserve enough to attain predictive validity. The percent of MHR at which symptoms or electrocardiographic evidence of myocardial ischemia occurs is an indicator of severity of the cardiac impairment, the individual's disability, and a rough index of prognosis. Studies suggest that attained METs may represent a better unit of measure of stress in quantifying exercise.

During graduated exercise performed by normal subjects, heart rate and systolic blood pressure increase progressively. The product of the achieved MHR and blood pressure is called the *double product* or *rate-pressure product* and also serves as an index of myocardial oxygen consumption. At rest, for example, the heart rate may be 70 and the systolic blood pressure 120 mm Hg, giving a double product of 8400. During exercise, the double product may exceed 30,000. When subjects cannot achieve a double product of 18,000 without signs or symptoms of cardiac disease, cardiac reserve is severely impaired, indicating a poor prognosis (Cintron, 1996; Fletcher, 1992).

A normal or negative test is one in which the end points are achieved without the appearance of symptoms, signs, or electrocardiographic findings that suggest the presence of cardiac disease. A negative test usually indicates a low statistical probability for the presence of clinically important cardiac disease.

The normal physiologic response to exercise may be altered by a number of cardiac diseases. Coronary atherosclerosis is the most common and limits the dilatory capacity of the coronary arteries. This restricts the amount of blood available to the myocardial tissues. Heart rate, blood pressure, myocardial contractility, and left ventricular chamber diameter and wall thickness all determine myocardial oxygen demand. The increase in heart rate, systolic blood pressure, and myocardial contractility induced by exercise is balanced by an increase in myocardial blood flow. Since myocardial oxygen extraction is almost maximal, even at rest, an imbalance between oxygen demand and blood supply quickly leads to myocardial ischemia and its clinical counterparts—angina, electrocardiographic changes, transient myocardial mechanical dysfunction, and, occasionally, cardiac rhythm disorders. The most common objective finding in patients with physiologically limiting coronary atherosclerosis who are subjected to exercise testing is electrocardiographic ST segment depression, with or without anginal symptoms (Fig. 11-2).

PATIENT PREPARATION

■ Explain the indications for and benefits and inherent risks of the test to the patient and assess for understanding.

■ The patient should have been given a physical examination and had a medical history taken that focused on cardiopulmonary and orthopedic systems before scheduling the test. Attention to the use of β-blocker therapy, cardiac glycosides, and medicines altering the patient's state of consciousness should be considered before testing. With the use of an imaging modality, it is not always necessary for the patient to discontinue β-blocker or digitalis therapy, although these medicines can alter the quality of the study by modifying the patient's MHR response or cause an abnormal baseline ECG. The physical examination should be directed toward eliciting signs or symptoms of orthopedic disease, peripheral

Phase name	Stage name	Time in Stage	Speed mph	Grade %	Workload METS	Heart rate bpm	BP mm Hg	RPP bpm*mm Hg	VE count ves/min
PRETEST	SUPINE	0:00	1.0	0.0	1.7	74	142/78	14500	0
EXERCISE	STAGE 1	3:00	1.7	10.0	4.6	102	158/74	17100	0
	STAGE 2	3:00	2.5	12.0	7.0	106	166/72	22700	0
	STAGE 3	3:00	3.4	14.0	10.1	137			0
	STAGE 4	3:00	4.2	16.0	13.4	162			0
RECOVERY		6:06	0.0	0.0	1.0	103			0

40 yr   White   Male   BRUCE   Total exercise time: 12:00
Wt: Ht: Max HR: 162 bpm 90% of Max Predicted 180 bpm   25 mm/sec
Med: Max BP: 166/72   Maximum workload: 13.7 METS   10 mm/mV
100 Hz

Reason for termination: Max HR attained
Comments:

BASELINE   MAX ST

EXERCISE STAGE 1   74 bpm   ST @ 10 mm/mV   Lead ST slope   EXERCISE STAGE 4   161 bpm   ST @ 10 mm/mV   Lead ST slope
00:00   1.7 METS   80 msec post-J   11:37   13.7 METS   80 msec post-J

I	aVR	V1	V4		I	aVR	V1	V4
0.0	0.3	0.0	−0.2		0.1	1.3	0.2	−2.1
−0.3	0.0	0.2	−1.3		0.3	−0.6	1.9	0.5

II	aVL	V2	V5		II	aVL	V2	V5
−0.7	0.3	0.0	−0.2		−2.8	1.6	0.2	−2.0
−1.6	−0.1	0.1	−1.4		0.6	0.3	1.7	0.8

III	aVF	V3	V6		III	aVF	V3	V6
−0.7	−0.7	−0.2	−0.2		−3.0	−2.9	−1.3	−1.3
−1.8	−1.8	−0.8	−1.4		−0.4	0.1	1.2	1.3

FIGURE 11-2. Examples of electrocardiographic changes indicative of a positive exercise stress test. Compare baseline ST segments (Bruce protocol—stage 1—1.7 METs) with exercise ST segments at 11:37 (Bruce protocol—stage 4—13.7 METs) in this 40-year-old man with a positive exercise stress test. ST segments are measured 0.08 seconds after the J point. Note significant ST segment depression of 0.2 mm in leads II, III, aVF, and V_2-V_6. BP, blood pressure; bpm, beats per minute; HR, heart rate; MAX ST, maximal ST; METS, metabolic equivalent; RPP, rate-pressure product.

vascular disease (claudication), or neurologic abnormalities that would limit the patient's ability to perform ergometry.

■ In an attempt to minimize patient anxiety and maximize performance in this patient-dependent test, written instructions that outline the patient's responsibilities and address common concerns and questions should be offered. A detailed description of the test procedure should occur before patient preparation, and questions should be solicited and addressed.

■ In preparation for the test, the patient should be told to abstain from smoking and to wear comfortable clothing and sturdy footwear.

■ Much information is gained when the examiner "walks the patient" back to the testing area. Information regarding gait, balance, respiratory reserve, and overall physical ability identifies individuals for whom treadmill testing is prohibitive and in whom pharmacologic stress might be considered.

 ## Materials Utilized for Performing Exercise Stress Testing

General Environment

Note: Treadmill testing is usually conducted in a laboratory environment; however, family practitioners and internists often use any extra available space for this type of procedure. The space should be adequate for the testing team who must attend the patient during the testing. This typically involves the test proctor and one or more technicians.

■ Temperature control and adequate ventilation essential to maximize patient performance

Note: Generally, temperatures between 22° and 26° C (72° to 79° F) are comfortable for exercise, especially if adequate air movement is present. In geographic locations where environmental humidity is greater than 50%, the testing environment temperature must be adjusted down to accommodate this. Often, a portable fan improves exercise performance.

■ Adequate lighting for patient assessment and patient comfort and safety

Note: In the setting of diagnostic imaging modalities, adjustable lighting, usually in the form of a dimmer switch, can be a useful feature.

■ Room for readily available emergency equipment

■ Crash cart

■ Portable defibrillator

■ Supplemental oxygen supply

■ Curtains to ensure patient privacy as well as provide enough separation between patients to allow for normal conversation and promote patient comfort and performance

■ A sink, supply of towels, and wash cloths for the patient to use after exercise

Testing Equipment

■ Treadmill

Note: Treadmill weight capacity should equal or exceed a patient weight of 350 pounds. The system should have a variable range of speeds and degree of incline (1 to 8 miles per hour and 0 to 20 degrees) and should optimally be electronically controlled by and in synchrony with the testing clock.

A dedicated electrical source should be used for the treadmill and electrocardiograph system to avoid interruption during studies. A standard treadmill platform should be equal to or exceed 50 inches in length and 16 inches in width (Pina, 1995). Padded handrails and emergency stop switches, which are readily visible and accessible to both patient and staff, afford added safety. The area directly behind the treadmill (often referred to as the run-out area) should be kept clear of obstruction and afford the patient safe egress from the treadmill at any time. Typically, a reclining chair or bed should be stationed proximal to the treadmill to afford the patient recumbence in the recovery period.

- Imaging equipment

- Echocardiogram

- Radionuclide camera

- Continuous oscilloscopic monitoring of a minimum of three leads, and preferably 12 leads, in the Mason-Likar configuration

- ST segment templates, baseline correction software, and automatic dysrhythmia alerts are helpful but not essential to the safe conduct of testing

- Machine-patient interface, specifically the electrocardiographic electrode placement

Note: Commercially available silver-silver chloride electrodes with adhesive attachment offer excellent electrocardiographic signal transmission.
- The addition of a "tube shirt," using elasticized medical mesh material, adds stability to electrodes

- The cable array should arise from a central module, which should be attached by a belt worn about the patient's waist

Note: Attention paid to confirming quality signals before testing will serve the examiner in ensuring good data for interpretation.
- Blood pressure monitoring equipment, which consists of a variety of available devices, ranging from automated systems that use oscillatory signaling to a standard manual mercurial sphygmomanometer and stethoscope

Note: In high-volume, experienced laboratories, manual cuff measurement is still the standard, offering reliable blood pressure monitoring but requiring specially trained personnel. Attention should be paid to using appropriately sized blood pressure cuffs in the variety of patients seen in a laboratory, as well as routine maintenance and calibration of manometers. Attention to basic details, such as placing the manometer at the level of the patient's heart, as well as routine cleaning and calibration, ensures accurate and reliable blood pressure monitoring.

Note: Laboratories using stationary bicycle ergometers for individuals with specific orthopedic, peripheral vascular, or neurologic limitations to weight bearing on a treadmill test should have similar automated resistance control features. Commercially available stationary bicycles use either mechanically braked or electronically braked flywheels for this purpose. Often, software that interfaces with the ECG and bicycle ergometer will "ramp" the degree of stress on a preprogrammed basis. As with treadmill testing, the cycle ergometer area must be free of other equipment and afford rapid egress from the bicycle for the recovery period. Attention to seat height and handlebar adjustments can improve the chances of maximal exercise performance and data quality. Numerous tables have been computed to project METs for cycle ergometry, but generally speaking, maximal oxygen uptake is lower on cycle ergometry than on treadmill testing.

An arm ergometer uses not only dynamic arm exercise but also the musculature of the chest, back, buttocks, and legs for body stabilization. Individuals with lower extremity impairment, such as those with orthopedic or vascular disease, can often be stressed safely with this equipment; however, difficulty often arises with electrocardiographic signal quality because of electrical or mechanical interference with upper body musculature activity. Close attention to detail in skin preparation for electrode placement can often overcome this technical limitation.

Imaging Equipment

In an effort to increase the sensitivity and specificity of exercise stress testing, an imaging modality is useful. Its typical application is in the patient with an abnormal baseline ECG for whom stress-related changes might not be quantifiable. Examples of this are left bundle branch block; prior myocardial infarction with Q waves; ST-T abnormalities of any cause, including digitalis effect; or individuals taking β-blockers in whom failure to achieve target heart rate may occur. Pacemaker-dependent patients may benefit from adjunctive cardiac imaging. Equipment ranges from scintigraphy cameras for radionuclide imaging to two-dimensional cardiac ultrasonography. Although beyond the scope of this discussion, cardiac ultrasonography or radionuclide imaging can be applied in patients undergoing ergometry or in those who are stressed with pharmacologic agents such as dobutamine, dipyridamole, or adenosine. In the application of stress echocardiography, an echocardiographic bed with a "cutaway" in the mattress—affording the sonographer apical access with the patient in the left lateral decubitus position (before and after exercise or during pharmacologic stress)—markedly improves image quality. A variety of commercially available systems afford continuous loop (rest and stress) imaging, as well as comparative (before and after) formatting.

Emergency Equipment

Exercise testing is a common and safe procedure, even in the outpatient setting, but still presents some risk. Accordingly, basic emergency

Table 11.2	**Emergency Equipment for Exercise Stress Testing**

Nasal cannula, non-rebreathing oxygen mask, airways (oral), oxygen tank (portable for transport)
Defibrillator (portable)
Bag-valve-mask hand respirator (Ambu bag)
Syringes and needles
Intravenous tubing, solutions, and stand
Suction apparatus and supplies (e.g., gloves, tubing)
Adhesive tape

Table 11.3	**Emergency Medications and Solutions**

MEDICATIONS	INTRAVENOUS FLUIDS
Atropine	Normal saline (0.9%)
Epinephrine	D5W
Isoproterenol	
Procainamide	
Verapamil	
Bretylium	
Lidocaine	
Dobutamine	
Adenosine	
Sublingual nitroglycerin	
Dopamine	

Adapted from Pina IL, Balady GJ, Hanson P: Guidelines for clinical exercise testing laboratories: A statement for healthcare professionals from the Committee on Exercise and Cardiac Rehabilitation, American Heart Association. Circulation 91:912-921, 1995.

equipment should be readily available to the testing team. Most diagnostic exercise stress tests are performed on a population with at least a moderate pretest probability of CAD. Thus, the testing facility must have appropriate emergency equipment, pharmaceuticals, and personnel trained in their use.

A written protocol that clearly outlines the responsibilities of each testing team member should be composed and periodically reviewed. Mock emergency drills should be carefully planned, executed, and critiqued, using a variety of scenarios on a regular basis in an effort to remain prepared for the inevitable medical emergency that affects all laboratories. At a minimum, the emergency equipment listed in Table 11-2 should be close to the testing area and considered "ready" on a regular basis.

When generating emergency protocols, the testing team must decide the limits of its response. In the outpatient setting, basic cardiac life support and early Emergency Medical Service (EMS) activation are the mainstays of the emergency response, whereas stress testing facilities within the confines of hospitals or medical centers may offer advanced cardiac life support procedures (endotracheal intubation), highly specialized personnel, and equipment. Emergency medications and solutions should also be available in these settings (Table 11-3).

Personnel

The exercise stress team often consists of nurses, physicians, physician assistants, an exercise physiologist or specialist, a physical therapist, and electrocardiography and nuclear medicine technicians. Members of the team should have appropriate training and periodic proficiency evaluation in the duties they perform routinely. All staff members should receive training in basic cardiac life support, with at least one member of the team being versed in advanced cardiac life support. Stress testing in the outpatient environment is usually conducted under the supervision of a clinic physician who should be available in the immediate area during the conduct of stress testing. A laboratory policy and procedure manual should be established in keeping with the policies of the health care facility and any state or local restrictions. An individual identified as the Medical Director of the testing facility should be active in the formulation of policies and procedures as well as proficiency evaluations of the staff members. Documentation of this duty should be ongoing and available for review. Requirements for physician competency in the exercise stress testing of patients with known or suspected cardiac pathology are well outlined in the American College of Physicians/American College of Cardiology/American Heart Association statement on clinical competence (Schlant, 1990).

Procedure for Exercise Stress Testing

Applying Electrodes and Obtaining Resting Electrocardiographic Tracings

1. Remove hair in the testing region of the electrode placement with battery-operated shaving equipment.

2. Remove lotions and skin oil from the area of electrode application with alcohol-saturated gauze. Allow the skin to dry.

3. Place commercially available electrodes in the proper location.

Note: In many laboratories, an abrasive (fine sandpaper or commercially available pads) is used to abrade the superficial layer of skin, thus decreasing skin resistance to 5000 Ω or less.

4. Attach lightweight ECG cables to the electrode array and secure the central module to the patient, usually with a holster-and-belt device around the waist.

5. Apply a flexible tube vest over the patient's trunk to help in decreasing electrical or mechanical interference associated with lead bouncing.

6. Perform a baseline ECG in the standard 12-lead configuration.

7. Perform a standard 12-lead ECG with the patient in the supine and standing positions and after 30 seconds of hyperventilation.

Note: ST segment depression occurring with hyperventilation, although uncommon, should be taken into account before initiation of the exercise test itself.

8. Evaluate the tracing for baseline ST-T abnormality or other rhythm

disturbances that would prohibit the performance of stress testing.

Note: When using an imaging modality, the baseline ECG is performed at this time. To afford adequate acoustical windows, often leads V_4, V_5, or V_6 must be altered to accommodate ultrasonographic transducer placement.

Data Collection

Note: Average individuals exercise between 8 and 12 minutes when tested on the appropriate exercise treadmill protocol. There is a variety of protocols available, each with its proponents. Most can be programmed with a typical electrocardiographic-treadmill system. The Bruce protocol is used most commonly, beginning with a low level of stress and increasing in speed and incline every 3 minutes (Bruce, 1977).

9. Demonstrate the proper technique for mounting the treadmill, handgrip placement, and body positioning for performing the exercise protocol.

10. Advise the patient that the protocols start the patient at a slow walking pace with a minor or no incline and then ramp up to the next level of work (speed and incline) at predetermined time intervals.

11. Have monitoring personnel or yourself obtain a 12-lead ECG at least every minute (depending on the patient's symptoms) and a blood pressure check just before advancement to the next stage.

Note: Because of the inaccuracy of data generated by automated systems, manual blood pressure measurement, using a mercury manometer, stethoscope, and

Modified Borg Scale		Original Borg Scale	
0	Nothing at all	6	
0.5	Very, very weak	7	Very, very light
1	Very weak	8	
2	Weak	9	Very light
3	Moderate	10	
4	Somewhat strong	11	Fairly light
5	Strong	12	
6	Somewhat hard	13	
7	Very strong	14	
8		15	Hard
9		16	
10	Very, very strong (almost maximum)	17	Very hard
		18	
		19	Very, very hard
	Maximum	20	

FIGURE 11-3. Borg scales. (Adapted from Pollock ML, Wilmord JH: Exercise in Health and Disease: Evaluation and Prescription for Prevention and Rehabilitation, 2nd ed. Philadelphia, WB Saunders, 1990, p 290.)

trained personnel, remains the preferred technique of monitoring (Froelicher, 1993).

12. Instruct the patient to communicate to the monitoring team his or her perception of exertion.

Note: Often, a hand-held card or sign (in large print), with various descriptions of perceived exertion (Borg scales [Borg, 1982]), is held before the patient by the monitoring team in preparing for test termination (Fig. 11-3).

   Note: Symptoms of general fatigue, dyspnea, leg fatigue, and pain are often difficult to quantify, and a system of quantifying perceived exertion can aid in stopping at an appropriate end point.

13. Counsel patients not to exit the treadmill while it is going; instead, the patient should signal to the testing team their impending exhaustion so that the test may be terminated in a safe manner.

continued

Note: The test should be stopped as indicated. End points for stress testing include, but are not limited to, the following:

- Progressive angina

- Persistent ventricular tachycardia

- Significant blood pressure blunting or decrease below baseline

- Significant and progressive ST-T depression or any ST-T elevation

- Progressive heart block

- Excessive blood pressure response greater than 250 mm Hg systolic and greater than 120 mm Hg diastolic

- Lightheadedness

- Confusion

- Ataxia

- Cyanosis or evidence of cerebral or peripheral circulatory collapse

- Sincere patient requests to stop the test

- Failure of critical monitoring equipment

14. On completion of the test, assist the patient into a supine position while serial ECGs and blood pressure data are collected every 1 to 2 minutes or until the patient's heart rate approximates baseline by 10%.

Note: Exercise stress testing using imaging requires special patient positioning, such as a left side lying position (stress ECG), thus resulting in a short delay in vital sign monitoring.

15. Record blood pressure, heart rate, and electrocardiographic data recording continually until patient is asymptomatic and near-baseline vital signs are present.

16. Observe any patient who manifests signs or symptoms of cardiac disease during or after testing (angina, hypertension, hypotension, ventricular tachyarrhythmias, or other clinical indications for continued monitoring) until those conditions stabilize.

Note: A typical monitoring period after exercise recovery is between 6 and 12 minutes.

17. While the patient is preparing for exit, review electrocardiographic, hemodynamic, and applicable imaging data before the patient's discharge from the testing facility.

18. Although a final report may require a more detailed analysis, in the interest of patient safety, make a preliminary evaluation of the collected data and inform the patient of these preliminary findings and, if appropriate, the referring provider.

SPECIAL CONSIDERATIONS

It is imperative that the test administrator monitor vital signs (blood pressure, heart rate, respiratory rate, and tissue perfusion) throughout the exercise protocol, which includes pre-exercise evaluation and continuous monitoring throughout the exercise test itself and throughout an appropriate recovery period. Symptom evaluation using the Borg scale serves as an important aid in the assessment of functional capacity, as well as dictating appropriateness of test termination. The testing team, directed by the test administrator, must be continuously vigilant for signs of cardiovascular compromise or deteriorating ambulatory ability. Scenarios in which test termination must occur abruptly should be practiced frequently by the testing team, with provisions for acute intervention in the setting of hemodynamic collapse. Most patients experiencing an abrupt inability to continue provide adequate warning to the testing team and afford them the opportunity to terminate the test and come to the aid of the patient without resultant injury.

- In the setting of abnormal cardiac rhythm, rapid intravenous cannulation and supplemental oxygen are essential to the patient's positive outcome.

- In patients in whom rhythm abnormality or hemodynamic deterioration is highly suspected, intravenous placement before testing affords the testing team a route for rapid drug administration.

- In the setting of ventricular tachyarrhythmias, immediate termination of the testing protocol and placement of the patient in a supine position with supplemental oxygen and establishment of intravenous access are important.

- Individuals who continue to manifest ventricular or atrial tachycardia, or both, benefit from antiarrhythmic therapy, typically lidocaine or adenosine, but may require elective or even emergent DC cardioversion.

- Individuals manifesting lightheadedness, confusion, pallor, cyanosis, or diaphoresis in the setting of profound ST-T abnormalities may be demonstrating acute ischemia and may benefit from oxygen therapy and nitroglycerin.

- Chronotropic impairment (i.e., relative bradycardia in the setting of increasing metabolic demands) is treated most successfully with termination of cardiac stress and rest.

- Patients manifesting severe bradycardia may benefit from instructions to cough until sinus node function returns.

- Patients demonstrating progressive angina on termination of stress testing are best treated with immediate supplemental oxygen therapy, nitroglycerin, and rest.

- Individuals who do not respond to the preceding measures in the setting of significant ST-T abnormality are likely to have multi-vessel CAD and should be considered unstable angina patients and managed accordingly.

FOLLOW-UP CARE

- Advise patients on discharge from the testing facility that it is not unusual to feel fatigued for the remainder of the day and counsel against activities that would compound this symptom.

- In individuals with findings suggestive of tachydysrhythmia or ischemia, the referring provider should be involved in making any further recommendations and in initiation of therapy.

- Provide printed literature that addresses findings as well as instructions on activity modifications, monitoring for and response to changes in symptoms, and contacts for further information or evaluation.

- Individuals demonstrating unstable responses to stress testing should be hospitalized (unstable angina; early, marked positive electrocardiographic changes; and hemodynamically unstable rhythms).

REFERENCES

Borg G: Psycho-physical bases of perceived exertion. Med Sci Sports Exerc 2:100-119, 1982.

Bruce RA: Exercise testing for ventricular function. N Engl J Med 296:671-675, 1977.

Cintron GB: Clinical exercise testing. In Chizner MA (ed): Classic Teachings in Clinical Cardiology, vol 1. Cedar Grove, N.J., Laennec, 1996, pp 378-392.

Fletcher GF, Blair SN, Blumenthal J, et al: Statement on exercise: Benefits and recommendations for physical activity programs for all Americans: A statement for health professionals by the Committee on Exercise and Cardiac Rehabilitation of the Council on Clinical Cardiology, American Heart Association. Circulation 86:340-344, 1992.

Froelicher VF: Exercise and the Heart, 3rd ed. St. Louis, CV Mosby, 1993.

Gianrossi R, Detrano R, Mulvihill D, et al: Exercise-induced ST depression in the diagnosis of coronary artery disease: A meta-analysis. Circulation 14:87-98, 1989.

Gibbons RJ, Balady GJ, Beasley JW, et al: ACC/AHA guidelines for exercise testing: A report of the American College of Cardiology/ American Heart Association Task Force on the Practice Guidelines (Committee on Exercise Testing). J Am Coll Cardiol 30:260-311, 1997.

Gordon NF, Kohl HW: Exercise testing and sudden cardiac death. J Cardiopulmon Rehabil 13:381-386, 1993.

Pate RR, Blair SN, Durstine JL, et al: Guidelines for Exercise Testing and Prescription: American College of Sports Medicine, 4th ed. Philadelphia, Lea & Febiger, 1991.

Pina IL, Balady GJ, Hanson P, et al: Guidelines for clinical exercise testing laboratories: A statement for healthcare professionals from the Committee on Exercise and Cardiac Rehabilitation, American Heart Association. Circulation 91:912-921, 1995.

Schlant RC, Friesinger GC, Leonard JJ: Clinical competence in exercise testing: A statement for physicians from the ACP/ACC/AHA taskforce on clinical privileges in cardiology. J Am Coll Cardiol 16:1061-1065, 1990.

Sox HC, Littenberg B, Garber AM: The role of exercise testing in screening for coronary disease [see comment]. Ann Intern Med 110:456-469, 1989.

Weiner DA, Ryan TJ, McCabe CH, et al: Exercise stress testing: Correlations among history of angina, ST-segment response and prevalence of coronary artery disease in the Coronary Artery Surgery Study (CASS). N Engl J Med 301:230-235, 1979.

BIBLIOGRAPHY

Darrow MD: Ordering and understanding the exercise stress test. Am Fam Phys 59:401-410, 1999.

Ladenheim ML, Kotler TS, Pollock BH, et al: Incremental prognostic power of clinical history, exercise electrocardiography and myocardial perfusion scintigraphy in suspected coronary artery disease. Am J Cardiol 59:270-277, 1987.

Pina IL, Chahine RA: Lead systems: Sensitivity and specificity. Cardiol Clin 2:329-335, 1984.

Vogel JA, Jones BH, Rock PB: Environmental consideration in exercise testing and training. In Resource Manual for Guidelines for Exercise Testing and Prescription. Philadelphia, Lea & Febiger, 1991, p 119.

Chapter 12

Endotracheal Intubation

Shepard B. Stone

PROCEDURE GOALS AND OBJECTIVES

Goal: To successfully insert an endotracheal tube while observing standard precautions and with a minimal degree of risk to the patient.

Objectives: The student will be able to …

- Describe the indications, contraindications, and rationale for performing endotracheal intubation.

- Identify and describe common complications associated with endotracheal intubation.

- Describe the essential anatomy and physiology associated with the performance of endotracheal intubation.

- Identify the materials necessary for performing endotracheal intubation and their proper use.

- Identify the important aspects of patient care after endotracheal intubation.

BACKGROUND AND HISTORY

Endotracheal intubation is the process by which a tube is inserted into the trachea. This may be accomplished through the larynx or through the skin of the neck. *Cricothyroidotomy* and *tracheostomy* are the terms for the latter approach. This chapter limits discussion to the former approach and refers to the translaryngeal intubation of the trachea simply as *intubation*.

Intubation is a procedure that is performed daily in many locations around the world—electively in the operating room and urgently in emergency rooms, in clinics, and in the field. Practitioners should be familiar with this lifesaving skill. Proficiency at intubation is a requirement for practitioners whose practices put them in an environment in which advanced cardiac life support, pediatric/neonatal advanced life support, and advanced trauma life support skills are used on a regular basis and in which advanced backup (an anesthesia care provider) is not rapidly accessible.

The technique has been performed since the 18th century (Roberts, 1983); however, its use as we know it today became more common in the 1940s. The value of intubation is well established. The ability to place an unobstructed conduit into a patient's airway to assist with ventilation and to protect the airway is potentially a lifesaving skill. Conversely, if performed improperly, endotracheal intubation can be life threatening. Providing the necessary knowledge and skills to master this technique successfully is the goal of this chapter.

INDICATIONS

Intubation, which provides a secure means of maintaining a patent air passage, should be used for the following situations:

- For a patient who has lost the ability to maintain a patent airway if other methods are ineffective or unreliable

- If a patient is at risk of losing the ability to ventilate adequately (e.g., airway edema, decreasing levels of consciousness, respiratory failure)

- For bypassing anatomic obstructions to clear airflow and provide a means to suction the lower airways of secretions and foreign materials; positive-pressure ventilation with a self-inflating reservoir bag (e.g., Ambu) is facilitated, as is the use of mechanical ventilators

CONTRAINDICATIONS

The only contraindication to translaryngeal intubation is laryngeal disruption itself. Airway compromise must never be tolerated, but intubation through the traumatized larynx may not succeed, may waste precious time, and may exacerbate the injury. In this situation, creation of a surgical airway (e.g., cricothyroidotomy) may be the more prudent choice.

POTENTIAL COMPLICATIONS

Complications of intubation may be anatomic, physiologic, or psychological. Anatomic complications, which may result from the intubation itself or from the presence of the tracheal tube, are as follows:

■ Nasal intubation may traumatize the nasal turbinates, the nasal mucosa, or the adenoids or may dissect into the retropharyngeal tissues.

■ Oral intubation may cause damage to the lips, teeth, tongue, tonsillar pillars, tonsils, or a combination of these structures. All intubations may damage the epiglottis, the laryngeal cartilages and mucosa, and the vocal cords.

■ Esophageal and tracheal perforations have occurred during intubation attempts.

■ Cervical spine injuries and ocular injuries have also been reported.

■ As in any instrumentation, bleeding may occur.

■ Late complications of intubation include vocal cord paralysis and a subsequent increased risk of aspiration and dysphonia, tracheal stenosis, and tracheomalacia.

■ The "anatomic" problems of tracheal tube malposition or kinking can also occur.

Physiologic complications of intubation include the following:

■ Hypoxia

■ Hypercarbia

■ Cardiac dysrhythmias (including cardiac arrest)

■ Hypertension

■ Hypotension

■ Intraocular hypertension

■ Intracranial hypertension

■ Vomiting and aspiration

■ Bronchospasm

■ Laryngospasm

Late complications include

■ Pain

■ Sore throat

■ Speech problems

■ Difficulty swallowing and breathing

■ Sinusitis

■ Pneumonia

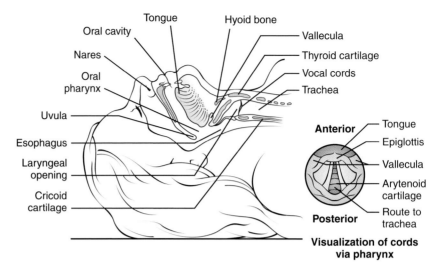

Cutaway side view of head and neck

FIGURE **12-1.**   Anatomy of the oropharynx, nasopharynx, and larynx. (Redrawn from Pfenninger JL, Fowler GC: Procedures for Primary Care Physicians. St. Louis, Mosby–Year Book, 1994, p 456.)

Psychological complications include
■ Posttraumatic stress disorder that may result from intubation of patients who have not been adequately prepared psychologically for the intubation procedure or have not been sufficiently anesthetized or sedated during or after the intubation, or both.

Prevention of all complications in all patients is not possible. However, proper preparations (physical, psychological, and pharmacologic) and gentle manipulations result in both the highest success and the lowest complication rates.

REVIEW OF ESSENTIAL ANATOMY AND PHYSIOLOGY

The successful performance of any procedure is enhanced by adequate knowledge of the relevant anatomy. Review of the structures of the oropharynx, nasopharynx, and larynx is essential (Fig. 12-1).

The nasotracheal tube traverses the nostrils, passing between the nasal septum and the nasal turbinates and bending around the posterior nasopharynx to arrive in the hypopharynx. The nasal mucosa is both friable and sensitive. Efforts must be made to reduce the likelihood of epistaxis before tube insertion.

Orotracheal intubation involves manipulation of the tongue to elevate the epiglottis, exposing the larynx. The lips and teeth are structures to avoid when manipulating the laryngoscope, as are all other tissues. Epiglottic manipulation is carried out either directly with the laryngoscope blade or indirectly by placing the laryngoscope blade in the vallecula. The vallecula is the point at which the epiglottis attaches to the tongue. Elevation of the tongue at this point causes the epiglottis to rotate anteriorly and expose the larynx.

When the epiglottis is elevated, the larynx is visualized. Note that in pediatric patients (younger than 3 years of age), the epiglottis is relatively long and floppy, and it must be manipulated directly for laryngeal exposure. The key landmark is the glottis, the opening into the larynx itself. The glottis is bordered laterally by the vocal cords, which are whitish structures originating at the 12 o'clock position and attaching at 5 and 7 o'clock (when the patient is supine). The arytenoid cartilages are the paired posterior laryngeal landmarks from the 3 to 9 o'clock positions. The vocal cords are located in the narrowest portion of the adult larynx. Deep to the larynx (which is formed anteriorly by the thyroid cartilage) is the cricoid cartilage. This is a complete cartilaginous ring attached to the thyroid cartilage via the cricothyroid membrane. This is important to remember when it is desirable to manipulate the larynx during intubation attempts or to occlude the esophagus. Also, the cricoid cartilage is the narrowest part of the pediatric airway. Distal to the cricoid is the trachea itself. The tracheal bifurcation results in the left main stem bronchus taking a more acute deviation to the left than the right main stem bronchus takes to the right. Overly enthusiastic tracheal tube insertion usually results in a right main stem bronchial intubation. The esophagus lies posterior to the airway structures.

The nasopharynx, oropharynx, and larynx are richly innervated by the sphenopalatine ganglion, anterior ethmoidal nerve, glossopharyngeal nerve, superior laryngeal nerve, and the recurrent laryngeal nerve (Sanchez , 1996). This must be considered when intubating a patient who is conscious. The placement of a tracheal tube or a laryngoscope, or both, in this circumstance will result in discomfort and autonomic nervous system stimulation. This is the cause of many of the physiologic complications mentioned earlier.

There are certain features assessable on physical examination that may predict difficulties in intubation. Narrow nostrils make nasal intubation difficult, as do narrow nasal passages. This can be ascertained by occluding one nostril and having the patient breathe in rapidly and deeply through the nonoccluded nostril. If there is occlusion, this is readily noted by the patient. Limited mouth opening may make laryngoscopy difficult. Limited intraoral visualization (often caused by a large tongue) is a risk factor for difficult laryngoscopy. Limited neck movement, especially extension, may be a predictor of intubation difficulty. A significant overbite or micrognathia may make intubation challenging. Another predictor of possible difficulty is if the distance from the chin to the larynx is less than three fingerbreadths (patient's), or 6 cm. None of these physical examination findings is completely reliable for accurately predicting difficult intubation. Their presence should not be ignored, however, and the presence of multiple risk factors must be considered as an increasing likelihood of difficult intubation (Mallampati, 1996).

Standard Precautions   Practitioners should use standard precautions at all times when interacting with patients. Determining the level of precaution necessary requires the practitioner to exercise clinical judgment based on the patient's history and the potential for exposure to body fluids or aerosol-borne pathogens (for further discussion, see Chapter 2).

PATIENT PREPARATION

Having a cooperative patient markedly facilitates intubation.
- In the patient who is capable of responding to the environment but requires intubation, it is important to explain why he or she needs to be intubated and what the procedure will entail, both during and after the procedure.

As always, it is important to consider historical information, including the patient's past medical history.
- If possible, query the patient or the patient's family about any prior difficulties with intubation.
- If time permits and previous medical records are available, look for an anesthesia record.
- If it is found that general anesthesia was administered, intubation may have taken place. If intubation was difficult, the anesthesia care provider should have noted it.

PHARMACOLOGY

Pharmacologic support can be useful. If intubation with the patient awake is desired, the process can be facilitated with the use of topical anesthetics; in fact, intubation may be performed using topical anesthetics alone. Intubation can also be performed without any pharmacologic support; if time is critical, this may be the only option. Providing adequate topical anesthesia requires approximately 10 to 20 minutes of preparation. The anesthetization itself takes no more than 10 minutes, but the drying of the airways that enhances absorption of the local anesthetics takes about 10 minutes after intravenous administration or 20 minutes after intramuscular administration. Glycopyrrolate, 0.2 mg intravenously in adults, is an adequate dose. The advantage of glycopyrrolate over atropine is that it does not cross the blood-brain barrier, decreasing the potential for causing confusion, which can be a major problem when patient cooperation is desired.

Local Anesthetics

Commonly used topical anesthetics include cocaine, benzocaine, tetracaine, lidocaine, or combinations thereof. These drugs are applied to the surfaces that are to be in contact with the laryngoscope and endotracheal tube, but they are not necessary for airway anesthesia. One nerve that must not be blocked is the recurrent laryngeal nerve, because sensory blockade anesthetizes the larynx and part of the epiglottis, and motor blockade results in vocal cord paralysis. A unilateral block causes hoarseness, dysphonia, and possible aspiration; a bilateral block causes complete airway obstruction. One may attain sensory blockade only by topical application of local anesthetics to the larynx and trachea (this may be carried out from above the larynx or by injecting through the cricothyroid membrane). If the patient is at risk for pulmonary aspiration of oral or gastric secretions, anesthesia should not be provided, some argue, so that the patient can sense the presence of aspirated material and be able to clear it by coughing.

Cocaine
Cocaine offers the unique advantage of also providing topical vasocon-striction. This is useful for reducing epistaxis when performing intubations via the nasal route. If used, no more than 3 mg/kg of body weight of a 4% or 10% solution should be used to avoid toxicity. It should also be avoided when tachycardia and hypertension are a concern. If vasoconstriction is desired, phenylephrine (Neo-Synephrine) or oxymetazoline (Afrin) may be used in conjunction with other local anesthetics.

Benzocaine
Benzocaine has a rapid onset and brief duration of action. The dose limit of 4 mg/kg is readily exceeded, because it comes in high concentrations of 10%, 15%, and 20%. Overdosage can result in methemoglobinemia.

Tetracaine
Tetracaine has a longer duration of action than benzocaine. It is available in dilute concentrations of 0.5%, 1%, and 2%, and the dose limit is 0.5 mg/kg.

Cetacaine
Cetacaine is a commercially available aerosolized mixture of 14% benzocaine and 2% tetracaine that has a rapid onset and reasonable duration. Be aware that the toxic effects of local anesthetics are additive, thus it is recommended to limit administration to no more than two one-second sprays. Cocaine, benzocaine, and tetracaine are all members of the amino ester group of local anesthetics. This group has a higher associated incidence of allergic reactions.

Lidocaine
Lidocaine is the most readily available local anesthetic. It is of the amino amide group, and allergic reactions to lidocaine itself are rare. It is available in 0.5%, 1%, 2%, and 4% solutions; 2% viscous solution; 2% jelly; 2.5% and 5% ointments; and a 10% aerosol spray. The dose limit is 5 mg/kg.

Sedatives
The intubation of the patient who is not obtunded (by pathologic or iatrogenic processes) is made easier by sedation. Drugs that have a rapid onset and

brief duration of action are best for this purpose. Surprisingly small amounts are necessary in the presence of a well-anesthetized airway; in fact, the anesthetization itself may be facilitated with judicious sedation. The most commonly used drugs are fentanyl and midazolam. These drugs also have the advantage of having an antagonist available—naloxone (Narcan) and flumazenil (Romazicon), respectively. Titrated to effect, they are not likely to produce adverse hemodynamics. Be aware that synergism may result from polypharmacy and undesired responses such as airway obstruction and respiratory depression may result. Any drug can be used as long as the desired effects are achieved, that is, a patient who breathes and is calm and cooperative. The advantage of intubation performed in a conscious patient is that the patient maintains airway patency, spontaneous ventilation, the ability to protect the airway, and the ability to verify neurologic function during and after intubation. This is particularly important with cervical spine injuries (Sanchez, 1996). It should always be considered in patients who are known to be difficult to intubate, those who are anticipated to be difficult to intubate, those who have airway or neck trauma, or those who are hemodynamically unstable (Sanchez, 1996).

Other Methods of Anesthesia

If performing intubation while the patient is awake is not required, performing intubation while the patient is unconscious is usually faster and easier for both the patient and the practitioner. Psychological stress is reduced, and the intubating conditions may be improved by general anesthesia. The risk of anesthized intubation is that it removes the patient's ability to maintain the airway and ventilate spontaneously. There is also the chance that the intubation will not succeed. If the patient cannot be ventilated by face mask or other device and cannot be intubated and the anesthetizing drugs cannot be cleared, the only recourse to save the patient's life is to create a surgical airway, which is not without risk. In the process of performing intubation, it is important to remember to "do no harm."

The practitioner can use the sedatives mentioned earlier in larger doses to obtain unconsciousness, or other drugs can be used. The intravenous agents that are used most commonly to induce rapid unconsciousness are thiopental, propofol, etomidate, and ketamine. All work within seconds. Thiopental and propofol may cause hypotension. Propofol and etomidate cause local pain on injection and sometimes cause myoclonic movements. Etomidate has a high incidence of nausea associated with its use. Ketamine is associated with auditory and visual hallucinations during the recovery phase that may be attenuated by benzodiazepines. It also causes bronchodilation, making it especially useful as an induction agent in status asthmaticus. Both etomidate and ketamine tend to maintain blood pressure and are the preferred induction agents in hemodynamically unstable patients in whom anesthetized intubation is desired. It should be noted that ketamine might cause hypotension in patients who are catecholamine-depleted (associated with long-term physiologic stress). Note that ketamine and etomidate may cause increases in cerebral metabolic rate and are not the agents of choice if cerebral ischemia is of greater concern than the ability to intubate the anesthetized patient. Usual induction doses are thiopental, 3 to 5 mg/kg; propofol, 2 to 2.5 mg/kg; etomidate, 0.3 to 0.5 mg/kg; and ketamine, 1 to 2 mg/kg. Doses should be decreased in elderly, hypovolemic, and hemodynamically unstable patients. There are no reversal agents for these drugs.

Neuromuscular Blocking Drugs

Rendering the patient unconscious may be helpful; providing neuromuscular blockade (NMB) or paralysis may be helpful or may result in death. By causing all the skeletal muscles to relax, the patient cannot cough or offer any physical resistance to intubation. The jaw muscles are lax, enabling easier mouth opening and facilitating laryngoscopy. The lack of coughing prevents spontaneous movement of an unstable cervical spine. Lack of coughing also prevents increases in intrathoracic pressure that can increase central venous pressure, which can result in increased intracranial pressure. The life-threatening complication of neuromuscular blockade is cessation of any spontaneous ventilatory efforts. If the patient cannot be intubated and/or ventilated and surgical access to the airway is not attained rapidly, the patient may die.

The other consideration when using neuromuscular blocking drugs is that they paralyze skeletal muscles only. They do nothing to suppress consciousness, pain, or the reception and interpretation of any sensory stimulus. When NMB agents are administered alone, the patient remains as awake as you are, with the ability to feel, hear, smell, taste, and see (if you open the patient's eyelids). The only way that the patient can protest is autonomically by becoming hypertensive, developing arrhythmias, becoming bronchospastic, or increasing intracranial pressure. Subtle clues are pupillary dilation, tearing, and diaphoresis. Administering sufficient amounts of sedating and anesthetizing drugs can prevent these undesirable effects. If this cannot be carried out because of hemodynamic status, the patient should be informed. Let the patient know that he or she will feel and hear everything that goes on.

The desirable characteristics of NMB agents to facilitate intubation include the rapidity of onset and brevity of duration; therefore, if intubation fails, breathing may return sooner. The absence of unwanted hemodynamic and other side effects is also desirable. The NMB agents are of two classes: depolarizers and nondepolarizers. The one depolarizer, succinylcholine, causes muscular depolarization at the neuromuscular junction. This is just like acetylcholine. Unlike acetylcholine, however, it takes minutes rather than seconds to be cleared from the muscle receptor. The depolarizers (all other NMB agents) are competitive inhibitors of acetylcholine, preventing depolarization by occupying the muscle receptor site where acetylcholine normally triggers the depolarization. Termination of effect takes minutes to hours, depending on the drug and the dose; a greater dose results in a longer duration of action. Anticholinesterases (e.g., neostigmine, pyridostigmine, and edrophonium) can be used to reverse nondepolarizing neuromuscular blockade when indicated. Note that this reversal may be neither rapid nor complete depending upon the intensity of the neuromuscular block.

Succinylcholine

Succinylcholine is effective at a dose of 1 mg/kg (in children 1 to 2 mg/kg). Its onset is within 60 seconds, and the duration of action is about 5 to 10 minutes. Increasing the dose increases the duration of action. Its mode of action, skeletal muscle membrane depolarization, results in a transient hyperkalemia of about 0.5 to 1 mEq/L. Patients who are paretic, those who have been burned, those who have sustained crush injuries, or those who are hyperkalemic for any reason may sustain a hyperkalemic increase of 5 to 10 mEq/L, resulting in cardiac arrest. Succinylcholine may also trigger malignant hyperthermia. It may also cause transient increases in intraocular and intracranial pressures, so it should be used with caution if the patient has an open globe injury and closed head injury unless the risk of a failed intubation is greater than the risk of increased intracranial pressure. Succinylcholine may cause bradycardia; therefore, its use in pediatric patients should be preceded by anticholinergic administration. Myalgias sometimes follow succinylcholine use; administering a small dose of a nondepolarizing agent prior to the succinylcholine may reduce the incidence of myalgias. If a nondepolarizing NMB agent is used to mitigate myalgias, the dose of succinylcholine should be increased to 1.5 mg/kg.

Nondepolarizing Neuromuscular Blockade Agents

The nondepolarizing NMB class includes curare, metocurine, pancuronium, vecuronium, atracurium, cis-atracurium, doxacurium, pipecuronium, mivacurium, and rocuronium. Rocuronium offers the fastest onset (within 1 minute and maximal effect within 3 minutes, with a duration of 30 minutes) at a dose of 1.2 mg/kg. The others have a slower onset. Increasing the dose enhances the onset of all these drugs, increasing their duration of action. Increasing the dose also increases the likelihood of unwanted side effects. Some of the drugs listed release histamine when given rapidly or in a large dose, which may cause flushing, hypotension, and bronchospasm.

PHYSICAL PREPARATION

Patient positioning is critical.
- Intubation is easiest if the patient is supine with the head as close to the practitioner as possible and at the level of the practitioner's xiphoid cartilage.

- The patient's head should be in the "sniffing" position: cervical flexion with C1-C2 extension.

- If cervical spine injury is a possibility, the patient should either be maintained in an appropriate cervical immobilization system or should

Figure 12-2. Axes in line with "sniffing" position. (Redrawn from Pfenninger JL, Fowler GC: Procedures for Primary Care Physicians. St. Louis, Mosby–Year Book, 1994, p 456.)

have axial stabilization maintained by an individual who does nothing else during the intubation sequence.

- In normal adults, the sniffing position is readily attained by placing a support under the head while displacing the occiput toward the patient's feet.

- In children and the obese, a more optimal position may be attained by placing support under the shoulders and neck.

Caution: The importance of this maneuver cannot be overstressed. The sniffing position aligns the axes of the oropharynx (mouth), hypopharynx (throat), and larynx, making the shortest distance from the "outside world" to the trachea (Fig. 12-2).

Materials Utilized to Perform Endotracheal Intubation (Fig. 12-3)

Adjuncts
- Emergency support equipment (More frequently than not, tracheal intubation is an urgent, if not an emergent, procedure.)

- An adequate source of suction to reduce the likelihood of pulmonary aspiration and to enhance laryngeal visualization

- Airway adjuncts such as oropharyngeal and nasopharyngeal airways

- An appropriately sized face mask, self-inflating reservoir bag, and oxygen source

- For patients in whom mask ventilation and intubation is unsuccessful, a laryngeal mask airway, which may be a lifesaving aid

FIGURE 12-3. Endotracheal intubation equipment. (Redrawn from Pfenninger JL, Fowler GC: Procedures for Primary Care Physicians. St. Louis, Mosby–Year Book, 1994, p 454.)

- Intravenous access and resuscitative medications as well as specific adjunctive medications (see later)

- Monitors for pulse oximetry, electrocardiography, and blood pressure

- If neuromuscular blocking drugs are to be used, a peripheral nerve stimulator to monitor the onset and duration of action of those drugs

Laryngoscopes

- The laryngoscope is a lighted tongue elevator (rather than depressor) and is a necessity for most oral intubations and some nasal intubations.

Note: The intubator should confirm that the laryngoscope is functioning. If the batteries are exhausted or the bulb is burned out, the intubation process will be significantly impeded. Other common causes of malfunction are loose bulbs and impurities between the contacts of the blade and the handle. Fiberoptic laryngoscopes are more reliable and often brighter than conventional devices.

- Appropriately sized blades for the patient: for adults, Macintosh No. 3 and No. 4 (curved blades) and Miller No. 2 and No. 3 (straight blades)

Curved blade   Straight blade

FIGURE 12-4. Curved and straight laryngoscope blades.

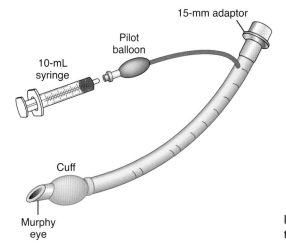

15-mm adaptor

Pilot balloon

10-mL syringe

Cuff

Murphy eye

FIGURE 12-5. An endotracheal tube.

(Fig. 12-4); for pediatric patients, straight blades in order to directly manipulate the relatively large and floppy epiglottis

■ Available backup equipment, such as additional handles, batteries, and blades

Tracheal Tubes

Tracheal tubes (or endotracheal tubes), constructed of a plastic that has been implant tested to prove it is not harmful to biologic tissues, are needed. They are for single-patient use. The tubes are described by their size, which is determined from the internal diameter in millimeters. Common sizes are from 2.5 to 10 mm. Sizes frequently used for orotracheal intubation in adults are 7 to 8 mm in women and 7.5 to 8.5 mm in men (Fig. 12-5). Tube size for nasotracheal intubation is limited by the size of the nasal passages; small nares or enlarged nasal turbinates may markedly limit the size of the tracheal tube that can pass.

Note: An often-used formula for calculating tube size in children is 18 + age in years/4; this is a rule of thumb, and adjustments are made as required (see below). Tracheal tubes of the expected size, as well as those a size larger and a size smaller, should be immediately available. The tubes have centimeter markings along the distal length.

Note: Tracheal tubes should be kept in the sterile wrapper until ready for insertion. Preparation of the tube includes confirming that the 15-mm external diameter adapter is securely in place—it is usually loosely in place in the unopened package. If the adapter is lost, conventional ventilation equipment will not be able to "mate" with the tracheal tube, and only "mouth-to-tube" ventilation or spontaneous ventilation will be possible.

Note: Other preparation includes confirming that the tube's inflatable cuff and its inflation valve are functional. First injecting a volume of air sufficient to distend the cuff into the inflation valve and then detaching the inflation syringe from the inflation valve accomplishes this. The cuff should be observed to maintain its inflated state. If it does, both the cuff and inflation valve are functional. If the syringe is not removed, the competence of the inflation valve has not been confirmed. It is more common to have a defective inflation valve than a defective cuff on a new tracheal tube.

Note: Tracheal tubes for children younger than 6 years of age are usually not cuffed (cuffed tubes are manufactured but are not commonly used). This is because of concerns of postextubation airway narrowing. The inflammation after intubation of the narrow pediatric airway can result in obstruction to airflow. Adult airways also develop inflammation, but because they are of much greater diameter, the effect of the inflammation usually is not clinically significant.

■ Lubrication for tracheal tubes

Note: This may be helpful in the presence of dry oral mucosa (oral intubation). Lubrication is essential for nasal intubation to reduce nasal trauma, bleeding, and pain. Water-soluble lubricants (sterile) or local anesthetics (e.g., lidocaine, 2% jelly) are useful. Use of tubes lubricated with local anesthetics is associated with an increased incidence of sore throat, although the cause is unknown.

Stylets

The final step in tube preparation is preparing a lubricated stylet for the tracheal tube.

■ Stylets are made of a malleable metal, often coated with polymeric silicone (Silastic). They serve to provide a means of modifying the tube's innate mild curve to the shape desired by the intubator.

■ Stylets should be lubricated before insertion into the tracheal tube. The lubricant must not be harmful if inhaled into the lungs. A sterile, water-soluble jelly is used most often. Care should be taken to avoid getting the lubricant on the outside of the 15-mm adapter because it can interfere with mating to self-inflating bag-valve units, ventilator tubing, or anesthesia circuits.

■ Stylet should be placed for all oral intubations. During intubation, removing an unneeded stylet is easier than placing a needed one.

Magill's Forceps

- Magill's forceps are used to help pass nasotracheal tubes when laryngoscopes are used to facilitate nasal intubation.

Confirming Tube Placement

- Tools for confirming correct placement of tracheal tubes must be immediately available.

- A stethoscope to confirm breath sounds and a carbon dioxide detector (a capnograph is ideal; colorimetric is acceptable) to confirm placement in a perfused, ventilated airway

Note: Other devices are advocated but are not yet in common use.

Medications

- See "Patient Preparation."

Other Equipment

Note: The equipment described is sufficient for most intubations. If it is insufficient, specialized assistance should be sought. If this assistance is unavailable, transcricothyroid jet ventilation or cricothyroidotomy should be considered. Tracheostomy specifically is not recommended.

A failed intubation is likely due to anatomic abnormalities such as a short, thick neck; airway edema and bleeding; and cervical immobilization. Emergently "cutting down" into this anatomy to search for the trachea while striving to avoid the carotid arteries, the jugular veins, and the thyroid gland while the patient is becoming increasingly distressed is not recommended. Many patients have died in such a circumstance. The specialist consultant may have more experience, "tricks of the trade," and special equipment. Examples of this equipment include (but are not limited to) fiberoptic laryngoscopes, fiberoptic bronchoscopes, specialized laryngoscope blades, antegrade and retrograde intubating stylets, and intubating laryngeal mask airways.

Procedure for Oral Endotracheal Intubation

1. Reliable intravenous access should be in place before beginning the procedure. Cardiac and respiratory monitors should be applied (electrocardiogram, pulse oximetry, and blood pressure, at a minimum). The patient must be breathing 100% oxygen, and suction and intubating equipment must be immediately available in close proximity.

2. On completion of the preceding preparations, open the patient's mouth as wide as possible, with the right thumb displacing the mandible toward the patient's feet and the right index finger pushing against the patient's maxillary teeth (thumb being anterior to index finger).

continued

Note: This is best accomplished at the level of the molar teeth, which are flat and will not injure the fingers as incisors might. Additionally, molars are closer to the temporomandibular joint, so displacement there will yield greater mouth opening, and by having a hand off to the patient's right, there will be ample room to place the laryngoscope in the mouth.

3. Hold the laryngoscope in the left hand and place it in the right side of the open mouth. Slide along the tongue, displacing the tongue anteriorly and to the left.

4. Keep the tongue from falling over the right side of the blade, which will obscure visualization.

5. Keep an eye on the tip of the blade as it is being manipulated.

Note: As the blade is advanced, the epiglottis comes into view.

6. When a fair amount of the epiglottis is visualized (curved blade; Fig. 12-6), apply force along the axis of the laryngoscope's handle. This lifts the tongue and rotates the epiglottis, exposing the larynx (Fig. 12-7).

Note: When using a straight blade (Fig. 12-8), the epiglottis is directly elevated with the tip of the blade, again exposing the larynx.

Note: A common mistake is inserting the blade too far. This can be disorienting, as the ensuing esophageal visualization is unanticipated. Another common error is not applying the force vector along the laryngoscope handle's axis but "levering" the laryngoscope. This tends to cause it to pivot on the patient's upper incisor teeth, sometimes breaking them. More importantly (in a lifesaving situation), it makes laryngeal visualization more difficult because it tends

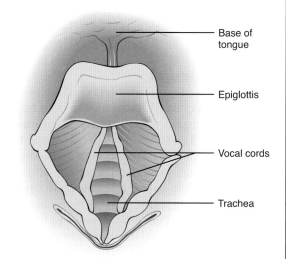

Base of tongue

Epiglottis

Vocal cords

Trachea

Figure 12-7.

Figure 12-6.

Figure 12-8.

to lift the larynx anteriorly out of the view of the intubator. The goal is to raise the structures above the larynx, leaving the larynx in the field of vision. Assistance may be obtained by displacing the cricoid cartilage posteriorly; this displaces the larynx for a better view. A cephalad and rightward displacement may also be helpful—*b*ackward, *u*pward, *r*ightward, *p*osteriorly (BURP) describes this combination maneuver (Knill, 1993).

7. Take the tracheal tube in the right hand, held as one would hold a writing instrument, and pass it from the right side of the mouth into the laryngeal inlet, medial to the vocal cords and anteromedially to the arytenoid cartilages.

8. If the patient is breathing spontaneously, the vocal cords will be moving. Time the tube insertion to correspond to the end of inspiration. This is when the vocal cords are farthest apart.

Note: Be aware that at the moment of tube insertion, the view into the larynx is lost. If the tube is not properly aligned with the larynx, it is possible for it to be deflected into the esophagus. The key to this potential problem is to keep one's eye on the larynx during and after the tube insertion. If the tube is visualized between the vocal cords and anterior to the arytenoids after tube insertion, the tube is in the correct position. If it is visualized posteriorly in the esophagus, it is not in the correct position and should be removed and placed properly.

9. Pass the tube so that the cuff just passes the vocal cords; more is neither necessary nor better.

Note: There is a great tendency among practitioners who intubate infrequently to advance the tube much too far. In most adults, the depth of insertion is in the range of 18 to 24 cm at the level of the upper incisor teeth; the depth is less in shorter patients and more in taller patients. As long as the cuff is just beyond the vocal cords, tube placement is adequate.

10. Pass the uncuffed pediatric tube so that the heavy black marker line just passes the vocal cords.

11. At this point, remove the laryngoscope from the patient's mouth, holding the tube securely while the stylet is removed.

12. Inflate the cuff at this time with just enough air to cause a seal within the trachea.

Note: The volume of air depends on the size of the tube relative to the size of the trachea: large tube, small trachea, small volume; small tube, large trachea, large volume. It is usually in the range of 5 to 10 mL. More is not better, because excessive pressure is exerted on the tracheal mucosa. This causes ischemia that may predispose to tracheal scarring and stenosis or tracheomalacia. Just enough air should be administered so that during positive-pressure ventilation one does not hear air leaking around the tube out of the patient's mouth.

    Note: In children, a leak should be heard at 20 cm of water pressure. If there is no leak at this level of positive pressure, replace the tube with a smaller one. If, conversely, the leak is so large that one cannot effectively ventilate the child, replace the tube with a larger one.

    Note: A recommended technique to change the tube is to repeat the laryngoscopy and, under direct vision, withdraw the wrong-sized tube and replace it with another.

13. Confirm tube placement by auscultating breath sounds bilaterally at the lung apices (either in the axillae or supraclavicularly)—first the right, then the left. If tube placement is in question, radiographic confirmation may be helpful.

Note: Auscultating the right side first confirms placement in the airway; if there

continued

are sounds, there is either a tracheal or right main stem bronchial intubation. No sounds indicate esophageal intubation. If there are sounds on the left, it confirms tracheal intubation. This sequence verifies correct placement. Another approach is to disprove *incorrect* placement. One auscultates over the stomach first, then the right hemithorax, and finally the left hemithorax.

14. Assess if the expiratory gas contains the appropriate amount of carbon dioxide.

Note: This is highly desirable, especially if a capnographic waveform is available for analysis. This enables one to rule out a false-positive determination, as is seen when a patient has recently consumed carbonated beverages. False-negative determinations occur when there is a total absence of blood flow to the lungs, as happens during either cardiac arrest or massive pulmonary embolus.

15. Also inspect for symmetrical chest expansion, fogging of the tube with airway moisture, and absence of gastric distention. If the tube is seen in the larynx after tube placement, it is in place (unless it gets displaced afterward). The tube must now be secured.

16. Degrease the patient's skin and prepare the skin with tincture of benzoin or other skin adherent/protector. Use of some commercially available tube holders makes this step unnecessary.

Note: The tube can be secured by circumferentially wrapping the tape around the patient's neck and then the tracheal tube. If performed properly, it is almost impossible for the tube to "fall out." The tube can also be secured circumferentially with cloth umbilical tapes or commercial tube holders.

Procedure for Nasal Endotracheal Intubation

Note: Nasal intubation is most easily performed in the spontaneously breathing patient who is placed in a sitting position. Topical vasoconstrictors are essential to reduce the chance of epistaxis. If both nostrils are equally patent, the right nostril is preferred, as the bevel of the tube is less likely to "scoop" the nasal turbinates as it passes them.

1. Lubricate the tube; an easy way is to place water-soluble jelly or anesthetic jelly in the nostril, and the tube will "pick up" the jelly as it is inserted.

2. Exert firm, steady pressure along the axis of the nasopharyngeal floor (just as one would do during insertion of a nasogastric tube).

3. As the tube reaches the posterior nasopharynx, some resistance is felt; continue the steady pressure, and the resistance decreases as the tube "turns the corner."

4. As the tube is advanced further, breath sounds are audible. It may be helpful to occlude the other nostril and the patient's mouth so that all ventilation is via the tube.

5. Advance the tube during inspiration.

Note: If the tube is aligned with the larynx, it will pass into the trachea. This is often marked with a cough and, if the patient is conscious, the loss of the ability to phonate.

6. If alignment is off in the midline, flex the patient's neck and advance the tube. This may attain success.

7. If the tube is misaligned laterally (the tube causes a bulge laterally), rotate it to remedy the situation.

Note: Because of the resistance of the tube in the nose, a much greater rotation is necessary than would be expected. It might be necessary to rotate the tube 180 degrees to get 30 degrees of rotation at the tube's tip.

8. If these maneuvers are ineffective, place the patient supine as for oral intubation and perform laryngoscopy and advance the tube under direct vision.

Note: The Magill's forceps is often helpful at manipulating the tube into the larynx.

Caution: Do not grab the tube's cuff with the forceps, as it may tear. An assistant should advance the tube as the intubator guides it.

9. Once in place, confirmation should be obtained and the tube secured.

FOLLOW-UP CARE AND INSTRUCTIONS

Having succeeded in this therapeutic maneuver, the patient must be protected both physically and psychologically.

PHYSICAL PROTECTION

■ Provide an adequate amount of humidified oxygen.

■ Prevent the tube from kinking and becoming dislodged.

PSYCHOLOGICAL PROTECTION

■ Administer sedation and analgesia. If drugs are used to facilitate intubation, the patient will experience pain and anxiety after their effects have dissipated. It is both cruel and dangerous not to treat these symptoms. It is dangerous because self-extubation is likely, and hypertension, tachycardia, arrhythmias, and increased intracranial pressure may occur. NMB agents are an inappropriate means of keeping the tube in place in the absence of sedatives and analgesics.

■ There are infrequent circumstances when the patient's hemodynamic status is so precarious that administration of sedatives and analgesics is inadvisable, and the patient must be pharmacologically paralyzed to prevent him or her from self-harm or harming others, to facilitate evaluation and treatment, or to allow mechanical ventilation at safe airway pressures.

■ When these circumstances exist, all personnel must remember that the patient is *awake* and *sensate* and must be treated appropriately. Speech must be appropriate, and comfort and explanations offered to the patient. It is my opinion that NMB agents are overused both inside and outside the operating room.

REFERENCES

Knill RL: Difficult laryngoscopy made easy with a "BURP." Can J Anesth 40:279-282, 1993.

Mallampati SR: Recognition of the difficult airway. In Benumof JL (ed): Airway Management: Principles and Practice. St. Louis, CV Mosby, 1996.

Roberts JT: Overview in Fundamentals of Tracheal Intubation. New York, Grune & Stratton, 1983, p 4.

Sanchez A, Trivedi NS, Morrison DE: Preparation of the patient for awake intubation. In Benumof JL (ed): Airway Management: Principles and Practice. St. Louis, CV Mosby, 1996.

BIBLIOGRAPHY

Applebaum EL, Bruce DL: A short history of tracheal intubation. In Tracheal Intubation. Philadelphia, WB Saunders, 1976.

Benumof JL (ed): Airway Management: Principles and Practice. St. Louis, CV Mosby, 1996.

Mallampati SR: Airway management. In Barash PG, Cullen BF, Stoelting RK (eds): Clinical Anesthesia, 3rd ed. Philadelphia, Lippincott-Raven, 1997, pp 573-594.

Chapter 13

Office Pulmonary Function Testing

Gary R. Sharp, Daniel L. O'Donoghue, Roger A. Elliott, and Daniel L. McNeill

PROCEDURE GOALS AND OBJECTIVES

Goal: To perform office pulmonary function testing (PFT) on a patient successfully.

Objectives: The student will be able to …

- Describe the indications, contraindications, and rationale for performing office PFT.

- Identify and describe common complications associated with office PFT.

- Describe the essential anatomy and physiology associated with the performance of office PFT.

- Identify the materials necessary for performing office PFT and their proper use.

- Identify the important aspects of patient care after office PFT.

BACKGROUND AND HISTORY

The first explanation of the working of the body in mechanical terms dates back more than 300 years, and PFT has been used for more than 150 years. Thackrah, in 1832, was the first to present data on lung function in human subjects. He was investigating the effects of occupation on lung size. His initial study revealed that workers who stooped at work tended to have smaller lungs than those who did not. Hutchinson's work, in 1844, is typically identified as the founding work in spirometry and includes the first accurate description of the use of spirometry to measure vital capacity. The first measurement of dynamic lung function was proposed in 1933 by Hermannsen, who recorded maximal voluntary ventilation. Tiffeneau and Pinelli first proposed the measurement of a timed forced expiratory volume (forced expiratory volume in 1 second [FEV_1]) in 1947 (Miller, 1998).

Objective measurements of pulmonary function were developed initially in the 1940s with the advent of spirometry. Improvements in spirometric design, along with the development of complex procedures such as body plethysmography and gas dilution techniques, continue to provide valuable physiologic data on lung function. Because of the complexity of performing and interpreting the techniques, PFT remained within the domain of hospital-based laboratories (Ferguson, 1998). Currently, advances in spirometer design have enabled the primary care provider to conduct PFT testing in the office setting. Office-based spirometry has been made even more reachable by the adoption of standards for testing and interpreting results (American Thoracic Society, 1991, 1995).

When adding PFT to a practice, the provider must determine if it will be used simply to manage or assess disease or if it will be used to quantify pulmonary function for impairment ratings or for meeting Occupational Safety and Health Administration (OSHA) requirements. For impairment or OSHA uses, the examiner must undergo certification training through a National Institute of Occupational Safety and Health (NIOSH)–approved course and must adhere to stringent requirements for testing. Because of the governmental regulations that apply to the use of spirometry in occupational medicine, this chapter focuses on using the technique in a primary care setting. The terms *PFT* and *spirometry* are used interchangeably.

INDICATIONS

Spirometry alone does not establish the diagnosis of a specific disease. Spirometry aids in differentiating pulmonary dysfunction as having an obstructive, restrictive, or a mixed cause (Bosse, 1993). The provider must take into account the patient's complaints, a medical history, and physical examination before making a diagnosis. PFT provides objective measures of respiratory function that along with the clinical presentation aid the provider in establishing a diagnosis, which leads to proper disease management and prognosis (Bosse, 1993). Common indications for the use of office-based spirometry include the following:

- Evaluating patients with pulmonary complaints such as wheezing and dyspnea

- Determining the degree and reversibility of impairment in airflow

- Assessing preoperative pulmonary risk

- Establishing the impact of related risks on lung function, such as smoking or occupational exposures

- Assessing abnormalities of chest wall motion

- As a component of periodic physical examination testing for individuals requiring certification in respirator use—for example, emergency personnel, carpenters, and many industrial workers (OSHA, NIOSH)

- As a component of a Social Security disability examination (Social Security Administration, 2005)

Bronchodilator and medication use just prior to testing needs to be evaluated. Withholding short- and long-acting bronchodilators and steroids may be necessary to establish baseline lung function. If the goal is to determine bronchodilator response, simply discontinuing short-acting agents may be needed. Lastly, there is no need to discontinue drug therapies if the goal is to establish a new baseline for patients with long-standing pulmonary disease. If patients are to withhold medication, explaining the risk of encountering bronchospasm during the test is a prerequisite.

CONTRAINDICATIONS

Accurate spirometry is physically and mentally challenging, yet there are no absolute contraindications for performing the procedure. Despite the absence of absolute contraindications, the examiner should exercise common sense and not perform spirometry on a patient unable to tolerate the physical demands of the procedure. The American Association for Respiratory Care (1996) defined the following as relative contraindications:
- Hemoptysis of unknown origin

- Pneumothorax

- Unstable cardiovascular status

- Thoracic, abdominal, or cerebral aneurysm

- Recent eye surgery

- Recent surgery involving the thorax or abdomen

ECONOMICS

Given the number of patients who are encountered routinely with indications for spirometry, each clinic must determine the economic prudence of adding spirometry to the practice or continuing the referral of patients to a PFT laboratory. To aid in this decision, one must realize that the cost of a reliable and completely computerized and automated spirometer starts at about $1500, with replacement mouthpieces and supplies costing about $1.75 per test. Generating a spirogram takes approximately 10 minutes. Using Medicare and the author's home state of Oklahoma as examples, reimbursement under Part B for performing spirometry (CPT 94010) is approximately $28.72, and reimbursement for the technical component (e.g., interpretation, CPT 94010TC) is approximately $20.59. Thus, one could anticipate a total reimbursement from Medicare of about $49 per spirometry examination (U.S. Department of Health and Human Services, 2004). CPT code 94060, *Bronchodilation responsiveness, spirometry as in 94010, pre- and post-bronchodilator administration*, is reimbursed at approximately $79. Reimbursements vary by state and insurance carrier.

POTENTIAL COMPLICATIONS

Common complications of spirometry usually are related to the physical condition of the patient.
- Individuals with cardiopulmonary disease—for example, asthma, emphysema, chronic obstructive pulmonary disease (COPD), or unstable angina—may suffer an exacerbation of symptoms related to their disease when spirometry is performed.

- Paroxysmal coughing, bronchospasm, and chest pain have been reported after spirometry, even in a "normal patient."

- A more commonly occurring untoward effect of the procedure is lightheadedness or, on rare occasions, syncope brought on by the momentary change in intrathoracic pressure.

- Patient fatigue or lack of understanding of the test may compromise the results of the procedure.

For optimal results, the patient must be well motivated and understand that spirometry is a patient effort–dependent procedure. Consequently, providing patient education and instructions before the procedure begins is important. This is particularly useful in avoiding patient fatigue resulting from an incomplete understanding of instructions regarding performing the test. Finally, a well-trained staff is essential for maximizing the quality of the procedure and reliability of the data.

REVIEW OF ESSENTIAL ANATOMY AND PHYSIOLOGY

From a practical viewpoint, the lungs may be divided into the following:
- Large airways consisting of the trachea and bronchi

Table 13.1 **Pulmonary Disorders That Commonly Yield an Abnormal Spirogram**

DISORDERS RESULTING IN OBSTRUCTIVE DYSFUNCTION	DISORDERS RESULTING IN RESTRICTIVE DYSFUNCTION
Asthma	Fibrosis
Emphysema	Pneumonitis
Chronic bronchitis	Pneumoconiosis
Neoplasm	Granulomatosis
Foreign body	Pulmonary edema
Tracheal stenosis or malacia	Neoplasm
Vocal cord paralysis	Atelectasis
	Pleural effusion or fibrosis
	Kyphoscoliosis
	Neuromuscular disease
	Obesity
	Abdominal distention

- Small airways, which include bronchi and bronchioles down to less than 2 mm in diameter

- The respiratory component consisting of the alveoli

Although the diameter of the airways becomes progressively smaller over the 23 or so generations of divisions, the total cross-sectional area of the small airways actually increases (Brooks, 1981). Thus, resistance to airflow decreases as one proceeds from the lung hilum to the parenchyma. Because small airways contribute only about 15% to total airway resistance, significant disease must be present before evidence of small airway dysfunction is measurable by spirometry.

OBSTRUCTIVE DISEASE

Disorders that present with an obstructive pattern by spirometry are noted in Table 13-1. Congenital or mechanical impediments to airflow in the large airways obviously result in an obstructive dysfunction. However, in the smaller airways, the cause of obstructive dysfunction may be due to a decrease in the elastic recoil of the lung or an increase in airway resistance, or both. For example, a decrease in recoil is observed in emphysema, in which breakdown of alveoli and loss of lung stroma contribute to a decrease in elasticity. The increase in airway resistance observed in chronic bronchitis and asthma is produced by a decrease in small airway diameter secondary to mucosal edema, hypersecretion, spasm, or a combination (Brooks, 1981).

Obstructive diseases reduce the ability of the lungs to move air, whereas lung volumes and capacities remain normal or increase. Abnormalities in air movement become most obvious by spirometry during forced expiration (Fig. 13-1). As such, obstructive diseases result in a decrease in the volume of air a patient is able to move during the first second (FEV_1) and in midphase ($FEV_{25\%-75\%}$) of forced expiration (Table 13-2).

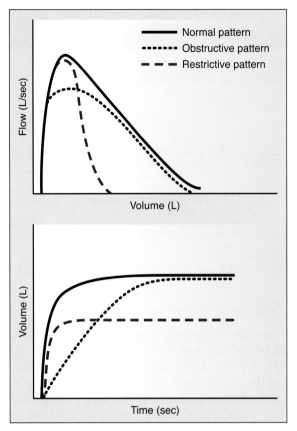

FIGURE 13-1. Normal and abnormal spirographic patterns.

Table 13.2	**Volumes and Flows in Obstructive and Restrictive Disease**				
INTERPRETATION	FEV$_1$	FORCED VITAL CAPACITY*	FEV$_1$/FVC RATIO	VITAL CAPACITY	TOTAL LUNG CAPACITY†
Normal	NL	NL	NL	NL	NL
Obstruction	Low	NL/low	Low	NL/low	High
Restriction	NL	Low	NL/high	Low	Low
Mixed	Low	Low	NL/low	Low	Low

FEV$_1$, forced expiratory volume, the volume of air *forcefully* exhaled in 1 second; FVC, forced vital capacity, the volume of air that can be exhaled *forcefully* after full inspiration; NL, normal.
*Vital capacity is the maximal volume of air exhaled from the point of maximal inspiration.
†Total lung capacity is vital capacity plus the total volume of inspired air.

RESTRICTIVE DISEASE

The pathologic presence of fibrotic tissue in the lungs underlies the basic cause of restrictive diseases. As a result of pulmonary fibrosis, the lungs are stiffened. This increases the elastic recoil pressure with a reciprocal decrease in compliance. The net effect is that restrictive disease prevents the lungs from expanding fully. See Table 13-1 for disorders that result in a restrictive lung dysfunction pattern.

In pure restrictive disease, there is no obstruction to airflow. Therefore, FEV_1 and other parameters of flow remain relatively normal (see Fig. 13-1 and Table 13-2). Conversely, spirogram tracings from patients with restrictive disease reveal a decrease in lung volumes that may be identified by the forced vital capacity (FVC) (see Fig. 13-1 and Table 13-2).

MIXED DISEASE

A mixed pattern of obstructive and restrictive disease is typical in patients presenting with more than one disease—for example, asthma and pulmonary edema. More commonly, a mixed pattern is observed in smokers with some degree of COPD. Therefore, caution must be exercised when attempting to make a diagnosis of restrictive disease if the comorbid obstructive disease is severe (Brooks, 1981). The reason for caution is that in severe obstructive disease, the FVC may be decreased because of hyperinflation and air trapping from the obstructive process. If severe obstructive disease is suspected, the examiner may rely on other parameters of lung volume, such as vital capacity without forced effort and total lung capacity (vital capacity plus total volume of inspired air; Milhorn, 1981). In mixed diseases, FEV_1, FVC, vital capacity, and total lung capacity are all decreased (see Table 13-2).

Standard Precautions   Every practitioner should use standard precautions at all times when interacting with patients, especially when performing procedures. Determining the level of precaution necessary requires the practitioner to exercise clinical judgment based on the patient's history and the potential for exposure to body fluids or aerosol-borne pathogens (for further discussion, see Chapter 2).

PATIENT PREPARATION

- Patient education regarding the procedure is the primary preparation required for spirometry.

- Because the procedure requires the ability to follow instructions and give maximal effort, children younger than 5 years of age are not good candidates.

- Although a common cold usually does not affect the outcome of the test, individuals with acute bronchitis or pneumonia should wait 3 weeks for recovery in order to perform at their optimal level (Horvath, 1981b).

- Advise the patient to wear loose-fitting clothing and not to eat a meal within 1 hour of testing.

Table 13.3 Suggested Times Medications Should Be Withheld Based on Drug Half-life

AGENT	WITHHOLDING TIME
Short-acting inhaled bronchodilators (e.g., albuterol)	6-8 hr
Long-acting inhaled bronchodilators (e.g., salmeterol)	48 hr
Anticholinergic inhalers (e.g., ipratropium)	24 hr
Long-acting anticholinergics (e.g., tiotropium)	≤1 wk
Mast cell stabilizers (e.g., cromolyn sodium)	48 hr
Leukotriene modifiers (e.g., montelukast)	24 hr
Corticosteroids, inhaled or oral (e.g., fluticasone)	Unknown, long

■ If the patient is a smoker, instruct him or her not to smoke for at least 1 hour before spirometry.

■ Advise the patient on which medications should be withheld prior to the procedure. Note that withholding long-acting medications may cause acute bronchospasm during the test and that the purpose of the test should guide the practitioner in determining which medications to instruct the patient to withhold. Table 13-3 offers a guide for withholding medications based on drug half-life (American Thoracic Society, 2000).

■ At the time of the examination, ask the patient to loosen any tight clothing and remove dentures, if worn.

■ The use of a nose clip during the procedure is optional.

■ The patient may be seated or standing for the procedure. If the patient chooses to stand for the test, a chair should be placed behind the patient should lightheadedness ensue during the procedure.

Materials Utilized for Performing Pulmonary Function Testing

Spirometers on the market today fall into two main groups. There are those that measure volume, such as a rolling seal or bellows type, and those that measure flow directly, such as a rotating vane, hot wire anemometer, or pneumotachograph. Most instruments today are computerized for data collection and analysis. The spirometer of choice should be one that meets American Thoracic Society standards. The type of instrument should be selected based on the need to store patient data and load computerized measurements into databases, ability to transmit data, cost per procedure, and maintenance requirements.

Procedure for Pulmonary Function Testing

Note: It is important to read the instructions specific for the operation of each machine, because operation may vary from model to model.

Calibration

1. The rationale for calibration is to provide data to the spirometer that corrects for fluctuations in ambient atmospheric pressure. Therefore, before performing PFT, the machine should be calibrated daily or every 4 hours, or both, if multiple tests are administered in a day.

Note: Calibration involves using a 3-L syringe to blow air through a mouthpiece. The syringe usually is provided with the machine. In addition, results from each patient must be corrected to BTPS (body temperature, ambient pressure, saturation with water). The BTPS correction factor is necessary because volumes change when warm expired air rapidly cools to the lower ambient temperature. Modern machines, fortunately, provide the BTPS correction automatically.

2. To complete the calibration, the altitude above sea level and the temperature must be entered into the machine.

3. For each test, enter the patient's height (without shoes), weight, age, gender, and race.

4. Many modern instruments are programmed to input other patient information (e.g., smoking history, presence of chronic cough). Although not critical in terms of calculating the results, recording the patient's history may be informative when interpreting the spirogram.

Patient Instructions

Note: Providing patients with instructions and active coaching during the test are critical in obtaining an acceptable spirogram.

5. Instructing the patient "I want to see how hard and how fast you can breathe or exhale your air" is usually sufficient. Explain the maneuver by stating "Take in a deep breath, close your mouth around the mouthpiece, and then blow the air from your lungs into the mouthpiece as hard and as fast as you can" (Fig. 13-2).

6. The preferred patient posture for performing spirometry is standing. A sitting position is acceptable if the patient is unable to stand or if the risk of syncope is a concern.

FIGURE 13-2. (Redrawn from Pfenninger JL, Fowler GC: Procedures for Primary Care Physicians. St. Louis, Mosby–Year Book, 1994, p 489.)

continued

7. During the maneuver, it is important to provide active coaching. As the patient begins to exhale, enthusiastically say "Blow, blow, blow!" When it appears that the patient is nearing the end of expiration, say "Keep blowing!"

Note: Most machines have a signal that identifies when the patient has reached a plateau (a change of 25 mL or less in 2 seconds) or meets the length requirement (between 6 and 15 seconds), or both. A plateau signifies the end of an acceptable maneuver.

   Note: The maneuver may also be ended when the patient cannot or should not continue.

Obtaining a Meaningful Spirogram

Note: An acceptable maneuver is free from coughs, early termination, hesitant starts, or variable effort. Coughs typically show up as spiked notches on the volume-time curve.

- Early termination is defined as an inability of the patient to plateau or have a change of 25 mL or less within 2 seconds.

- A hesitant start is determined by back extrapolation from the volume-time curve.

- Variable effort is an inconsistent curve and is often a sign of poor compliance with the procedure.

- Many computerized instruments have a built-in algorithm program that looks for and reports any of the preceding flaws in technique.

- If possible, it is best to save each maneuver, even if flawed.

- An acceptable spirometry test is composed of at least three acceptable maneuvers, with the two best curves for FVC and FEV_1 being within 5% of each other.

- No more than eight maneuvers should be performed at any one session, because fatigue can become a factor in the quality of expiratory effort. Most instruments let the examiner know when an acceptable spirometry test has been accomplished.

- Individuals with disease may not fulfill all criteria for an acceptable test. In such circumstances, information gained from at least an attempt may be useful in the management of their disease.

8. Documenting the patient's effort in complying with the procedure aids in interpreting the spirogram and is useful when comparisons are made with subsequent tests as part of monitoring the progression of disease.

9. It is common for errors in technique to occur during spirometry. Frequently, the patient may give up too soon, resulting in a spirogram tracing lacking a plateau. Properly encourage the patient toward the end of the maneuver to correct this.

10. Air leakage around the mouthpiece can give erroneous readings. Have the patient wet his or her lips to obtain a better seal.

11. Look for pursed lips and obstruction with the tongue, which are errors readily correctable by proper technique.

12. At the conclusion of the test, computerized instruments allow you to print the results of the test (Fig. 13-3).

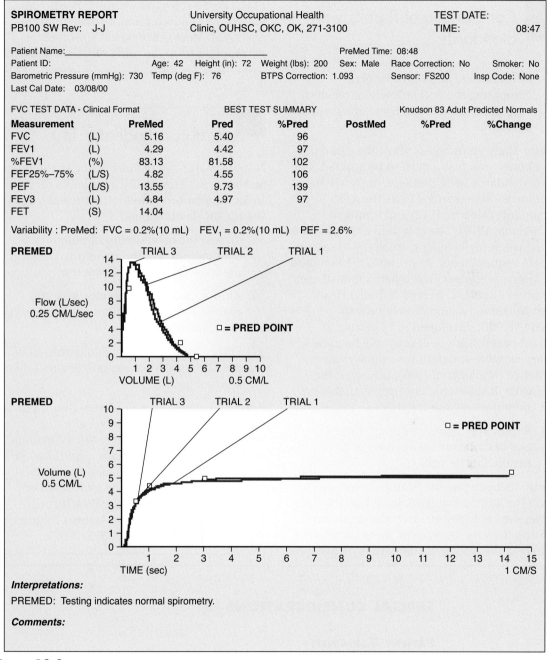

SPIROMETRY REPORT   University Occupational Health   TEST DATE:
PB100 SW Rev: J-J   Clinic, OUHSC, OKC, OK, 271-3100   TIME: 08:47

Patient Name:_____   PreMed Time: 08:48
Patient ID: Age: 42   Height (in): 72   Weight (lbs): 200   Sex: Male   Race Correction: No   Smoker: No
Barometric Pressure (mmHg): 730   Temp (deg F): 76   BTPS Correction: 1.093   Sensor: FS200   Insp Code: None
Last Cal Date: 03/08/00

FVC TEST DATA - Clinical Format   BEST TEST SUMMARY   Knudson 83 Adult Predicted Normals

Measurement		PreMed	Pred	%Pred	PostMed	%Pred	%Change
FVC	(L)	5.16	5.40	96			
FEV1	(L)	4.29	4.42	97			
%FEV1	(%)	83.13	81.58	102			
FEF25%–75%	(L/S)	4.82	4.55	106			
PEF	(L/S)	13.55	9.73	139			
FEV3	(L)	4.84	4.97	97			
FET	(S)	14.04					

Variability : PreMed: FVC = 0.2%(10 mL) FEV_1 = 0.2%(10 mL)   PEF = 2.6%

PREMED   TRIAL 3   TRIAL 2   TRIAL 1

Flow (L/sec)
0.25 CM/L/sec

□ = PRED POINT

VOLUME (L)   0.5 CM/L

PREMED   TRIAL 3   TRIAL 2   TRIAL 1

□ = PRED POINT

Volume (L)
0.5 CM/L

TIME (sec)   1 CM/S

Interpretations:

PREMED: Testing indicates normal spirometry.

Comments:

FIGURE 13-3.

continued

Comparison of Results with Standards

13. Interpreting spirometry involves comparing the patient's actual results with predicted results from an accepted standard.

Note: Many spirometers allow the examiner to choose which standard to be applied. The two standards used predominantly are those of Morris (also referred to as the ATS Standard) (Morris, 1971) and Knudson (Knudson, 1976). The standard of Knudson is used when performing spirometry to satisfy OSHA requirements. At present, the standard of Morris is applied in all other circumstances. Another standard, termed National Health and Nutrition Examination Survey III (NHANES III), developed in 1999 from a broad-based study, will probably become a more suitable standard for primary care practice (Hankinson, 1999). However, the NHANES III standard is not yet available on all computerized spirometers.

14. Report the highest values obtained from any of the three maneuvers as the results for the test.

Note: Using the highest values is consistent with the Morris standard. In fact, a principal difference between the two standards is that Morris uses the best of the three maneuvers, whereas the Knudson standard is an average of the three spirogram results. Predicted values for children are not consistently accepted. Most office-based spirometers extrapolate from the adult Morris standards.

Postbronchodilator Test

Note: A major use of spirometry in the office setting is in determining a patient's response to an inhaled bronchodilator, thus aiding in the diagnosis of asthma.

15. To test for reversibility of pulmonary dysfunction, ask the patient to perform prebronchodilator spirometry.

16. After collecting the results, give the patient two puffs of albuterol by metered dose inhaler.

17. Fifteen minutes after administration of the albuterol, perform postbronchodilator spirometry.

Note: The general agreement is that a 12% to 15% increase in FEV_1 and FVC after bronchodilator use is diagnostic of asthma or reversible airway disease. Additional PFT testing in asthma is not usually performed. Instead, patients should be instructed on monitoring peak expiratory flow through personal testing (National Asthma Education and Prevention Program, 1997, 2002).

SPECIAL CONSIDERATIONS

PATIENT VARIABILITY

Normal values for spirometric results vary with body habitus and gender. Height and age are of particular concern and must be considered with all spirometry examinations. Interestingly, airflow in liters per minute increases linearly with increased height. However, age has an opposite effect on airflow, with a decline of approximately 4% to 5% in FEV_1 and FVC occurring every 5 years after age 25 (Knudson, 1983). Gender also must be taken into consideration, with FEV_1 and FVC being approximately 10% less in women than in men of comparable height and age (Horvath, 1981a).

Another patient-related variable is race. Specifically, FEV_1 and FVC are observed to be consistently 15% less in nonwhites. Differences in thoracic configuration and diaphragm position are speculative explanations for the race-related decreases in flow and volume (Horvath, 1981a).

Finally, children are extremely variable due to the puberty growth spurt and a larger effect of race on predicted values.

UNDERSTANDING WHAT IS NORMAL

The actual, predicted, and percent of predicted values are presented in Figure 13-3. Regardless of which standard is applied, there is great variability in the normal values. For example, a patient's FEV_1 and FVC can fall between 80% and 120% of predicted and still be considered normal. This range represents two standard deviations from the mean. Other values frequently reported have an even larger range. One example is the $FEV_{25\%-75\%}$, which has an individual daily variability of 20% versus a 3% daily change in FEV_1 or FVC.

Despite the variability, a workable guideline for identifying the degree of pulmonary dysfunction (American Medical Association, 1993) is described in Table 13-4. Note that when following disease progression by spirometry, it is more prudent to document changes in the patient's actual values than to compare them with predicted values.

FOLLOW-UP CARE AND INSTRUCTIONS

In the management of pulmonary disease in the outpatient setting, it is crucial to be able to stabilize the airway using various pharmacologic approaches and to have rescue medications available in the event that stabilizing modalities fail.

Table 13.4 American Medical Association Guidelines for Determining the Degree of Pulmonary Dysfunction

CHARACTERIZATION	FEV_1, FVC, OR BOTH (PERCENT OF PREDICTED VALUES)
Normal	80%
Mild disease	60-79%
Moderate disease	41-59%
Severe disease	40%

FEV_1, forced expiratory volume, the volume of air *forcefully* exhaled in 1 second; FVC, forced vital capacity, the volume of air that can be exhaled *forcefully* after full inspiration.
From American Medical Association: Guides to the Evaluation of Permanent Impairment, 4th ed. Chicago, American Medical Association, 1993, pp 153-167.

- Provide patients with instruction on the mechanism of action for each medication, monitoring the progress of therapy, and follow-up care.

- Encourage patients to call if they are confused or if they have questions concerning medications. For patients with multiple medications, a simple outline may alleviate confusion and prevent exacerbations due to noncompliance.

- For patients who smoke, an unambiguous statement of the continued health risks of smoking should be emphasized at every visit.

The success of treating pulmonary disease depends largely on patient compliance with regimens. Providing patients with a peak flowmeter is a useful means of helping them to monitor their lung function at home. Cardio-pulmonary exercise testing is useful in trying to identify how pulmonary or cardiac factors are contributing to a patient's shortness of breath. For such advanced testing, an electrocardiographic stress test is performed with pulmonary function measurements including $\dot{V}O_2max$. Referral for single breath-hold carbon monoxide diffusing capacity (DLCO) may also be useful in pulmonary fibrosis and Social Security disability determinations. Patients will be more compliant if they understand the different treatment modalities and the central role of monitoring pulmonary function.

REFERENCES

American Association for Respiratory Care: Clinical Practice Guideline: Spirometry. Respir Care 41:629-636, 1996.

American Medical Association: Guides to the Evaluation of Permanent Impairment, 4th ed. Chicago, American Medical Association, 1993, pp 153-167.

American Thoracic Society: Standardization of spirometry: 1994 update. Am J Respir Crit Care Med 152:1107-1136, 1995.

American Thoracic Society: Lung function testing: Selection of reference values and interpretative strategies. Am Rev Respir Dis 144:1202-1218, 1991.

America Thoracic Society: Guideline for methacholine and exercise challenge testing—1999, Am J Respir Crit Care Med 161:309-329, 2000.

Bosse CG, Criner GJ: Using spirometry in the primary care office: A guide to technique and interpretation of results. Postgrad Med 93:122-148, 1993.

Brooks SM: Pulmonary anatomy and physiology. In Horvath EP (ed): Manual of Spirometry in Occupational Medicine. Washington, DC, U.S. Department of Health and Human Services, 1981, pp 3-11.

Ferguson GT: Screening and early intervention for COPD. Hosp Pract 33:67-84, 1998.

Hankinson JL, Odencrantz JR, Fedan KB: Spirometric reference values from a sample of the general U.S. population. Am J Respir Crit Care Med 159:179-187, 1999.

Horvath EP Jr: Calculations. In Horvath EP (ed): Manual of Spirometry in Occupational Medicine. Washington DC, U.S. Department of Health and Human Services, 1981a, pp 17-33.

Horvath EP Jr: Technique. In Horvath EP (ed): Manual of Spirometry in Occupational Medicine. Washington, DC, U.S. Department of Health and Human Services, 1981b, pp 13-16.

Knudson RJ, Lebowitz M, Holberg CJ, et al: Changes in the normal maximal respiratory flow-volume curve with aging. Am Rev Respir Dis 127:725-734, 1983.

Knudson RJ, Slatin RC, Lebowitz MD, et al: The maximal expiratory flow-volume curve: Normal standards, variability, and effects of age. Am Rev Respir Dis 113:587-600, 1976.

Milhorn HT Jr: Understanding pulmonary function tests. Am Fam Phys 24:139-145, 1981.

Miller MR: Chronic obstructive pulmonary disease and 150 years of blowing. Hosp Med 59:719-722, 1998.

Morris JF, Koski A, Johnson LC: Spirometric standards for healthy nonsmoking adults. Am Rev Respir Dis 103:57-67, 1971.

National Asthma Education and Prevention Program, Expert Panel Report 2. Guidelines for the Diagnosis and Management of Asthma. National Institutes of Health, National Heart, Lung and Blood Institute. NIH Publication No. 97-4051.Washington, DC: U.S. Government Printing Office, 1997.

National Asthma Education and Prevention Program, Expert Panel Report. Guidelines for the Diagnosis and Management of Asthma: Update on Selected Topics 2003. National Institutes of Health, National Heart, Lung and Blood Institute. NIH Publication No. 02-5075. Washington, DC: U.S. Government Printing Office, 2002.

Social Security Administration, 2005. Available at: http://www.ssa.gov/disability/professionals/bluebook/ 3.00-Respiratory-Adult.htm#content

U.S. Department of Health and Human Services: Medicare Part B, Participation Program for Physicians. Oklahoma City, Okla, Health Care Financing Administration, 2004.

BIBLIOGRAPHY

Eaton T, Withy S, Garrett JE, et al: Spirometry in primary care practice: The importance of quality assurance and the impact of spirometry workshops. Chest 116:416-423, 1999.

King D: Asthma diagnosis by spirometry: Sensitive or specific? Aust Fam Phys 27:183-185, 1998.

Thiadens HA, de Bock GH, Dekker FW, et al: Identifying asthma and chronic obstructive pulmonary disease in patients with persistent cough presenting to general practitioners: Descriptive study. BMJ 316:1286-1290, 1998.

Chapter 14

Nasogastric Tube Placement

Dan Vetrosky

PROCEDURE GOALS AND OBJECTIVES

Goal: To perform nasogastric (NG) tube placement in a patient safely and accurately.

Objectives: The student will be able to …

- Describe the indications, contraindications, and rationale for performing NG tube placement.
- Identify and describe common complications associated with performing NG tube placement.
- Describe the essential anatomy and physiology associated with the performance of NG tube placement.
- Identify the materials necessary for performing NG tube placement and their proper use.
- Describe the steps for correctly inserting an NG tube.
- Discuss aspects of post-NG tube placement care and follow-up.

BACKGROUND AND HISTORY

The first recorded use of a tube placed into the esophagus for feeding was reported by His to have been by Capivacceus in 1598 when he introduced nutrient substances into the esophagus using a hollow tube with a bladder attached to one end. In 1617, Fabricius ab Aquapendente reported using a silver tube passed through the nostril into the nasopharynx for feeding a patient with tetanus. In 1867, Kussmaul introduced a flexible orogastric tube for gastric decompression, and Ewald and Oser introduced the soft rubber tube for gastric intubation in 1874 (Randall, 1990).

The passage of a hollow tube into the stomach has been used for research and medical-surgical purposes for many years. Sampling the gastric contents, decompressing a distended stomach, preventing aspiration during surgery, and performing gastric lavage are just a few of the current and past uses for the NG tube. This chapter covers the indications, rationale, and complications of NG tube placement as well as types of NG tubes and insertion techniques.

INDICATIONS

Indications for the insertion of an NG tube are many and range from severe diverticular disease to unrelenting vomiting. NG tubes are indicated as follows:

- Sampling gastric contents

- Removing air, blood, ingested substances, and gastric contents

- Providing nutritional support for patients who cannot eat but have a functional gastrointestinal (GI) tract

Table 14-1 outlines some of the indications and rationale for the insertion of the NG tube.

CONTRAINDICATIONS

NG tube placement is contraindicated when the intended path of the tube is obstructed or any of the structures the NG tube would traverse are damaged, as well as in the following situations or conditions:

- Choanal atresia

- Significant facial trauma or basilar skull fracture

- Esophageal stricture or atresia

- Esophageal burn

- Zenker's diverticulum

- Recent surgery on the esophagus or stomach

- History of gastrectomy or bariatric surgery

Table 14.1 **Indications and Rationale for Nasogastric Tube Insertion**	
INDICATIONS	RATIONALE
Diverticulitis (usually severe)	To rest the gastrointestinal tract, especially if bowel obstructive symptoms exist; relieves abdominal distention and vomiting if present
Gastric outlet obstruction	As above, and can be diagnostic if >200 mL foul-smelling fluid obtained in the presence of obstructive symptoms
Gastrointestinal bleeding	Diagnostic if bright red blood or "coffee grounds" material is aspirated; can intermittently suction to assess presence of active bleeding (should *not* perform lavage in these patients because it may increase the chance of aspiration)
Intestinal obstruction	To relieve abdominal distention and vomiting
Near drowning	To empty swallowed water and to prevent aspiration
Vomiting	To prevent aspiration and in intestinal obstruction, if present
Surgery (stomach, abdominal)	Decompresses stomach and may help lessen the chance for aspiration; can monitor postoperative bowel function return
Severe burns	Patients in the immediate postburn period are prone to develop ileus; nasogastric intubation helps empty the gastric contents and lessen the chance of aspiration
Nutritional support	Used in patients who cannot take in adequate amounts of nutrition orally; must be used only in patients who are able to sit up in bed and can protect the airway; aspiration is a concern
Gastrointestinal lavage-aspiration	Used in patients with suspected or known overdose to lavage and evacuate any residual medication or ingested agents

POTENTIAL COMPLICATIONS

▪ Trauma to the turbinates or nasopharynx, or both, during passage of the tube: Bleeding from the nares and spitting of blood from the mouth are signs of trauma to the nasopharyngeal region caused by NG tube placement. Proper insertion techniques, gentle pressure during the tube's passage, and ensuring patient cooperation will help to prevent these problems.

▪ Erroneously assuming that the tube is in the stomach: Irrigation of an NG tube that is in the lungs can cause serious complications, such as pneumonia.

▪ Placement of the NG tube into the trachea and lung: This can result in pneumothorax if the tube is advanced forcefully into the lung tissue.

The best way to avoid complications associated with NG tubes placed in anatomic locations other than the stomach is to obtain radiographic confirmation. If radiography is not available, placing the NG tube in a glass of water once it has been passed can confirm poor placement. If the tube is placed in the lung, submerging the end of the tube in water reveals bubbles during exhalation. When this occurs, the tube must be removed completely and another NG tube inserted.

Other potential complications are as follows:

■ Gastric erosion with hemorrhage

■ Erosion or necrosis of the nasal mucosa

■ Aspiration pneumonia

■ Sinusitis

■ An NG tube passed in a patient with significant head, neck, thoracic, or abdominal trauma: In this setting, the NG tube may traverse a break in the nasopharynx, larynx, esophagus, or stomach. Advancement of the tube in this setting may result in severe damage to the brain, lungs, or peritoneal cavity.

REVIEW OF ESSENTIAL ANATOMY AND PHYSIOLOGY

Insertion of the NG tube involves passing it through one of the nares into the nasopharynx. It is then passed into the posterior oropharynx and further inferiorly until it reaches the level of the larynx. At the level of the larynx, the tube may pass either anteriorly into the trachea or posteriorly into the esophagus (Fig. 14-1). Having the patient swallow greatly facilitates the passage of the NG tube into the esophagus. With swallowing, the vocal cords of the

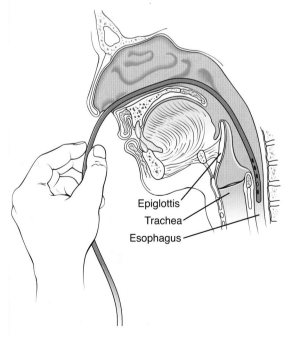

Epiglottis
Trachea
Esophagus

FIGURE 14-1. Passage of the nasogastric tube. (Adapted from Rosen P, Bankin RM, Sternback GL: Essentials of Emergency Medicine. St. Louis, CV Mosby, 1991, p 615.)

larynx are strongly approximated and the epiglottis swings backward, covering the opening of the larynx. These factors help prevent the passage of food (or in this case, the NG tube) into the trachea.

During swallowing, the entire larynx is pulled upward and forward by the muscles that are attached to the hyoid bone. This movement causes the opening of the esophagus to stretch. Simultaneously, the upper portion of the esophagus (upper 3 to 4 cm) relaxes and thus food moves more easily into the upper esophagus.

The esophagus is a muscular tube that begins at the level of the cricoid cartilage and is an average of 20 cm long and 3 cm in diameter in most adults. It courses through the posterior mediastinum, behind the heart and aorta, and penetrates the esophageal hiatus of the diaphragm. It then joins the cardia portion of the stomach just below the level of the diaphragm. Once the NG tube reaches the upper esophagus, rapid peristaltic waves are initiated, which assist in passing it down the length of the esophagus and facilitating its advancement into the stomach. The esophagus has two sphincters, one at each end, which serve to physically isolate the remainder of the GI system from the outside environment. The esophagus, like other organs in the thoracic cavity, undergoes negative pressure during inspiration, and without sphincters, gastric contents would be sucked into the esophagus with each breath.

Anterior flexion of the cervical spine during NG tube insertion also facilitates passage into the esophagus. This occurs by causing the tube to rest or press against the posterior portion of the oropharynx as the NG tube is advanced. Consequently, it is better aligned to pass into the esophagus when it reaches the level of the larynx.

Standard Precautions   Practitioners should use standard precautions at all times when interacting with patients. Determining the level of precaution necessary requires the practitioner to exercise clinical judgment based on the patient's history and the potential for exposure to body fluids or aerosol-borne pathogens (for further discussion, see Chapter 2).

PATIENT PREPARATION

- The patient should be alert and able to cooperate with the procedure.

- Informed consent typically is not required.

- Before beginning, explain and discuss the procedure to help facilitate patient cooperation.

- Explain to the patient the importance of keeping the neck flexed until the tube is in the esophagus. This is essential to avoid placement of the tube in the trachea.

- Patients should be informed that the introduction of the tube normally produces some degree of gagging.

■ Ask the patient to take small sips of water through a straw and swallow to facilitate placement of the tube into the esophagus.

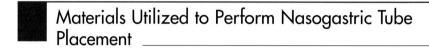

Materials Utilized to Perform Nasogastric Tube Placement

Note: Typical equipment needed for placement of an NG tube can include the following (equipment may vary slightly from setting to setting):

■ Nonsterile procedure gloves, goggles, and gown

■ Portable or wall suction equipment and connection availability

■ Hypoallergenic tape, an occlusive seal dressing, or a premanufactured NG tube holder (some hospitals keep them available)

■ Tincture of benzoin

■ Emesis basin

■ Cup of water and a straw

■ Stethoscope

■ 20- to 60-mL irrigation syringe (an irrigation-tip Toomey syringe, not a Luer syringe)

■ 100 mL of water (tap or sterile) for irrigation

■ Towels to protect patient gown and bed linen in case of emesis

■ Malleable stylet if small feeding tube is used

■ Appropriate size and type of NG (Levin) tube

Note: The most common type of NG tube used today is the Levin tube. These tubes range in size from 3 to 18 French (Fr). Tubes larger than 18 Fr should not be passed nasally because of the increased risk of trauma. Larger tubes, placed through the oral cavity, are reserved for extreme emergency procedures, and can be as large as 26 to 32 Fr.

The size of the NG tube used depends on the patient's age and size, purpose of the NG intubation, length of time the tube will be required, the viscosity of the fluids being instilled or evacuated, and disease processes present, if any. Neonates, infants, and patients with sinus or esophageal problems may require very small sizes (3 to 8 Fr), whereas typical, otherwise healthy adult patients require NG tubes from 10 to 18 Fr. Patients who require gastric lavage for medicine overdosage, ingestion of certain toxic substances, or evacuation of blood clots require larger bore NG tubes or may require oral gastric intubation.

Specialized NG tubes, such as those with weighted ends, are used to facilitate passage into the duodenum and small intestine. Double-lumen NG tubes that have one opening at the distal end (for feeding or instillation of fluids) and other openings along the distal sides of the tube allow for gastric decompression as well as jejunal feeding. NG tubes with multiple openings along the distal length, known as sump tubes, are used when it is necessary to irrigate or evacuate large amounts of fluids from the stomach.

Procedure for Performing Nasogastric Tube Insertion

1. Make sure the patient is sitting in a 45-degree angle or greater.

2. Ensure that all necessary materials and personnel are readily available before beginning the procedure.

3. Wash hands and don gloves, goggles, and gown.

4. Place protective sheet in place over patient's chest and abdomen.

5. Check for nasal patency and examine each nasal passageway. Choose the appropriate, most patent nostril for tube placement.

6. Using the tube to be inserted, measure from the tip of the nose to the ear lobe, and from the ear lobe to the patient's xiphoid to determine the appropriate tube insertion length and distance (Fig. 14-2).

Note: Either count the premade markings on the tube or place a small piece of tape at the measured insertion length. If the tube is to be placed below the stomach, add an additional 15 to 25 cm to the premeasured mark.

7. Lubricate the first 2 to 3 inches of the tube with lidocaine jelly lubricant.

8. Before inserting the tube, make sure the beveled opening or side of the tube is positioned toward the nasal septum to avoid trauma to the turbinates.

9. Have the patient flex the neck forward, bringing his or her chin toward the chest.

Figure 14-2. Measuring tube insertion length and distance. (Adapted from Potter PA, Perry AG: Fundamentals of Nursing: Concepts, Process, and Practice, 4th ed. St. Louis, CV Mosby, 1997, p 1407.)

10. Slowly and gently begin inserting the tube into the nostril straight back at a 90-degree angle to the long axis of the head.

11. Have the patient begin taking small sips of water through a straw and swallow as you gently advance the tube. Timing the advancement of the tube in conjunction with the patient swallowing greatly facilitates the passage of the NG tube into the stomach.

continued

Caution: **If any obstruction is encountered, do not force the tube, because you may cause damage to the turbinates.**

  Note: If resistance is met, withdraw the tube slightly and try placing the tube again. If continued resistance is met, try the other nostril.

12. If the tube advances without resistance, continue having the patient swallow while gently inserting the tube until the premeasured mark or tape is reached.

13. Have the patient slowly begin raising the chin from the chest as the tube passes, because this helps facilitate the tube's passage.

14. If the patient begins to gag, pause and have the patient take some deep breaths until the gagging has stopped or calmed down, and then continue with the insertion as already described.

15. If the tube curls up in the posterior pharynx, which typically causes the patient to gag, gently pull back on the tube until it uncurls.

Caution: **Do not pull the tube out completely. Wait until the patient has stopped gagging or has calmed down.**

16. Make sure the patient takes sips of water and swallows while gently advancing the tube again.

17. Check the position of the tube by:

• Making sure the tube is inserted the measured or calculated distance

• Injecting approximately 10 mL of air through the tube while listening over the left upper quadrant of the abdomen with the stethoscope for the "rush of air"

• Aspirating gastric contents and checking the pH: If the pH reading is less than 3, the tube is in the stomach.

• Obtaining radiographs: Because there is a radiopaque strip in all Levin tubes, radiography is the gold standard for determining placement of feeding tubes or NG tubes when there is a question of appropriate placement. When radiography is readily available and not contraindicated, all NG tube placements should be confirmed radiographically as soon as conveniently possible.

18. Tape the tube in place; this is important for ensuring maintenance of proper tube placement.

19. Use tincture of benzoin to facilitate the adherence of the tape, premanufactured NG tube holder, or occlusive seal dressing.

Caution: **Taping the tube so that no torsion or pressure is placed on the nares while the tube remains in place is paramount** (Fig. 14-3).

FIGURE 14-3.   Proper taping technique. (Adapted from Rosen P, Bankin RM, Sternback GL: Essentials of Emergency Medicine. St. Louis, CV Mosby, 1991, p 615.)

SPECIAL CONSIDERATIONS

Patients with impaired mentation or who are comatose and cannot assist with important aspects of the procedure may present technical challenges. In this instance, placing the NG tube in an ice bath before insertion may help by causing the tube to become temporarily somewhat more rigid and less likely to kink. Also it may be necessary to pass the tube to the level of the oropharynx and then pass the tube into the esophagus using a Magill forceps.

Insertion of an NG tube in patients with endotracheal tubes can be challenging. In some instances, deflating the cuff on the endotracheal tube is necessary to pass the NG tube into the esophagus.

FOLLOW-UP CARE AND INSTRUCTIONS

- Ensure that the NG tube is functioning properly.

- The tubes are ineffective when they are not patent. To ensure the patency, disconnect the tube from the suction device.

- Using a large syringe, inject 20 to 30 mL of air through the NG tube. Free flow of air through the tube indicates that the tube is functioning properly.

- It is important to assess the nares and nasopharynx periodically to ensure that no pressure ulcer or tissue necrosis is occurring from irritation or pressure from the NG tube.

- Remove the NG tube as soon as it is no longer needed or indicated.

REFERENCES

Randall HT: The history of enteral nutrition. In Rombeau JI, Caldwell MD (eds): Clinical Nutrition. Philadelphia, WB Saunders, 1990.

BIBLIOGRAPHY

Feldman M, Scharschmidt BF, Sleisenger MH (eds): Sleisenger & Fordtran's Gastrointestinal and Liver Disease: Pathophysiology, Diagnosis, and Management, 6th ed, vol 1. Philadelphia, WB Saunders, 1998.

Chapter 15

Lumbar Puncture

Virginia F. Schneider

PROCEDURE GOALS AND OBJECTIVES

Goal: To obtain a high-quality sample of cerebrospinal fluid (CSF) while observing standard precautions and with the minimal degree of risk for the patient.

Objectives: The student will be able to ...

- Describe the indications, contraindications, and rationale for performing a lumbar puncture.

- Identify and describe common complications associated with a lumbar puncture.

- Describe the essential anatomy and physiology associated with the performance of a lumbar puncture.

- Identify the necessary materials and their proper use in performing a lumbar puncture.

- Properly perform the actions necessary to collect a CSF sample.

- Identify the important aspects of post-procedure care following a lumbar puncture.

BACKGROUND AND HISTORY

The first lumbar puncture is attributed to Heinrich Quincke, who performed it in December 1890 on a 21-month-old boy with fever, stiff neck, coma, and pneumonia. It was adopted and widely used within a few years as a diagnostic and therapeutic procedure. By 1900, Quincke had also reported the technique of spinal anesthesia, using the same procedure with cocaine as a local anesthetic (Evans, 1998). Complications of the procedure quickly became apparent and ranged from self-limited post-procedure headache to tonsillar herniation in the presence of increased intracranial pressure. Recognition of complication risk factors and the development of new equipment and techniques have resulted in a procedure that is relatively simple, safe, and commonly used in the diagnosis of a variety of conditions today.

INDICATIONS

- Lumbar puncture is performed in adults, children, and infants to obtain CSF for cell count, glucose, protein, culture, and other specialized analyses.

- It is frequently used in the evaluation of infection of the meninges, subarachnoid hemorrhage, and demyelinating diseases.

- CSF analysis results may also be helpful, although nonspecific, in diagnosing systemic lupus erythematosus with central nervous system involvement, central nervous system malignancy, and subdural or epidural hematoma (Evans, 1998; Martin, 1986).

- In infants and children, the procedure may be used serially as a way to relieve increased intraventricular pressure from hydrocephalus while the patient is awaiting a more definitive procedure (Hood, 1996).

- Lumbar puncture may serve as a route of administration for various pharmacologic agents, including antibiotics and chemotherapeutic agents for the treatment of disease (Martin, 1986).

- Evaluation for bacterial meningitis is the most common reason for lumbar puncture, and characteristically it is suggested by a CSF sample with an elevated white blood cell count, elevated polymorphonuclear cell count, and a low glucose level.

- Organisms may also be tentatively identified by Gram staining the CSF specimen.

- Patients with viral meningitis typically have CSF mononuclear pleocytosis, a normal glucose level, an elevated protein level, and a negative Gram stain result.

- Neurosyphilis is a difficult clinical and laboratory diagnosis and is most commonly manifested by a CSF pleocytosis, elevated protein level, and positive treponemal-specific antibody test.

■ Fungal meningitis should be suspected in immunocompromised or hospitalized patients on long-term, broad-spectrum antibiotics. In these patients, CSF analysis is usually somewhat abnormal but nonspecific.

■ Central nervous system tuberculosis may have similar findings. Identification depends on a high index of suspicion and specific microscopic, serologic, or culture testing for tuberculosis (Martin, 1986).

■ Subarachnoid hemorrhage is generally characterized by CSF with a xanthochromic color at the time of the lumbar puncture and an elevated erythrocyte count in the fluid. In contrast, a traumatic lumbar puncture is usually characterized by initially red CSF with subsequent clearing of the fluid as collection progresses (Martin, 1986).

■ In the evaluation of demyelinating diseases, lumbar puncture is primarily used in the diagnosis of multiple sclerosis and Guillain-Barré syndrome. In multiple sclerosis, analysis of the proteins by electrophoresis and the identification of specific band patterns is useful as a diagnostic measure. The CSF of patients with Guillain-Barré syndrome has an isolated, very high protein concentration (generally greater than 200 mg/dL), which is specific enough to this condition to be nearly diagnostic (Martin, 1986).

CONTRAINDICATIONS

■ The primary contraindication for lumbar puncture is increased intracranial pressure. Signs and symptoms of increased intracranial pressure include progressive headache, focal neurologic signs or symptoms, progressive deterioration of mental status over hours to weeks, and papilledema on funduscopic examination. Lumbar puncture and the associated removal of CSF fluid results in a corresponding area of decreased pressure in the spinal column. In patients with increased intracranial pressure, creation of this area of lower pressure may result in herniation of the brain through the foramen magnum. Any patient suspected of having increased intracranial pressure should be evaluated by computed tomography before a lumbar puncture is attempted.

■ Lumbar puncture is also contraindicated in the presence of suspected or known coagulation disorders. This may include hemophilia, leukemia, liver disease, or a patient receiving anticoagulant therapy. It is only a relative contraindication in the event of suspected meningitis in a patient with a coagulopathy, because the benefits of the procedure may outweigh its risks.

■ Local infection overlying the site of the lumbar puncture risks direct inoculation of organisms into the CSF.

■ Abnormalities such as nevi, hair tufts, sinuses, or palpable bony abnormalities may be associated with spinal column structural abnormalities.

■ Lumbar puncture is contraindicated in any patient who is severely ill or medically unstable.

POTENTIAL COMPLICATIONS

Several potential complications exist for the lumbar puncture procedure:

■ Postdural puncture headache (PDPH) is the most common complication of lumbar puncture and may occur in as many as 30% to 50% of patients. The headache is always bilateral but varies in location and is usually described as "throbbing" or "pressure." Intensity is increased in the upright position and by movement, coughing, straining, or sneezing. It is relieved by lying supine. Patients may also have neck stiffness, nausea, vomiting, dizziness, or visual symptoms (Evans, 1998). Management of this complication is discussed later (see "Follow-Up Care and Instructions").

■ Herniation into the foramen magnum may occur when lumbar puncture is performed in the presence of increased intracranial pressure. In the presence of tumors or hematoma, herniation is relatively uncommon. It can be difficult to determine if the lumbar puncture or the underlying pathologic condition is ultimately responsible for subsequent neurologic deterioration or death. The absence of papilledema and focal neurologic symptoms does not guarantee normal intracranial pressure. The patient's presentation and differential diagnosis should guide the need for computed tomography or magnetic resonance imaging before lumbar puncture.

■ Nerve damage occurs when the needle inadvertently moves laterally, contacting the dura and penetrating a segmental nerve in the extradural space, causing pain, electric shocks, and dysesthesias. Transient cranial nerve dysfunctions have been reported, including cranial nerves III, IV, V, VI, VII, and VIII. Up to one third of patients complain of back pain and discomfort for several days after lumbar puncture because of local trauma. Disk herniation or infection is a rare complication but has been reported.

■ Bleeding (e.g., hematoma of the spine and subdural, epidural, or subarachnoid space) is rare and occurs almost exclusively in patients with blood dyscrasias or those receiving anticoagulant therapy. In infants, inquire about a family history of blood dyscrasias, routine vitamin K administration, or signs and symptoms of disorders predisposing to thrombocytopenia, such as cytomegalovirus infection.

■ Intraspinal epidermoid tumors are rare but may be induced by lumbar punctures in which epidermal fragments are carried in by the needle and implanted into the spinal canal. Use of a stylet minimizes this risk. Symptoms, occurring months later, consist of pain at the site or neurologic symptoms in the lower extremities.

■ Infection may be introduced by improperly preparing the skin, contaminating the needle, performing the procedure through an area of local infection, or introducing blood into the subarachnoid space in the presence of bacteremia. Consequences may range from local cellulitis to meningitis and empyemas of the epidural or subdural space. Sterile technique and selection of an infection-free puncture site significantly reduce the risk of infection.

■ Needle breakage is an unusual event. If the needle breaks and the fragment is beneath the skin surface, leave the stylet in place, if possible, and use it as a guide to perform a small incision. Once the end is found, it can be removed with a hemostat. If this is not quickly and easily accomplished, a neurosurgeon should be consulted.

REVIEW OF ESSENTIAL ANATOMY AND PHYSIOLOGY

CSF is produced almost exclusively in the choroid plexus. Fluid formed in the lateral ventricles flows through the interventricular foramen of Monro and mixes with the fluid produced in the third ventricle. It passes through the aqueduct of Sylvius to the fourth ventricle, where another choroid plexus adds its component, and it flows into the cisterna magna. From there, the fluid is directed anteriorly under the base of the brain and then up over the sulci between the cortical convolutions.

Although the cisterns at the base of the brain communicate freely with the spinal subarachnoid space, the main circulation continues in the cerebral subarachnoid space. The CSF is transferred back into the blood stream by filtration and osmosis chiefly through arachnoid villi and granulations in the supratentorial region.

The spinal cord terminates at the L1 level in an adult (Fig. 15-1). Lumbar puncture is performed usually at the L4-L5 or L3-L4 interspace by inserting a

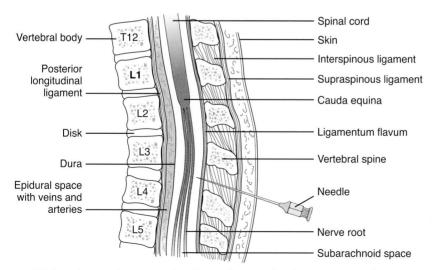

FIGURE 15-1. Anatomic orientation for performing lumbar puncture. (Redrawn from Taft JM: How to perform a lumbar puncture. JAAPA 3:473-476, 1990.)

needle into the subarachnoid space via percutaneous puncture. In the absence of spinal abnormalities, there is little danger of injuring the spinal cord. In infants, however, the spinal cord terminates at the L3 level. More care should be used to ensure appropriate interspace identification, and use of those above L3-L4 should never be attempted.

Standard Precautions   Practitioners should use standard precautions at all times when interacting with patients. Determining the level of precaution necessary requires the practitioner to exercise clinical judgment based on the patient's history and the potential for exposure to body fluids or aerosol-borne pathogens (for further discussion, see Chapter 2).

PATIENT PREPARATION

■ Because this procedure involves placing a relatively large-appearing needle into the spinal column, it can be very anxiety-producing for patients and parents. Frequently, patients and families have heard negative anecdotal experiences about the procedure from acquaintances, friends, or family members. Therefore, it is important to establish a good rapport by thoroughly explaining the procedure, answering questions, and addressing any concerns of the patient and family before beginning.

■ Explain the steps of the procedure and include the use of drawings to illustrate the anatomy of the spine to emphasize the low risk of spinal cord damage associated with the procedure when properly performed.

■ It is important to emphasize that although complications are possible and can be serious, this is a commonly performed procedure. The risk of complication is low in contrast to the benefit to be gained from the information received from the CSF sample.

■ When the procedure is performed on an outpatient basis, the patient is typically retained for observation and monitoring for at least 1 to 2 hours after the procedure has been performed.

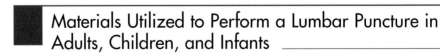

Materials Utilized to Perform a Lumbar Puncture in Adults, Children, and Infants

The standard lumbar puncture tray contains the following:
■ Three sterile skin swabs or sponges

■ 1% lidocaine solution

■ 20- and 25-gauge skin infiltration needles

■ 3-mL syringe

■ Four sample collection vials, numbered and capped

Stylet (obturator)   Needle

FIGURE 15-2. Spinal needle with stylet.

- Sterile bandage or dressing
- Sterile gauze pads
- Pressure manometer with three-way stopcock
- 20-gauge (adult) or 22-gauge (child) spinal needle with stylet (Fig. 15-2)
- Spare spinal needle with stylet
- Povidone-iodine solution
- Sterile gloves
- Fenestrated sterile drapes

An assistant is also required (O'Brien, 1999).

Procedure for Lumbar Puncture in Adults

1. Have an assistant present.

2. Position the patient.

- Position the patient in the lateral recumbent position with the knees flexed toward the chest and the chin touching the knees.

Note: It is helpful if an assistant gently holds the patient at the upper back and behind the knees in a flexed position. The assistant can help the patient avoid sudden movements during the lumbar puncture. The patient's back should be just at the edge of the table, with the vertical plane of the back perpendicular to the table surface.

- For an alternative position, place the patient in an upright sitting position with the legs hanging over the side of the bed and the trunk flexed forward over a pillow or bed table. The head is flexed toward the chest, and the arms are brought

forward for support. One cannot assess opening CSF pressure with the patient in this position.

Note: Again, it is helpful if the assistant holds the patient in this position during the procedure.

3. Put on sterile gloves.

4. Open the lumbar puncture tray using sterile technique.

5. Pour povidone-iodine solution into the well of the tray or over the skin preparation sponges.

6. Set up the four collection tubes and unscrew the tops. Preassemble the manometer and attach the three-way stopcock.

7. Partially remove the stylet from the spinal needle to check for smooth

continued

function and then return it to its fully inserted position.

8. Check to make sure all necessary equipment is in the tray before beginning the procedure.

9. Using two sterile drapes, place one under the patient and the second on the table.

10. Clean the patient's back with povidone-iodine solution. Start at approximately the L3 level and work in a circular fashion outward three times, cleansing upward to the lower thoracic spine, downward over the buttocks and sacroiliac area, and sideways over the iliac crests. Repeat this procedure a total of three times.

11. Place the fenestrated, sterile drape over the patient's back, with the circular opening centered over the L3-L4 area.

Note: The second drape allows you to touch the area around the immediate field while maintaining sterile technique.

12. Identify the level of L4, which is usually lying on an imaginary line created by joining the iliac crests with a straight line. This imaginary line crosses the spine at the level of L4. Anesthetize the skin with 1% lidocaine solution in this area.

13. Once local surface anesthesia has been achieved at the L4 level, slowly insert the spinal needle (see Figure 15-2) with the stylet into the L3-L4 intervertebral space. The needle should be precisely in the midline and directed toward the patient's umbilicus (Fig. 15-3). Advance the needle slowly.

Note: Removal and replacement of the stylet allows you to determine if the subarachnoid space has been reached. There is usually a "popping" sensation appreciated when the

Figure 15-3. Needle placement. (Redrawn from Pfenninger JL, Fowler GC: Procedures for Primary Care Physicians. St. Louis, Mosby–Year Book, 1994, p 1112.)

needle passes through the ligamentum flavum. When this occurs, remove the stylet and CSF should flow.

14. Attach the manometer as soon as fluid appears in the hub of the needle and measure the opening pressure. Have the patient gently relax the legs and breathe slowly.

15. Collect approximately 1 mL in each of the four collection bottles provided, using them in numerical order.

16. When sufficient fluid is collected, replace the stylet and, with a quick, smooth motion, remove the needle from the spine. Use sterile gauze to apply pressure to the site, holding the pressure for several minutes at a minimum. When no bleeding or fluid leakage can be detected at the lumbar puncture site, cleanse the area, removing the povidone-iodine, and place a sterile bandage over the site (O'Brien, 1999).

SPECIAL CONSIDERATIONS

■ Traumatic lumbar punctures are extremely common and are estimated to occur in up to 40% of lumbar puncture attempts. If vessels are punctured during needle insertion with a return of bloody fluid, several maneuvers can be attempted. First, rotate the needle 45 degrees from the original orientation. This may move the needle bore away from the site of bleeding and allow clearing of the fluid. Second, be patient and allow a few minutes with the stylet in place to see if the bleeding site seals over and allows clearing of the fluid. Finally, if these maneuvers are unsuccessful, you may attempt to repeat the lumbar puncture at the next higher interspace if that is an appropriate site within usual guidelines for the patient's age.

■ Nerve root pain may occur during insertion if the needle disrupts small nerve fibers in the area. This is usually described by the patient as paresthesias or the sensation of mild shooting pains locally or with radiation down the leg, or both. Repositioning the needle slightly often eliminates the symptoms.

■ Occasionally, no fluid is obtained at lumbar puncture—a "dry tap." The most common reason for this is that the epidural space was not pierced, and repositioning of the needle is indicated. Other things to consider are dehydration, blockage to fluid circulation, and congenital anomalies.

Procedure for Lumbar Puncture in Children

1. The same precautions and positioning description outlined for adults apply to children (Fig. 15-4). A 22-gauge spinal needle is commonly used for infants and children.

2. The most important component in performing a successful lumbar puncture in a child is to take the necessary steps to ensure adequate restraint of the patient. With the child in the lateral recumbent position, have an assistant hold the child securely at the knees and shoulders.

3. Depending on the child's clinical state, a mild, short-acting sedative may be administered (Hughes, 1996; Rowe, 1994).

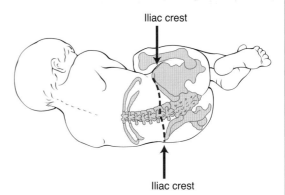

Iliac crest

Iliac crest

FIGURE 15-4. Patient positioning. (Redrawn from Hughes WT, Buescher ES: Pediatric Procedures, 2nd ed. Philadelphia, WB Saunders, 1980, p 180.)

Procedure for Lumbar Puncture in Infants

Note: Maintenance of body temperature, positioning, and an open airway must be taken into account when performing a lumbar puncture in an infant.

1. Bring the baby to an infant treatment warmer. Attach a skin temperature probe and set the warmer to maintain the baby at normal body temperature during the procedure.
2. Position the infant on the warmer. Two positions can be used. The infant may be placed in the sitting position, with the holder flexing the thighs on the abdomen, allowing him or her to grasp the right knee and elbow with the right hand and the left knee and elbow with the left hand.
3. Gently flex the spine, using care not to cause excessive abdominal pressure or to overflex the neck and occlude the infant's airway (Fig. 15-5). Alternatively, the assistant may place the infant on his or her side, using one hand to flex the thighs to the abdomen and secure the extremities while the other hand flexes the neck and spine (Fig. 15-6). The second position is useful with small premature and term infants who may not be well enough to tolerate the sitting position.

Note: An infant with a distended abdomen may have difficulty breathing when flexed into a lumbar puncture position and become bradycardic and apneic, requiring cardio-pulmonary resuscitation. When performing a lumbar puncture on any ill or premature infant, electronically monitor the heart and respiratory rate during the procedure. Also, be sure an assistant observes the baby during the lumbar puncture for respiratory movements and the development of cyanosis.

FIGURE 15-6. Flexing of the thighs to the abdomen and flexing of the neck and spine. (Redrawn from Hughes WT, Buescher ES: Pediatric Procedures, 2nd ed. Philadelphia, WB Saunders, 1980, p 181.)

FIGURE 15-5. Flexing of the spine. (Redrawn from Hughes WT, Buescher ES: Pediatric Procedures, 2nd ed. Philadelphia, WB Saunders, 1980, p 181.)

FOLLOW-UP CARE AND INSTRUCTIONS

Contrary to conventional wisdom, study data indicate that bed rest and hydration do not reduce the risk of postdural headache, the most common complication of lumbar puncture (Evans, 1998). Follow-up care and instructions should include the following:

■ Observation of the patient to ensure that the lumbar puncture site has sealed over, and no leakage of CSF persists.

■ Recommendations for treatment of postdural headache:

For initial or mild headache
  ■ Bed rest

  ■ Over-the-counter analgesia

  ■ Caffeine, 300 mg orally every 6 to 8 hours *or*

  ■ Theophylline, 300 mg orally every 8 hours

For moderate to severe headache that is present more than 24 hours
  ■ Return to the clinic for evaluation

  ■ Although bed rest does not prevent PDPH, it is a recommended treatment once it has developed. Methylxanthines may relieve PDPH through their action as an intercerebral vasoconstrictor, resulting in decreased cerebral blood flow and intracranial pressure. If the PDPH persists beyond 24 hours, an epidural blood patch is the most effective treatment. This is accomplished by drawing 10 to 20 mL of the patient's blood and then slowly injecting it into the lumbar epidural space near the prior puncture site. The patient should remain in the decubitus position for 1 to 2 hours after the procedure for maximal benefit. The epidural blood patch works by exerting a mass effect and compressing the dural sac, sealing any continued CSF leak (Evans, 1998).

REFERENCES

Evans RW: Complications of lumbar puncture. Neurol Clin N Am 16:105, 1998.

Hood BR: Lumbar Puncture in Procedures in Infants and Children. Philadelphia, WB Saunders, 1996, pp 202-205.

Hughes WT, Buescher ES: Central Nervous System: Pediatric Procedures. Philadelphia, WB Saunders, 1996, pp 178-185.

Martin KI, Gean AD: The spinal tap: A new look at an old test. Ann Intern Med 104:840-848, 1986.

O'Brien J: Lumbar Puncture in Primary Care Practice Procedures. Philadelphia, WB Saunders, 1999, pp 1109-1114.

Rowe PC: Pediatric Procedures in Principles and Practice of Pediatrics. Philadelphia, JB Lippincott, 1994, pp 2206-2207.

Chapter 16

Urinary Bladder Catheterization

Dan Vetrosky

PROCEDURE GOALS AND OBJECTIVES

Goal: To perform urinary bladder catheterization on a patient safely and accurately.

Objectives: The student will be able to ...

- Describe the indications, contraindications, and rationale for performing urinary bladder catheterization.

- Identify and describe common complications associated with performing urinary bladder catheterization.

- Describe the essential anatomy and physiology associated with the performance of urinary bladder catheterization.

- Identify the materials necessary for performing urinary bladder catheterization and their proper use.

- Discuss aspects of post–urinary catheter placement care and follow-up.

BACKGROUND AND HISTORY

Disease processes that require urinary bladder catheterization have existed since ancient times. Urethral strictures, bladder stones, and prostatism are among the first diseases that necessitated urinary bladder decompression by catheterization. The approach to urinary catheterization remains the same today as it was in ancient times. It is the technique of passing a hollow tube through the urethra into the urinary bladder for purposes of circumventing an obstructed urinary bladder or obtaining a sample of urine for analysis, or both.

The first known urologic instruments would be considered somewhat barbaric by today's standards. Ancient and medieval "urologists-lithotomists" used perineal incision and metal and glass tubes to circumvent urinary obstruction. Today's approach often uses a local anesthetic and urethral catheters made of rubber, latex, polytetrafluoroethylene (Teflon), or silicone polymers. Urethral catheterization is used currently for relief of bladder outlet obstruction or when measurement of urinary output must be precise (e.g., in multiple trauma, surgery, intensive care, renal failure).

INDICATIONS

Reasons for passing a catheter into the urinary bladder are many. The most common uses of bladder catheterization are as follows:

■ To obtain a sterile urine sample, especially in the female patient

■ To monitor urinary output closely in critically ill patients

■ To facilitate urinary drainage in patients who are incapacitated (e.g., due to stroke, advanced Alzheimer's disease, spinal transection)

■ To bypass obstructive processes in the urethra, prostate, or bladder neck caused by disease or trauma until surgical repair can be performed

■ To hold urethral skin grafts in place after urethral stricture repair

■ To act as a traction device for the purpose of controlling bleeding after prostate surgery

■ Specialized three-way Foley catheters are used after bladder or prostate surgery to allow for continuous bladder irrigation. Continuous irrigation as well as drainage helps prevent the formation of blood clots, which can occlude a catheter and cause bladder obstruction. Three-way Foley catheters also allow for easier evacuation of formed blood clots (Fig. 16-1).

The main reasons for using the "one time," "straight," or Robinson catheter are as follows:

■ To obtain a sterile urine sample or to decompress a distended bladder caused by an acute obstructive process

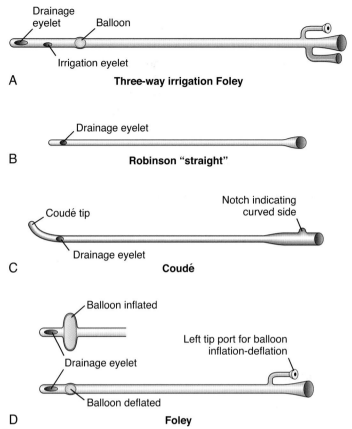

FIGURE 16-1.   **A,** Three-way Foley irrigation catheter. **B,** Robinson catheter. **C,** Coudé catheter. **D,** Foley catheter.

- As a protocol of intermittent catheterization in persons with neurogenic bladders: Catheterizing patients with neurogenic bladders at regular intervals with the Robinson catheter facilitates complete bladder emptying, routine urine sampling, and "bladder training." Some of these patients may be able to decrease the frequency of their catheterization or may regain complete bladder control, or both, after a time.

- To deliver topical antineoplastic medication to the bladder in patients who have bladder cancer or to deliver other topical medication to patients who suffer from interstitial cystitis

- To assess post-void residual urine in circumstances where ultrasound equipment is unavailable.

CONTRAINDICATIONS

The only contraindication to inserting a catheter (either Robinson or Foley) is the appearance of blood at the urethral meatus in a patient who has sustained pelvic trauma. This finding can be an indication that the urethra has been partially or totally transected. Attempting to pass a catheter in this situation could cause a partial urethral transection to become total. It is advised that a urologist be consulted when blood at the urethral meatus is present in a patient with pelvic trauma. Allergy to materials used in the procedure, such as latex, rubber, tape, and lubricants, is also a contraindication.

POTENTIAL COMPLICATIONS

Most of the complications with catheterization are seen in the male patient. Female patients rarely have urethral stricture, and because the female urethra is comparatively short, false passages are rarely created. Complications can include the following:

- Urethral dilation due to placement of a long-term indwelling Foley catheter in women. Leaking can occur because of bladder spasm. Instead of treating the spasm, progressively larger diameter catheters are placed causing urethral dilation and continuation of leaking.

- Urinary structural trauma

- Urinary tract infection

- Inflammation of the urinary tract secondary to the procedure

- Catheterizing a male patient with urethral stricture disease, bladder neck contracture, or an enlarged prostate; this may present some technical difficulties for the unsuspecting health care provider

- Passage of a Robinson or Foley catheter in a patient with urethral stricture disease or an enlarged prostate: This increases the danger of creating false passages in the urethra if excessive force is applied when resistance is met during the catheterization. The mechanism of injury occurs when the obstructive process deflects the catheter into the side wall of the urethra. If the clinician meets these types of obstructive processes and continues to apply excessive pressure in an attempt to bypass the blockage, the catheter can act like a drill and undermine the lining of the urethra, thus creating a "false passage." The worst scenario in this situation would be pushing the catheter completely through the urethra into the surrounding tissue. This results in copious bleeding from the urethra and creates the possibility of urine and blood extravasating into the surrounding tissues.

- Having the catheter "double back" or make a "U-turn" at the site of obstruction: It is not uncommon to have the catheter tip reappear at the urethral meatus when there is a significant obstruction or bladder neck spasm.

- Improper securing/taping of the Foley catheter.

FIGURE 16-2. Anatomy of the female **(left)** and male **(right)** lower urinary tracts with catheters in place. (Redrawn from Potter PA, Perry AG: Fundamentals of Nursing, 4th ed. St. Louis, Mosby–Year Book, 1997, p 1324.)

■ Patient caused trauma: patients who are confused can pull out a fully inflated Foley catheter.

REVIEW OF ESSENTIAL ANATOMY AND PHYSIOLOGY

Urine is produced by the kidneys and transported to the bladder by the ureters, where it is stored for transport through the urethra during urination. Bladder catheterization involves the passage of a mechanical device into the bladder through the urethra. To accomplish this without damage requires an understanding of the anatomy of the lower urinary tract. Figure 16-2 illustrates the anatomy in relation to the location at which a urinary catheter would be placed for females and males.

In females, the distance from the distal end of the urethra to the bladder is relatively short (1.5 to 2 inches) and the course through the urethra is relatively unobstructed. Because of this, bladder catheterization in the female patient is typically accomplished faster and with less discomfort than it is in the male patient.

In males, the distance from the distal tip of the urethra to the bladder is longer (typically 6 to 7 inches; however, it can vary considerably) and is more circuitous than in females, thus making catheter insertion potentially more difficult. In males, the path to the bladder typically includes curves that may be encountered while traversing the penis as well as a sharp bend through the prostate. Occasionally, prostatic hypertrophy can make catheter insertion difficult because the pressure of the hypertrophic prostate can add a curvature to the urethra as well as produce urethral obstruction.

Standard Precautions   Practitioners should use standard precautions at all times when interacting with patients. Determining the level of precaution necessary requires the practitioner to exercise clinical judgment based on the patient's history and the potential for exposure to body fluids or aerosol-borne pathogens (for further discussion, see Chapter 2).

PATIENT PREPARATION

■ Inform the patient before the procedure how the catheterization will be performed and what he or she might expect to feel during the procedure. This will help secure the patient's trust and cooperation. Do not tell the patient that he or she will not feel anything, because this would be untruthful and counterproductive during the procedure. Inform the patient that the passage of the catheter may feel as though he or she must urinate and that it will be slightly uncomfortable.

■ Patient comfort must be a primary consideration if a sterile, atraumatic catheterization is to be accomplished.

■ Explain to the patient the importance of being reasonably still and not touching your gloved hands or sterile implements.

■ Typically, the patient is positioned in the supine position. Drapes should be placed to cover all but the genitalia. The female patient will need to abduct the legs laterally to allow easy access to the urethra.

▌ Materials Utilized to Perform a Urinary Bladder Catheterization

■ Sterile tray or working area

■ Vessel for collecting urine (sometimes included with tray)

■ Sterile gloves

■ Sterile lubricant or anesthetic jelly lubricant

■ Antiseptic cleansing solution (typically povidone-iodine [Betadine])

■ Sterile gauze or cotton balls for cleansing the external exit of the urethra and the surrounding skin

■ Sterile forceps

■ Syringe filled with sterile water for catheter balloon, 5 mL to 30 mL depending on the balloon capacity of the catheter selected

- Urine collection tubing, bags, hardware, and specimen collection containers

- Sterile drapes to protect the sterile field and nonsterile drapes to maintain patient modesty

- Catheter (see "Types of Catheters")

- Catheterization kits containing the following:

  - Sterile lubricant

  - Sterile drapes

  - Sterile gloves

  - Sterile cotton swabs

  - Povidone-iodine

  - Forceps to grasp the cotton swabs

  - Sterile specimen container for urinalysis and culture

  - Container to catch the urine

  - Robinson or Foley catheter, 14, 16, or 18 French: If a Foley catheter is used, the kit will also contain a prefilled 10-mL Luer-tipped syringe to inflate the Foley balloon and can contain a preattached drainage bag (attached to the Foley catheter). The advantage of a preattached drainage bag is that once in place, the Foley catheter and the drainage bag are considered a sterile "closed system." The disadvantage is the inability to obtain a specimen or irrigate the bladder without "breaking the seal" and making what was once a sterile closed system a "contaminated" open system.

TYPES OF CATHETERS

Urinary catheters (Robinson, coudé, and Foley types) are made of various materials and are soft and flexible (see Fig. 16-1). The most common catheter, Robinson or "straight" type, is made of rubber. Catheters can be made of pure rubber, rubber with synthetic coatings such as latex, or pure latex. Pure silicone and silicone-coated catheters are also manufactured, although they are much more expensive than rubber or latex catheters. These coated catheters are more commonly seen in indwelling or Foley catheter lines. The coatings are touted to resist encrustation when left in the bladder for prolonged periods. Patients with latex allergies should not be catheterized with rubber or latex catheters. In such cases, catheters made of pure silicone are an acceptable alternative.

ROBINSON CATHETER

The Robinson catheter is also known as the "straight" catheter and is sterile if the package seal is not broken. It has a soft, rounded tip and one or two drainage eyelets on the tip side walls. The catheter is hollow, and the distal end is flared to facilitate urinary drainage. These catheters are designed for one-time use, hence the term *in-and-out catheter* (see Fig. 16-1).

COUDÉ CATHETER

Coudé catheters have a bend at the distal tip that causes the catheter to follow the anterior surface of the male urethra. This bent tip facilitates the insertion of the catheter in patients with false passages, which typically occur on the posterior surface of the urethra.

FOLEY CATHETER

The Foley catheter is designed to remain in place in the bladder. It too is sterile, and its appearance is similar to the Robinson catheter, with a few exceptions. At the tip, behind the drainage eyelets, is an inflatable balloon. The balloon is inflated after the catheter is properly placed in the bladder to help keep the catheter seated in the bladder. The flared end of the catheter is located at the distal end, and it can be attached to a drainage bag. Also at the distal end is an elbow with a Luer-Lok cap attached. This elbow is the end of an extremely small lumen, which traverses the length of the catheter and ends in the balloon at the tip. The Luer-Lok cap allows the balloon to be inflated once the catheter is in place and deflated once the catheter needs to be removed. The balloon is typically inflated with sterile water. Use of saline is discouraged because of the possibility of crystal formation along the balloon's lumen. Should this occur, the balloon might not deflate when the catheter needs to be removed.

There are two sizes of Foley catheter balloons: a 5-mL balloon and a 30-mL balloon. The most common balloon size used is 5 mL, and it is typically inflated with 10 mL of sterile water, which accounts for the lumen volume and the balloon volume; 30-mL balloons are used to ensure that the Foley catheter does not migrate into the prostatic fossa or out of the urinary bladder altogether. In addition, the 30-mL balloon can be inflated with 50 mL of sterile water and used as a traction stent after certain urologic procedures (e.g., radical prostatectomy, transurethral prostatectomy).

CATHETER SIZE REQUIREMENTS

Urinary catheters come in various sizes and are measured according to the Charrière French scale (0.33 mm equals 1 French [Fr]). A 3-Fr catheter is

1 mm in diameter, whereas a 30-Fr catheter is 10 mm in diameter. The French size of the catheter depends on the patient and the catheter's purpose. As an example, pediatric boys need a French size between 5 and 12 Fr. Adult men should be catheterized with a 16- or 18-Fr catheter. These sizes are slightly stiffer and will follow the anatomic curvature of the male urethra easier and better than the smaller French catheters (14 Fr or smaller). Smaller French catheters have a tendency to "turn around" in the male urethra if the slightest resistance is met (especially at the bladder neck). The adult woman should also be catheterized with 16- or 18-Fr catheters, although a 14 Fr should be used most of the time to facilitate comfort. Larger French catheters (20 to 30 Fr) are used to evacuate blood clots in postoperative prostate surgery patients or in patients who are bleeding from the kidney or bladder.

Procedure for Performing a Urinary Bladder Catheterization on a Male Patient

Note: Male patients are more prone to sustaining damage to the urethra during the catheterization procedure. Improper lubrication and excessive force used to "overcome" an obstruction are the most common offending factors causing urethral trauma. The steps outlined here will help reduce the chances of inflicting excessive pain, causing urethral damage, or introducing infection.

1. Obtain the Robinson or Foley catheter that is sized commensurate with the procedure or purpose. Make sure it is sterile (packaging must be intact).

2. Obtain the appropriate catheterization kit or supplies.

3. Follow aseptic techniques and standard precautions by washing hands and putting on sterile gloves.

4. Open the kit in a sterile manner.

5. Prepare the patient by draping him in sterile drapes (found in the kit) and exposing the genital area, making sure to allow for the patient's privacy and comfort.

6. Open the catheter, if not contained in the kit, and place on the sterile drape using sterile technique.

7. Even if a package of sterile lubricant is contained in the kit, obtain a sterile 15- to 20-mL syringe and place it on the sterile drape.

8. Once the operator is gloved, an assistant is needed to squirt some lubricant into the syringe. Water-soluble lubricant can be substituted for sterile anesthetic jelly (lidocaine [Xylocaine] *jelly,* not ointment, or Anestacon [a prepackaged anesthetic jelly]).

Note: If there is a prefilled sterile syringe with water-soluble lubricant in the kit, this step can be omitted.

9. Open the package of povidone-iodine and pour onto the cotton swabs.

10. Inform the patient that you are going to hold his penis and clean it with the povidone-iodine. Assure him that it will not stain the skin permanently. Swab the head of the penis, making sure to clean the meatal opening first and wiping out

continued

to the glans with the povidone-iodine soaked cotton swabs. (Use your nondominant hand to hold the penis.) Use all the cotton swabs.

Note: If the patient is uncircumcised, the foreskin needs to be drawn back before beginning the cleansing and catheter insertion process.

11. Once the penis is clean, do not let go and position the penis at a 90-degree angle from the abdomen and instill the lubricant or anesthetic agent into the urethra. Gently occlude the urethra so that the lubricant or anesthetic agent does not come back out the urethra. If using anesthetic jelly, wait for approximately 1 minute before proceeding so that the anesthetic jelly has time to work.

12. Position the urine container near the patient's leg or between the patient's legs, as appropriate.

13. Grasp the catheter with your dominant hand about three quarters of the way toward the catheter tip. Inform the patient that you are now going to insert the catheter. Gently begin inserting the catheter into the urethral meatus and continue the insertion without stopping (Fig. 16-3). When the sphincter is encountered, you will feel slight resistance. Ask the patient to take a deep breath, which might assist in relaxing him somewhat, but continue to insert the catheter, applying gentle pressure if necessary.

Note: When a stricture or obstruction is encountered during catheterization, the clinician has some techniques and tools that may facilitate atraumatic bladder catheterization. The first technique is to make sure the urethra is well lubricated by instilling sterile, water-soluble lubricating jelly or topical anesthetic jelly into the

Figure 16-3.   Catheter insertion in a male patient. (Adapted from Potter PA, Perry AG: Fundamentals of Nursing, 4th ed. St. Louis Mosby–Year Book, 1997.p 1323.)

urethra. Once this is accomplished, a 16- or 18- Fr coudé-tipped catheter (see Fig. 16-1) can be used to facilitate bypassing false passages or bladder neck obstruction. The coudé tip is fashioned to follow the normal curve of the urethra and should be passed with the tip facing the anterior portion of the patient's urethra. If the clinician continues to meet obstruction and is unsuccessful using the coudé catheter and the techniques outlined, a urologist should be called. The urologist will most likely try using a filiform bougie and followers in order to bypass and dilate urethral structures or bladder neck contractures. If these techniques or tools are not successful, a flexible cystoscope or suprapubic catheterization may be used.

14. Once the sphincter is passed, continue to pass the catheter until almost to the hub of the catheter. Urine should begin to flow, although it may take some time for the lubricant, which will be in the

catheter after you pass it into the bladder, to "melt." Place the end of the catheter into the urine container and empty the bladder.

15. Obtain a specimen at this point if needed.

16. Once the bladder is empty, remove the catheter in one continuous motion, making sure to pinch off the distal end so that the column of urine left in the catheter does not pour onto the patient.

17. Make sure to measure the amount of urine obtained and record it.

Note: This is important in any situation, but especially when trying to measure a post-void residual. Having the patient void immediately before catheterizing him allows for the measurement of residual urine in the bladder. The amount voided must be measured, and then the post-void residual left in the bladder can be measured following catheterization. In many practices, ultrasound measurement of post-void residual urine in the bladder is replacing the in-and-out catheterization.

18. If this is a Foley catheter placement, once the catheter is in the bladder and urine begins to flow, get the prefilled syringe (with sterile water) and inflate the Foley balloon.

19. Make sure the Foley catheter is inserted almost to the hub.

Note: This ensures that the balloon is not blown up in the prostate, bladder neck, or urethra.

20. Once the balloon is blown up, pull the Foley catheter out gently until it stops. The Foley catheter is now in the proper position.

21. Attach the drainage bag if it is not already in place.

22. Tape the Foley catheter to the abdomen.

Caution: **Taping the Foley catheter is an important step. The penis should be pointing toward the umbilicus and the catheter taped just below the hub.**
Note: Taping the Foley catheter in this manner prevents it from eroding through the urethra by eliminating the first curve of the "S" formed by the male urethra. Maintenance of the Foley catheter includes daily cleaning, retaping in the proper position when necessary, and appropriate meatal care.

23. Apply bacitracin ointment to the urethral meatus one to three times a day as needed. This helps keep the catheter from irritating the meatus excessively and prevents infection.

Note: If the patient is uncircumcised, the foreskin needs to be placed back into its original position.

Procedure for Performing a Urinary Bladder Catheterization on a Female Patient

Note: Female patients can be difficult to catheterize because of the placement of the urethral meatus. If the female patient has a normal anatomy and is not excessively obese, the urethral meatus should be superior to the vaginal introitus and inferior to the clitoris. Some women's urethral meatus is located just inside the superior aspect of the vaginal introitus. This can make catheterization difficult, as identification of the urethral orifice can be obscured by vaginal tissue.

continued

1. Obtain a Robinson or Foley catheter in a size commensurate with the procedure or purpose, making sure that it is sterile (the packaging must be intact).

2. Obtain the appropriate catheterization kit or supplies.

3. Wash your hands.

4. Open the kit in a sterile manner.

5. Put on sterile gloves.

6. Prepare the patient by draping her in sterile drapes (found in the kit) and exposing the genital area, making sure to allow for the patient's privacy and comfort.

7. Open the catheter, if not contained in the kit, and place on the sterile drape using sterile technique.

8. Instead of instilling lubricant into the female urethra, lubricate the catheter well, about one third of the way from the tip of the catheter up.

9. Open the package of povidone-iodine and pour onto the cotton swabs.

10. Inform the patient that you are going to swab the urethral opening with povidone-iodine once you separate the labia majora and labia minora. Using the nondominant hand, spread the patient's labia. Wipe the urethral opening with the cotton swabs from an anterior to a posterior direction. If the urethral opening is at or in the vaginal opening, the vaginal opening must be swabbed as well.

11. At this point, you can anesthetize the urethra if desired. To do this, apply lidocaine jelly or aqueous cocaine to a cotton-tipped swab and gently insert it into the urethra. Leave it in place for approximately 1 to 2 minutes before placing the catheter.

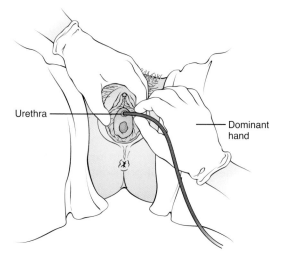

FIGURE 16-4. Catheter insertion in a female patient. (Redrawn from Potter PA, Perry AG: Fundamentals of Nursing, 4th ed. St. Louis, Mosby–Year Book, 1997, p 1323.)

12. Place the urine container between the patient's legs.

13. Grasp the catheter with your dominant hand, making sure that the catheter is still well lubricated, and gently insert the tip of the catheter into the urethral opening until urine starts to flow or approximately one third of the catheter has been inserted into the bladder (Fig. 16-4).

Note: If you have missed the urethral opening or inserted the catheter into the vagina, you must obtain a new catheter and try again. (A helpful technique is to leave the catheter you missed with temporarily in place. This helps you identify where *not* to place the new catheter.)

14. Once the bladder is empty (and you have obtained your specimen), remove the catheter in one continuous motion, making sure to pinch off the distal end of the catheter so that the column of urine left in it does not pour onto the patient.

15. If this is a Foley catheter placement, once the catheter is in the bladder and urine begins to flow, get the prefilled syringe (with sterile water) and inflate the Foley balloon.

16. Make sure the Foley catheter is inserted at least one third of the way into the bladder.

Note: This ensures that you do not blow the balloon up in the bladder neck or urethra.

17. Once the balloon is blown up, pull the Foley catheter out gently until it stops. The catheter is now in the proper position.

18. Attach the drainage bag if it is not already in place.

Caution: **Taping the Foley catheter is an important step.**

19. Tape the Foley catheter to the inner thigh. Leave some slack so that it is not taut and pulling against the bladder neck. This can cause bladder spasms. Tape just below the hub.

Note: Maintenance of the Foley catheter includes daily cleaning, retaping in the proper position when necessary, and appropriate meatal care. Typically, povidone-iodine ointment is applied to the urethral meatus one to three times daily as needed. This helps keep the catheter from irritating the meatus excessively and helps prevent infection.

FOLLOW-UP CARE AND INSTRUCTIONS

SHORT-TERM OR IN-AND-OUT CATHETERIZATION

- Complications are unlikely.

- The most common complications include irritation of the urinary tract and infection.

- Patients will most likely "burn" the first few times they urinate following catheterization. Reassurance is usually all that is needed.

- Instruct the patient to monitor urination for continuous dysuria, urinary frequency, hematuria, and pyuria, as well as for systemic signs of urinary tract infection such as fever or back pain.

INDWELLING CATHETERIZATION

- The two major risks associated with an indwelling urinary catheter are trauma and infection. After successful catheter placement, trauma is typically a result of not protecting the catheter properly.

- Instruct the patient that the catheter should be secured with tape at all times and that care should be taken not to snag the tubing on clothing or furniture in a way that would pull on the catheter.

Infection prevention measures include the following:

- Advise the patient always to position the drainage bag below the bladder to prevent urine from flowing back into the bladder.

- Instruct the patient to be careful to avoid kinks in the tubing system.

- Instruct the patient to monitor the bag often to make sure that it is emptied before it becomes completely full.

- Caution the patient to be careful when emptying the bag or manipulating the drainage system, to avoid introducing contaminants.

- Instruct the patient to wash hands frequently and to use latex gloves (if not allergic; if allergic to latex, indicate which type of gloves to obtain).

- Instruct the patient to be careful not to have the drainage system come into contact with contaminated objects such as toilet bowls.

- Caution the patient to be aware of signs of infection, such as changes in the appearance of the urine or symptoms of a urinary tract infection, and to call the office.

BIBLIOGRAPHY

Potter PA, Perry AG: Fundamentals of Nursing, 4th ed. St. Louis, Mosby–Year Book, 1997.

Tanagho EM, McAninch JW (eds): Smith's General Urology, 14th ed. Norwalk, Conn, Appleton & Lange, 1995.

Chapter 17

Clinical Breast Examination

Patricia Kelly

PROCEDURE GOALS AND OBJECTIVES

Goal: To perform a thorough breast examination on a female patient in a manner that preserves the patient's modesty while maximizing the likelihood of identifying abnormal findings.

Objectives: The student will be able to ...

- Describe the indications, contraindications, and rationale for performing a breast examination.
- Describe the essential anatomy and physiology associated with the performance of the breast examination.
- Describe the logical order of the steps used to perform the breast examination.
- Describe normal and abnormal findings associated with the breast examination.

BACKGROUND AND HISTORY

The clinical breast examination (CBE) is a universally taught ambulatory care skill. As part of a physical examination, CBE complements but does not replace mammography. The CBE is both a screening and diagnostic procedure. As a screening procedure, its purpose is to detect cancer in asymptomatic women. As a diagnostic procedure, it is part of a comprehensive evaluation for patients with symptoms related to the breasts.

Breast cancer is diagnosed in more than 170,000 women annually in the United States. Established risks for breast cancer include age older than 50 years, family history of breast cancer in first- and second-degree relatives, a younger age at menarche (<12 years), older age at menopause (>55 years), older age at first birth (>30 years) or nulliparity, some types of benign breast disease (particularly atypical hyperplasia), and hormone replacement therapy. Societal, demographic, and medical trends have markedly increased the number of women at risk.

Before the introduction of cancer screening as an integral part of generalized preventive medical services, most breast cancer was discovered by women themselves or as an incidental finding during the evaluation of other complaints. Frequently, breast cancer was advanced at the time of diagnosis. Specific techniques to increase the sensitivity of the examination, therefore, were not generally thought to be important. In its later stages, the alterations caused by breast cancer were evident on physical examination.

Historically, breast cancer has been a fearful entity. Before 1970, the diagnosis of breast cancer called for "automatic" radical mastectomy, a disfiguring procedure with substantial postoperative morbidity. Because many newly diagnosed women had advanced disease, the prognosis was considered poor. Breast cancer also carried with it a social stigma; therefore, it was not widely discussed. Women were frequently not told of female relatives who had succumbed to the disease. Risk factors for the disease had not been clearly described. Most patients, and many physicians, had incomplete or erroneous knowledge concerning the disease. Adjuvant chemotherapy and hormonal therapy were unavailable until the latter half of the 20th century, and breast cancer generally carried with it an aura of hopelessness. Many women died in excruciating agony. The concepts of palliative therapies or hospice care were not well explored until recent decades.

More recently, societal change and medical progress have correctly imbued us with the notion that breast cancer is a relatively common—and treatable—malignancy. Unfortunately and concomitantly, longevity, decreased rates of childbearing, and younger age at menarche have raised the incidence of this illness. Increased public awareness, however, along with growing emphasis on screening techniques such as CBE and mammography, have improved detection efforts.

Although breast cancer is still frequently a systemic disease at the time of diagnosis, therapeutic advances and earlier detection have rendered it, in many or most cases, a "curable" entity. More than 60% of breast cancer victims now survive and succumb to other diseases. Less radical surgical interventions, increased consumer knowledge and empowerment, and "gender shift" in the ranks of clinicians have all undoubtedly played an important role in subduing this disease.

INDICATIONS

The value of CBE is not universally supported. The American Cancer Society recommends CBE every 3 years in women of reproductive age until 40 years of age and annually after that. The U.S. Preventive Services Task Force (2002) states that there is insufficient evidence to recommend for or against the examination. The National Cancer Institute recommends annual screening examinations in women age 40 years or older. Recent studies indicate that screening CBEs discover a small number of cancers that are missed by routine mammography (Elmore, 2005). The effect on disease end-outcome, however, is uncertain.

The following guidelines seem reasonable:

■ CBE is performed on an annual basis for women who are age 40 years or older.

■ Women who have a strong family history of early breast cancer should undergo annual examination at a younger age. Although traditionally performed in all women of reproductive age, whether annual CBE for women younger than age 40 who are at normal risk confers any survival advantage is unclear. The positive predictive value (the chance that an abnormality discovered on examination is malignant) increases with age and with the presence of other risk factors for breast cancer. Barton and coworkers (1999) estimate the specificity and sensitivity of CBE at 54% and 94%, respectively.

■ The current legal standard of care strongly suggests that CBE be combined with screening mammography in women age 40 years or older. Neither procedure alone is sufficient. Masses apparent on physical examination require further evaluation even in the face of negative or normal mammographic findings. Informed consent regarding the potential benefits and limitations of various screening modalities, including CBE, should always be documented in the patient record.

The CBE, when used as a screening procedure, has legal as well as medical importance. Failure to diagnose breast cancer is a leading source of malpractice litigation. Providers who fail to perform or document adequate examinations are at high risk for adverse legal consequences.

CONTRAINDICATIONS

There are no medical contraindications to the performance of this procedure.

POTENTIAL COMPLICATIONS

There are no reported medical complications associated with the performance of this procedure. Legal or practical complications may arise when the examination is omitted or improperly documented, or if adequate informed consent regarding the benefits and limitations of the procedure is not obtained. Since this is a sensitive examination, many providers may wish to have the procedure chaperoned or assisted by another clinician or office staff person. Patient education regarding the breast self-examination, necessity of the examination by a clinician, and the presence of any assistants should be documented in the medical record.

REVIEW OF ESSENTIAL ANATOMY AND PHYSIOLOGY

The average female breast is somewhat "lumpy" to palpation and contains glandular tissue, fibrous tissue, supporting ligaments, and fat. Glandular tissue, intended to produce breast milk, radiates centrally from the nipple. Each glandular lobe terminates in a milk sinus and an excretory duct in the nipple area. The nipple is slightly inferior and lateral to the center of each breast. The skin of the nipple generally extends outward to form the areola. Small sebaceous glands also terminate in the areola. These serve to secrete a protective substance during nursing. Smooth muscles in the subcutaneous tissue under the areola control the erection of the nipple. Small supernumerary nipples, often mistaken for moles, can sometimes be found along the embryological milk lines. These are of no clinical consequence.

Fibrous tissue provides support to the breast, which is connected to the underlying muscle by fascial suspensory structures called Cooper's ligaments. The breasts overlie the pectoral muscles of the chest. Nerves, blood vessels, and lymphatic structures are also contained within the breast. Fatty tissue intermingles with breast tissue in the breast itself. Lymphatic drainage of the breast provides the primary pathway for cancer spread (Fig. 17-1).

The area requiring visual inspection and manual palpation extends inferiorly (vertically) from the clavicle, or second rib, to the seventh rib and laterally from the sternal border to the midaxillary line. The "tail" of the breast extends well into the axilla and must not be omitted during examination. The upper outer quadrant of the breast has the greatest amount of breast tissue and is frequently the site of malignant processes. Peripheral and superficial breast structures are predominantly fatty; deep, central areas contain the greatest percentage of glandular and fibrous tissue. The breasts are usually slightly unequal in size; the left is frequently larger.

The breasts change during maturation and pregnancy and in a cyclic fashion dependent on the menstrual cycle. The glandular breast tissue typically increases in size and tenderness in a pattern conforming to normal hormonal fluctuations. Increased tenderness and engorgement coincide with

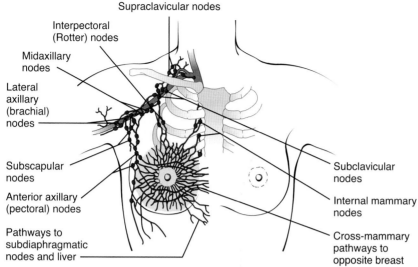

FIGURE 17-1. Lymphatic drainage of the breast. (Redrawn from Seidel HM: Mosby's Guide to Physical Examination, 4th ed. St. Louis, Mosby–Year Book, 1999.)

the immediate premenstrual period and with pregnancy. The premenstrual period, therefore, is not the optimal time for screening CBE.

Women in their reproductive years have "denser" and "lumpier" breasts than postmenopausal women. The latter frequently have some diminution of breast tissue that increases with age. Women who are obese have excess adipose tissue and, hence, larger breasts.

Lactation, or milk production, is influenced by prolactin, which is present secondary to parturition, drug effect, or abnormalities of the pituitary. During nursing, the breasts become markedly engorged.

Abnormalities that are commonly present in the breast may be of the breast tissue itself or of overlying skin. Edema of the skin, characterized by unusually prominent pores (sometimes called peau d'orange because of its orange peel appearance), is an important sign of carcinoma of the breast. Inflammatory breast carcinoma can appear as an eczematous eruption. Erythema can also signify malignancy, although it is more often indicative of infection. Scars may mark the presence of previous biopsies. Retraction or dimpling of skin, although not truly a superficial phenomenon, signifies underlying fibrotic tissue changes that are frequently due to cancer.

Many findings on breast examination are the consequence of stimulating hormones on breast tissue. Both estrogen and progesterone affect breast tissue; progesterone causes more cell division than does estrogen. As previously stated, breast tissue therefore "swells and shrinks" in a relatively predictable fashion during the menstrual cycle. However, sometimes this effect can cause discrete, although benign, abnormalities. Fibroadenomas—characterized by firm, rubbery, nontender, freely movable but solid masses—can be caused by hormonal influences on one component of breast tissue, the stroma. Breast cysts, which are fluid-filled, tender, benign entities, are also largely due to hormonal fluctuations. As such, they are rare (as initial presentations) in postmenopausal women, who are the group at most risk for breast cancer. Although both these benign entities are fairly characteristic on physical examination, further studies, including ultrasonography, mammography, and tissue cytologic studies, are almost always indicated. The diagnostic evaluation of a breast mass is beyond the scope of this chapter.

Other solitary, nontender breast masses that may be mistaken for carcinoma are chronic abscesses and fat necrosis. These, too, generally must be subjected to biopsy for definitive diagnosis.

Inflammatory breast changes (tender, red) can represent acute mastitis, which generally occurs during lactation or pregnancy. If the cause is not evident (i.e., if this occurs in a 65-year-old, nonlactating woman), inflammatory carcinoma must be ruled out. If not promptly treated, mastitis can lead to an acute abscess, which can present as a localized, fluctuant, exquisitely tender mass.

The classic presentation of breast cancer is a hard, irregular, fixed mass. Evidence of metastatic disease is denoted by enlarged, fixed, hard lymph nodes (pectoral, subscapular, or central groups) in the axilla. If the suspending ligaments are involved, dimpling or retraction may occur. Bloody or clear discharge indicates invasion of the milk ducts. Lymphatic obstruction, as previously stated, can produce skin edema.

Standard Precautions   Practitioners should use standard precautions at all times when interacting with patients. Determining the level of precaution necessary requires the practitioner to exercise clinical judgment based on the patient's history and the potential for exposure to body fluids or aerosol-borne pathogens (for further discussion, see Chapter 2).

PATIENT PREPARATION

As discussed later, the duration of CBE is important. It is likely that many patients have never received an adequate examination and might be surprised by the length of time required to perform the examination and its thoroughness.

- The examination should be conducted in a room that is climate controlled and ensures privacy. Cold examination rooms deter clinicians and patients; hot rooms cause patients and providers to perspire, inhibiting optimal technique.

- The patient must be relaxed for an adequate examination, and cloth gowns enhance comfort. Pillows provide comfort while improving positioning.

Materials Utilized to Perform a Breast Examination

Note: The CBE can be considered a low-cost examination in that it uses only the time and expertise of the clinician to screen for disease. Basic equipment is as follows:

- Powder
- Lotion
- Gloves
- Sufficient light
- Pillow

Procedure for Performing a Breast Examination

Note: Recommendations for performance of the CBE are derived predominantly from Barton and colleagues (1999). These researchers thoroughly reviewed the literature and specified components of the examination that have been validated in independent investigations.

    Note: Some clinicians prefer that a female assistant be present for this sensitive examination.

Inspection

Note: Inspection has been traditionally advised but has not been demonstrated to add additional specificity or sensitivity to an examination with palpatory components alone.

1. Inspect the breasts with the patient sitting, hands by her side (Fig. 17-2).

2. Note the condition of the skin: any eczematous changes, "enlarged pores" (peau d'orange), or erythema.

Note: Tangential light may aid this portion of the examination.

FIGURE 17-2. (Redrawn from Seidel HM: Mosby's Guide to Physical Examination, 4th ed. St. Louis, Mosby–Year Book, 1999.)

3. Look for retraction, dimpling, displacement, nipple inversion, or obvious mass defect. Also note scars from previous biopsies.

continued

Note: Since retraction and dimpling are phenomena that result from underlying tissue compression or displacement, the patient may be examined in several different postures. Pressing the hands against the hips contracts the pectoralis muscles (Fig. 17-3); bending at the waist to let the breasts hang free can also be useful (Fig. 17-4).

FIGURE 17-3. (Redrawn from Seidel HM: Mosby's Guide to Physical Examination, 4th ed. St. Louis, Mosby–Year Book, 1999.)

FIGURE 17-4. (Redrawn from Seidel HM: Mosby's Guide to Physical Examination, 4th ed. St. Louis, Mosby–Year Book, 1999.)

Palpation in the Axillary Area

4. Palpate the axillae for enlarged nodes (see Fig. 17-1).

Note: Many clinicians conduct this portion of the examination with the patient in a supine position; others support the sitting patient's arm with one hand and examine the axilla with the other. However, palpating the axillae with the patient lying down facilitates a smooth segue into the remainder of the supine breast examination.

Note: Since the axillary areas are frequently damp, the clinician may want to don gloves for this procedure. After the axillary examination, the gloves should be removed, leaving a powder residue on the hands. This substance, or lotion, may enhance the ease of the palpatory breast examination.

Palpation of the Breast

Note: Palpation is emphasized because inspection, although traditionally included, has not been demonstrated to substantially increase diagnostic yield.

Note: Most authorities advise that palpation is optimally performed on women who are supine. Some classic references on physical examination technique recommend conducting the examination with the patient sitting and supine. This has not proved to increase sensitivity or yield and would be very time consuming if done with sufficient thoroughness.

Note: Women, especially those with larger breasts, can improve examination efficacy by flattening the breast (e.g., by raising the ipsilateral hand, rotating the shoulder externally, placing a pillow behind the back).

Technique

5. With the patient supine, and the hands behind the head, use the finger pads of the middle three fingers of the dominant hand to palpate breast tissue. These fingers are held together; the hand may flex slightly at the knuckles.

Note: If the proximal interphalangeal joints are flexed, the clinician will examine the patient with the fingertips instead of the fingerpads; this is incorrect and must be avoided. The proximal interphalangeal joints and the distal interphalangeal joints should be held in hyperextension for this delicate maneuver (Fig. 17-5).

6. For optimal palpation, "rock" the fingers back and forth in the horizontal and vertical planes, producing an almost circular "rotatory" movement from a central axis located at the fingerpad of the third digit.

Note: The diameter of this rotation, as measured from each fingertip, should be no greater than 1.5 cm. Light, medium, and deep palpation are used sequentially.

7. Never lift the fingerpads completely from the skin, but advance very slightly (≤1 cm) by sliding along the skin, still exerting traction, after each area is thoroughly palpated. Again, maintain palpatory pressure at all times.

Note: In order for this maneuver to be successful, the fingerpads and breast tissue must be either powder "dry" or moistened with lotion. Otherwise, the fingerpads stick to the skin surface and cannot be rotated or advanced smoothly.

   Note: "Walking" fingertips are to be avoided.

Pattern of Palpation

8. Begin palpation laterally at the midaxillary line and extend inferiorly in a straight line until approximately the level of the seventh rib, where the breast tissue stops.

9. Shift the finger pads medially and continue palpation superiorly, again in a straight line, back to the midaxilla or clavicle, depending on how far medially the examination has progressed.

Note: Some examiners palpate the area around the nipple in exactly this same manner; some, however, also traditionally "squeeze" the nipple to check for fluid. The validity of this technique in cancer detection is uncertain.

   Note: This technique, called the *vertical strip pattern,* is analogous to "lawn mowing." Much as in cutting grass, rows need to overlap to avoid skipping areas. The vertical strip pattern has been found to be more thorough and reproducible than the

Figure 17-5. (Redrawn from Seidel HM: Mosby's Guide to Physical Examination, 4th ed. St. Louis, Mosby–Year Book, 1999.)

continued

traditional concentric circumferential technique or the radial spoke method (Fig. 17-6). However, it is certain that any uniformly practiced, sequential technique is better than "random" palpation, which, unfortunately, is the method used by many busy clinicians.

Examination of the breast

Vertical stripping Concentric circles Radial spokes

FIGURE 17-6.

SPECIAL CONSIDERATIONS

Training and practice enhance diagnostic capability. Silicone breast models, demonstrating common benign and malignant abnormalities as well as the consistency of "normal" breast tissue, have demonstrated efficacy when used with lay and professional populations. Although experience with previous abnormalities does enhance the diagnostic efficacy of a provider, the single most important determinant of examination sensitivity is duration of the procedure. The other vital component is a sequential palpation plan with well-defined landmarks, ensuring that no area of breast tissue is inadvertently overlooked. The attention, thoroughness, and diligence of the examiner are more predictive of screening sensitivity than the examiner's specific professional role (physician assistant, nurse, physician), level of training, or previous experience.

FOLLOW-UP CARE AND INSTRUCTIONS

- A breast examination not recorded is a breast examination not performed. The clinician should clearly document the performance and findings of the CBE and the plan of action.

- If referral for further diagnostic or screening studies is warranted or recommended, "tickler" files or computer reminders to ensure and document patient compliance and the results obtained are essential. Written documentation of all patient contacts regarding referral or recommended further diagnostic or screening studies is vital. Patients who do not keep referral appointments should be contacted by telephone and certified mail.

- Patient education concerning the CBE should include information on the sensitivity and specificity of the examination and information about why the duration of the examination is important.

■ Education must also include accurate information concerning breast cancer prevalence.

■ Information concerning current recommendations for other breast cancer screening modalities, such as mammography and breast self-examination, should be provided as well.

■ The patient education provided must be accurately documented in the medical record.

■ Most clinicians include information and education concerning the breast self-examination during the annual CBE. The effect of breast self-examination on breast cancer mortality is uncertain. Self-reported frequency of breast self-examination has never been correlated with improved outcome. Appropriate teaching of technique, however, has been shown to improve the efficacy of breast self-examination in the discovery of smaller, and hence more treatable, masses. Many studies of this practice have provided contradictory results; the evidence is not considered strong enough to make a clear recommendation for or against breast self-examination by many governmental health authorities. Private organizations, however, including the American Cancer Society, recommend this procedure. As a result, women should be instructed in appropriate technique, frequency, and duration of breast self-examination. These examinations, however, should not substitute for CBE.

Many clinicians traditionally included information and education concerning the breast self-examination during the annual CBE. However, breast self-examination has not been demonstrated to decrease breast cancer deaths; it does increase the number of negative invasive diagnostic procedures without providing a corresponding survival benefit. Although some prominent organizations continue to recommend the procedure and it is widely publicized, its risks and lack of demonstrated positive outcomes should be discussed with each patient thoroughly.

REFERENCES

Barton MB, Harris R, Fletcher SW: Does this patient have breast cancer? The screening clinical breast examination: Should it be done? How? JAMA 282:1270-1280, 1999.

Elmore JG, Armstrong K, Lehman CD, Fletcher SW: Screening for breast cancer. JAMA 293:1245-1256, 2005.

U.S. Preventive Services Task Force: Guide to Clinical Preventive Services: Breast Cancer Screening. Rockville, Md., Agency for Healthcare Research and Quality, 2002.

BIBLIOGRAPHY

Armstrong K, Eisen A, Weber B: Primary care: Assessing the risk of breast cancer. N Engl J Med 342:564-571, 2000.

DeGowin RL, Brown DD: DeGowin's Diagnostic Examination, 7th ed. New York, McGraw-Hill, 2000.

Elmore JG, Reisch LM, Barton MB, et al: Efficacy of breast cancer screening in the community according to risk level. J Natl Cancer Inst 97:1035-1042, 2005.

Fletcher SW, Black W, Harris R, et al: Report of the international workshop on screening for breast cancer. J Natl Cancer Inst 85:1644-1656, 1993.

Hortobagyi GN: Drug therapy: Treatment of breast cancer. N Engl J Med 339:974-984, 1998.

National Cancer Institute and American Cancer Society: Joint statement on breast cancer screening for women in their 40s. Press release of March 27, 1997.

Physician Insurers Association of America Breast Cancer Study. Washington, DC, Physician Insurers of America, 1995.

Roy JA, Swaka CA, Prichard KI: Hormone replacement therapy in women with breast cancer: Do the risks outweigh the benefits? J Clin Oncol 14:997-1006, 1996.

Schwartz MH: Textbook of Physical Examination, 3rd ed. Philadelphia, WB Saunders, 1998.

Chapter 18

The Pelvic Examination and Obtaining a Routine Papanicolaou Smear

L. Gail Curtis

PROCEDURE GOALS AND OBJECTIVES

Goal: To perform a thorough pelvic examination (PVE) in a female patient in a manner that preserves the patient's comfort while maximizing the likelihood of identifying abnormal findings and obtaining a sample for a Papanicolaou (Pap) smear.

Objectives: The student will be able to …

- Describe the indications, contraindications, and rationale for performing a PVE.

- Describe the essential anatomy and physiology associated with the performance of a PVE.

- Describe the logical order of the steps used to perform a PVE.

- Describe normal and abnormal findings associated with a PVE.

BACKGROUND AND HISTORY

Many women dislike having a PVE performed. The lithotomy position makes some women feel vulnerable. This examination may invoke feelings of anxiety or embarrassment. It is the examiner's responsibility to put the patient at ease while conveying the importance of the examination. The challenge is to make this experience educational, comfortable, and not to be feared in the future.

The PVE is an extension of the abdominal examination in the female patient. The Pap smear is one aspect of the PVE and was developed in the 1920s by Dr. George Nicolas Papanicolaou, an anatomist and cytologist in the United States. Dr. Papanicolaou identified characteristic cellular changes associated with cervical cancer. The original technology allowed for cytologic evaluation of cervical cells exfoliated from the female genital tract. Approximately 20 years elapsed before the technique named for him, the Papanicolaou smear, was accepted as a cancer screening procedure. The Pap smear was initially used to detect asymptomatic invasive cervical cancer; as time passed, the importance of preinvasive disease was recognized. The Pap smear remains a screening test. It does not provide a diagnosis. Current standard of care requires further workup of any abnormality found on a Pap smear. This work-up typically includes a screening for human papilloma virus (HPV), a colposcopy, and biopsy of cervical samples.

INDICATIONS

Pap smear screening has been documented to decrease the incidence and mortality rate of cervical cancer. In the United States there are approximately 20,000 new cases of cervical cancer per year, with an annual mortality rate of roughly 7600. American women have a 0.83% chance of developing cervical cancer in their lifetime, and death from the disease is estimated at 0.27%. Debate exists on recommended standards for obtaining a Pap smear, such as age to begin screening, how frequently to screen, and at what age to cease screening.

The American Cancer Society (ACS) updated their recommendations in 2002 and the U.S. Preventive Services Task Force (USPSTF) guidelines were updated in 2003. These are summarized and contrasted in Table 18-1.

Factors thought to increase the risk for an abnormal Pap smear can be divided into two broad categories: those related to coitus and those related to nonsexual factors. Coitus-related factors include a young age at first intercourse, multiple sexual partners, sexually transmitted disease, and HPV. Nonsexual factors include tobacco smoking, illicit drug use, diet, oral contraceptive use, a prior history of abnormal Pap smears, poor personal hygiene, and an uncircumcised partner. Though all these factors may play a part, the presence of or exposure to HPV is now accepted as the leading risk factor for an abnormal smear and development of cervical cancer. HPV types 16 and 18 seem to be the most oncogenic. The natural history of how HPV infection progresses to cancer is still poorly understood.

Table 18.1 **Comparison of USPSTF and ACS Guidelines on Screening for Cervical Cancer**		
CRITERIA	USPSTF GUIDELINE	ACS 2002 GUIDELINE
Age to initiate screening	Optimum age unknown; within 3 years of onset of sexual activity or age 21	Three years after the onset of sexual activity; no later than age 21
Screening frequency	At least every 3 years	Annually with conventional cytology or every 2 years with liquid-based cytology. After age 30, women with three consecutive normal tests may be screened every 2 to years.3
Screening after hysterectomy	No cytologic testing after total hysterectomy for benign condition	No cytologic testing after total hysterectomy for benign condition
Discontinuation	After age 65 (see below)	After age 70 (see below)
Routine screening for HPV infection	Insufficient evidence	Not yet FDA approved. If approved, conventional or liquid-based cytology combined with test for DNA from high-risk HPV subtypes should be performed not more often than every 3 years

ACS, American Cancer Society; FDA, U.S. Food and Drug Administration; HPV, human papillomavirus; USPSTF, U.S. Preventive Services Task Force.

From U.S. Preventive Services Task Force: Screening for cervical cancer: Recommendations and rationale. AHRQ Publication No. 03-515A. Rockville, Md, Agency for Healthcare Research and Quality, 2003; and Saslow D, Runowicz CD, Solomon D, et al: American Cancer Society guideline for the early detection of cervical neoplasia and cancer. CA Cancer J Clin 52:342-362, 2002.

CONTRAINDICATIONS

There are no absolute contraindications to performing a routine PVE. Permission to perform the examination should be obtained.

POTENTIAL COMPLICATIONS

False-negative Pap smear results do occur. Common causes of a smear being interpreted as normal when the cervical epithelium is abnormal include the following:

■ Sampling error: due to poor sampling technique or small, peripherally located lesions missed on sampling

■ Lesions that do not shed cells well

■ Interpretation error

The most common cause is sampling error. The error that is most publicized is misinterpretation. Using the proper technique to obtain the Pap smear can significantly decrease the incidence of false-negative results due to sampling error. New technologies have been developed to decrease the false-negative rate from errors in interpretation. Other sources of Pap smear screening

FIGURE 18-1. External anatomy of the vulva.

errors are failure of the clinician to understand or respond appropriately to Pap smear results or failure of the patient to follow the clinician's recommendations.

REVIEW OF ESSENTIAL ANATOMY AND PHYSIOLOGY

EXTERNAL ANATOMY (Fig. 18-1)

The vulva consists of the mons pubis, the labia majora, the labia minora, the clitoris, and the glandular structures that open into the vagina. The shape, size, and color of the various structures vary among individual women and racial groups. Normal hair distribution is in the shape of an inverted triangle centered over the mons pubis.

The labia majora are two mound-shaped structures composed primarily of adipose tissue originating at the mons pubis and terminating in the perineum. They form the lateral boundaries of the vulva. Underlying the skin is a poorly developed muscle layer: the tunica dartos labialis. There are also numerous sweat glands in the labia majora. The internal and external pudendal arteries and a branch of the perineal artery provide the arterial blood supply to the labia majora. The venous drainage is extensive and provided primarily by the perineal, posterior labial, external pudendal, and saphenous veins. Lymphatic drainage occurs through two systems: one superficial and one deep within the subcutaneous tissue primarily draining into the inguinal nodes.

The labia minora are two skin folds medial to the labia majora that begin at the base of the clitoris and extend posteriorly to the introitus. The arterial supply is from the superficial perineal artery. The venous drainage is to the perineal and vaginal veins. Lymphatics pass to the superficial and deep subinguinal nodes. The innervation is supplied from branches of the pudendal nerve, which originates from the perineal nerve.

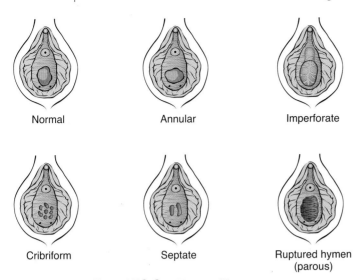

FIGURE 18-2. Types of hymens.

The clitoris is the homologue of the dorsal aspect of the penis. Blood supply is rich, with the dorsal and pudendal arteries supplying arterial blood. Venous drainage consists of a rich plexus draining into the pudendal vein. The lymphatics coincide primarily with those of the labia minora. Innervation to the clitoris is from the terminal branch of the pudendal nerve. Nerve endings in the clitoris vary, from woman to woman, from total absence to a rich supply.

The vestibule is the space bordered by the labia minora and includes the entrance to the vaginal canal or the introitus. The vaginal opening can be obscured by the hymenal ring or hymen. The hymen is a membrane that partially or wholly occludes the introitus. The shape and opening of the hymen can vary greatly (Fig. 18-2), but only a completely imperforate hymen is pathologic. The arterial supply to the vestibule and hymen is from an extensive capillary plexus from the perineal artery. The venous drainage is also extensive and involves the same areas as the arterial network. The lymphatic drainage terminates in the superficial inguinal nodes and the external iliac chain. The urethra is positioned between the clitoris and the vaginal opening and is not difficult to visualize.

Skene's glands are posterior to the urethral orifice and are often difficult to locate. Bartholin's glands lie inferior and lateral to the posterior vestibule, are less superficial, and are usually not visible. The arterial supply and venous drainage is along the pudendal vessels. The lymphatics drain directly via the perineum into the inguinal area. The innervation of Bartholin's glands is a small branch of the perineal nerve.

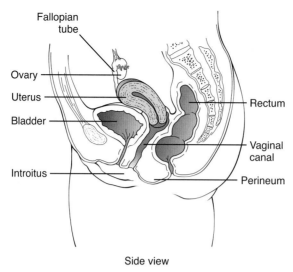

Fallopian tube

Ovary

Uterus

Bladder

Introitus

Rectum

Vaginal canal

Perineum

Side view

FIGURE 18-3. Female internal anatomy.

INTERNAL ANATOMY (Fig. 18-3)

The vagina is a muscular canal that is lined with mucosa or rugae and is approximately 7 cm long, extending from the uterus to the vestibule. It meets the cervix of the uterus at an angle of 45 to 90 degrees. The cervix projects into the upper portion of the anterior vaginal wall, thereby making the anterior vaginal wall slightly shorter than the posterior vaginal wall. The vaginal arterial supply is from the vaginal branch of the uterine artery, and the veins follow the course of the arteries. The lymphatics drain into the external iliac and inguinal nodes. Both sympathetic and parasympathetic nerves innervate the vagina. The perineum is the tissue between the vaginal opening and the anus.

The uterus is a pear-shaped, thick-walled muscular organ about 7 to 8 cm in length and 4 to 5 cm at its widest in the nonpregnant adult woman. It consists of three parts: the fundus, the body, and the cervix (Fig. 18-4). The uterine cavity opens into the vagina below and into the fallopian tubes above. It is supported by ligamentous attachments to various pelvic structures, including the vagina. The cervix is the portion of the uterus that can be visualized during the PVE and is the structure sampled to obtain the Pap smear. When viewed during the PVE, the cervix appears as a round bagel-like mound with a circular or slit-type opening that varies with parity (Fig. 18-5) and leads to the endocervical canal.

The fallopian tubes extend from the lateral portions of the uterine fundus and terminate in a fringed, cone-shaped conduit that arches toward the ovaries (Fig. 18-6). The ovaries are oval organs measuring about 2.5 to 5 cm in length, 1.5 to 3 cm in breadth, and 0.7 to 1.5 cm in width. The fimbriated ends of the fallopian tubes overhang the upper part of each ovary. The

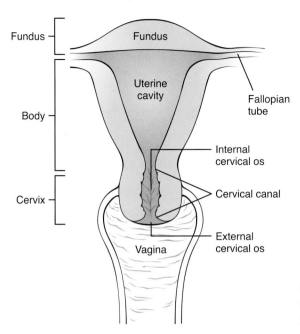

FIGURE 18-4. The uterus consists of three parts: the fundus, body, and cervix.

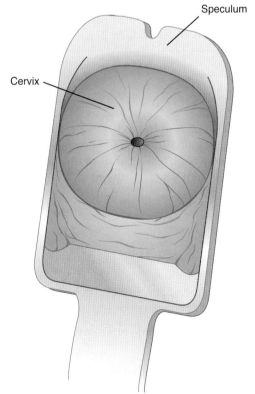

FIGURE 18-5. The cervix as viewed during pelvic examination.

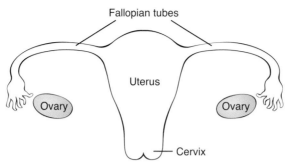

FIGURE 18-6. The fallopian tubes.

ovarian artery is the chief source of blood for the ovary, and the ovarian veins follow the course of the arteries. Lymphatic channels drain retro-peritoneally to the lumbar lymph nodes. The lymphatic channels in the ovaries are extensive and may provide additional fluid to the ovary during periods of preovulatory swelling. The ovaries produce ova and hormones, including estrogen and progesterone.

All the pelvic organs are supported within the lower abdominal cavity by a system of muscles, ligaments, and fascia.

Standard Precautions   Practitioners should use standard precautions at all times when interacting with patients. Determining the level of precaution necessary requires the practitioner to exercise clinical judgment based on the patient's history and the potential for exposure to body fluids or aerosol-borne pathogens (for further discussion, see Chapter 2).

PATIENT PREPARATION

As noted previously, some women may be reluctant to have a PVE performed. If a patient has had several previous examinations, she knows what to expect. If this is her first, she has most likely heard about it from others. Your responsibility as the examiner is to explain what is ahead and provide education in order to decrease anxiety.

FIRST PELVIC EXAMINATION EXPERIENCE

This examination will set the tone for all that follow.
- Schedule enough time to allow a complete explanation of the PVE from beginning to completion.

- It is helpful to have a diagram or model of the female anatomy to aid the explanation.

- Have the actual equipment to be used on hand to show your patient. Explain all aspects of the PVE and the Pap smear.

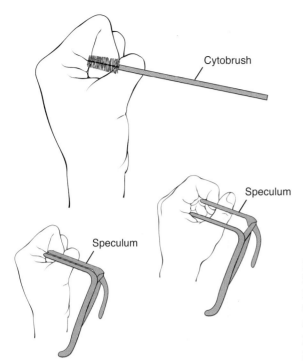

Cytobrush

Speculum

Speculum

FIGURE 18-7. **Top,** Closed fist, simulating the cervix. **Bottom,** Closed fist simulating the vaginal opening for speculum insertion in tensed position **(left)** and relaxed position **(right).**

- Show your patient, using your closed fist to simulate the cervix, how you will sample her cervical cells (Fig. 18-7). Explain that relaxing her pelvic muscles eases the insertion of the speculum (again, demonstrate with your fist; see Fig. 18-7).

- Allow and encourage your patient to ask questions.

- Explain terms she may have heard and been fearful about such as: "blades," "scraping," and "stirrups."

- Educate her about the lithotomy position: why it is necessary, including how it allows visualization of the cervix.

- Offer opportunities that empower the patient, such as the semi-sitting position and a hand-held mirror if she desires to observe the examination and visualize her own anatomy while the examination is in progress.

- Assure your patient that this examination is indicated and that the PVE should not be painful. Tell her you will be gentle and that if she wants you to stop at any time during the examination, you will.

THE RETURNING PATIENT

- Always ask the patient if she has any particular concerns about this examination.

Plastic   Graves   Pedersen

FIGURE 18-8.   Types of vaginal speculums.

- Reassure her that you will be gentle and that there should be no pain associated with the PVE.
- Assure her that she can ask questions at any time during the examination.
- Tell her that if she should experience any discomfort to alert you immediately and you will stop and redirect your attempt.
- Explain every step of the examination as it unfolds.

CHAPERONE IN ATTENDANCE FOR ALL PATIENTS

Having a chaperone in attendance is important for this examination. This is advised even if the provider is female. In addition to providing assistance with the examination, the presence of another member of the staff helps reduce the likelihood of a patient filing an unfounded accusation regarding inappropriate conduct of the clinician during the examination. Explain that the chaperone is in attendance to assist with any needs during the examination. Avoid statements such as "he (or she) is here to watch and observe."

Materials Utilized for Performing the Pelvic Examination and Obtaining Cells for a Routine Pap Smear

The Vaginal Speculum (Fig. 18-8)
Several types of speculums are available:
- Pedersen speculum, metal and reusable: This type of speculum comes in short and long sizes. It should be used if at all possible because it has a narrow blade and is more comfortable for most women.

- Graves speculum, metal and reusable: This speculum also comes in short and long sizes. The Graves has a "duckbill-shaped" blade and is a better choice for viewing the cervix if the patient is significantly overweight, has a lot of redundant skin surrounding the introitus, or has a severely retroverted uterus.

- Disposable speculum: This type of speculum is made of hard, clear plastic, usually has the Graves-type blades, and makes a loud click when locked into place. Warn patients about the upcoming click, and use great care not to pinch the patient's surrounding skin on insertion.

- Pediatric speculum: This speculum is useful for children and virginal or geriatric women. This speculum is also preferable when explaining a first PVE to a patient. Its small size reduces undue anxiety and fear of pain about the pending examination.

Note: It is all right to switch speculums during the examination if there is trouble viewing the cervix. Avoid comments such as "I have to get a bigger speculum." Women may feel sensitive to implications that their anatomy is too large. Rather state, "I am having difficulty visualizing your cervix and I don't want you to experience any discomfort, so I am going to change speculums to make this examination more comfortable for you."

Whichever speculum is chosen, be sure that you understand how to open it, insert it, and lock it into place before you begin.

Other equipment needed to complete the examination may include the following:

- Cytobrush (Fig. 18-9)

- Wooden spatula (see Fig. 18-9)

- Plastic broom (see Fig. 18-9)

- Pap smear slide or vial of preservative solution

- Good light source

- Water-soluble lubricating jelly

- Latex gloves

Note: The choice of a wooden spatula, a cytobrush, or a plastic broom to collect samples is dictated by the sampling system that is available. The spatula or cytobrush is typically used with fixation of the specimen on a slide. The plastic broom is preferred for liquid-based preparation of the specimen.

Cytobrush   Wooden spatulas   Plastic broom

FIGURE 18-9. Instruments used for gathering cervical cells.

Procedure for the Pelvic Examination and Obtaining Cervical Cells

Note: The examination itself is divided into three parts: inspection of the external genitalia; the internal examination, which includes obtaining the Pap smear; and the bimanual examination.

1. Before beginning the examination, have all your equipment ready and your chaperone in the room.

2. Extend the foot stirrups. Keep in mind the stirrups are often cold and uncomfortable. If possible, have the stirrups covered with a soft, warm material or allow the patient to keep her socks on. When prepared, ask the patient to lie back in the lithotomy position (hips flexed and abducted, feet in stirrups and buttocks slightly beyond the edge of the examining table). Place a sheet as a drape over her. Most women will indicate if they prefer to be fully draped with the sheet to their knees blocking their view of the examination or if they prefer to be able to see you throughout the examination.

Note: Although most examiners have patients lay flat on the examining table, some women prefer to be in a semi-sitting position (Fig. 18-10). The semi-sitting position works just as well for the examiner and makes some women feel more comfortable.

Be prepared to explain each step to the patient as it is being performed. Encourage her to ask any questions she may have. Continue to talk to her, and monitor her status throughout the examination. If she

FIGURE 18-10.

tenses her abdomen or buttocks, ask her to relax them. Once the patient is as comfortable as possible, the examination of the external genitalia should begin.

External Examination

3. Put on gloves and be seated comfortably on a rolling stool at the table end, adjust the light source, and begin inspecting the external genitalia.

4. First examine the mons pubis, labia, and perineum. Note the pubic hair for its pattern, for any lice or nits, infected hair follicles, or any other abnormality, and then inspect for any lesions, erythema, swelling, nodules, or discharge on the skin.

5. Expose the clitoris, urethral orifice, and the vaginal opening by gently retracting the labia minora. Inspect for any cysts or other lesions. Inspect the area of Bartholin's glands. Normal Bartholin's glands cannot be seen or felt.

6. If enlargement or redness is noted, or if indicated by symptoms, examine Bartholin's glands by inserting your index finger into the vagina and your thumb outside (Fig. 18-11), and palpate

Figure 18-11.

the tissue between the internal and external fingers. Check for any discharge from the duct. If discharge is noted, a culture should be obtained using the appropriate medium.

7. Next, ask your patient to perform the Valsalva maneuver or bear down while you check for cystocele, rectocele, or uterine prolapse.

Note: Take care during the external examination to avoid unnecessary contact with the clitoris.

Internal Examination

8. Warm the previously selected vaginal speculum under running water. Water warms the instrument and acts as a lubricant to ease insertion. Other lubricants cannot be used because they may interfere with the cytologic studies.

9. A digital examination performed by inserting a finger into the vaginal canal helps locate the cervix (it has a consistency similar to the end of the nose). Insertion of the speculum can then be directed toward the cervix for easy visualization and comfort of the patient. This technique eliminates the need to "search" for the cervix with the speculum, a maneuver which can be uncomfortable for the patient.

10. To insert the speculum, withdraw your internal finger while applying gentle pressure to the perineum in a downward motion. Ask the patient to relax this muscle as you press downward. Insert the speculum over your withdrawing finger with the blades closed and at a 45-degree angle (Fig. 18-12A).

continued

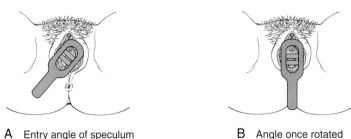

A Entry angle of speculum

B Angle once rotated

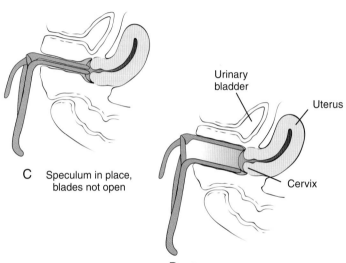

Urinary
bladder

Uterus

C Speculum in place,
blades not open

Cervix

D Speculum in place, blades open.
Ready for Pap smear

Figure 18-12.

11. Once the blades are fully inserted, rotate the speculum to the appropriate angle and open blades to allow visualization of the cervix (see Fig. 18-12B). Avoid pressure on the more sensitive anterior wall, urethral orifice, or clitoris.

12. If there is still a problem locating the cervix, withdraw the speculum and reposition it (usually more posteriorly). Apply gentle pressure to the posterior vaginal wall and try again.

13. Avoid excessive movements of the speculum while searching for the cervix, as this can be uncomfortable.

14. Once the cervix is visualized, lock the speculum in place. Your hands are now free to obtain the Pap smear sample and any other needed cultures or samples.

15. Collecting the Pap smear sample—spatula: A wooden spatula can be used to obtain cells from the cervix and the vaginal wall (Fig. 18-13).

- Use the pointed or longer end of the spatula and insert it into the external cervical os.

- Apply mild pressure while turning the spatula 360 degrees to obtain cells from the squamous-columnar junction or the transformation zone.

- Use the opposite, rounded end of the spatula to sample cells from the vaginal wall.

- Apply the obtained cells to a slide by gently dragging the spatula with the

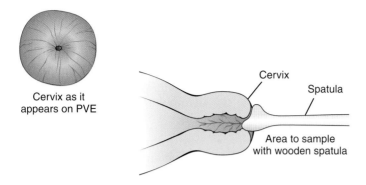

Cervix as it
appears on PVE

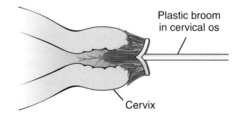

FIGURE 18-13.

samples from the external cervix and the vaginal wall down the slide.

16. Collecting the Pap smear sample—cytobrush: The cytobrush (see Fig. 18-13) is used to obtain cells from the endocervical canal.

- Insert this brush into the cervical os until the bristles are no longer seen and turn two full revolutions.

Note: Always warn the patient that this may induce uterine cramping and mild bleeding.

- Immediately place obtained cells on a slide by rotating the brush counterclockwise while moving the brush from left to right on the slide (Fig. 18-14).

17. Collecting the Pap smear sample—plastic broom:

continued

Side 1

Side 2

FIGURE 18-14.

- Insert the long central bristles into the os until the lateral bristles bend against the ectocervix. Rotate the broom three to five times in both directions.

- Transfer the material onto a slide with a stroke of both sides of the broom placing the second stroke exactly over the first.

- Or if using a vial of preservative solution, place the entire broom tip into the solution and stir vigorously to transfer material. Then remove tip and discard broom, or leave in solution based on lab preference.

18. Transfer cells collected from the Pap smear quickly to the appropriate transport medium:

- The object is to quickly but evenly spread the cellular material in a monolayer on the slide or into the vial of preservative solution.

- When using a slide, thin out large clumps of material as much as possible, while avoiding excessive manipulation, which can damage cells.

- Transfer material from both sampling instruments to the slide within a few seconds.

- Immediately fix the specimen by either immersing the slide in 95% ethanol or coating the slide with a surface fixative.

- Label the Pap smear slide or vial of preservative solution with the patient's name.

Be sure to obtain an adequate sample to avoid having to repeat the examination and to reduce the false-negative rate. In a woman with a uterus, endocervical cells must be obtained. If the cytologic report comes back stating "no endocervical cells seen," inadequate sampling is indicated, and the patient will need to have the examination repeated in order to obtain the adequate sample. Therefore, it is important to sample adequately the first time.

Note: If a wet mount or cultures are to be obtained, do so only after the Pap smear cells have been obtained.

19. After collecting the sample or samples, unlock the speculum and slowly withdraw the instrument while inspecting the vaginal wall for any abnormalities. Allow the speculum blades to close naturally as they are withdrawn.

20. Once the speculum is removed and the samples are preserved, proceed to the bimanual examination.

Bimanual Examination

21. Inform the patient that you are going to examine her uterus and ovaries. Tell her this includes a digital rectal examination.

Note: Lubricating jelly can be used during this portion of the examination, as the cytologic samples have been procured. This lubricant makes this portion of the PVE more comfortable for your patient.

22. Insert two lubricated fingers into the vagina while applying pressure to the abdomen in a sweeping motion toward the mons pubis.

23. Push upward on the cervix with your internal fingers while pushing downward on the uterine area of the abdomen with the external hand. Palpate the uterine fundus as it rises toward your external fingers.

24. Then palpate the ovaries by moving the internal fingers to the right and left of the cervix while sweeping down on either side of the uterus with the external hand.

Note: Ovaries should be palpable in women until menopause. A palpable ovary in a postmenopausal woman needs further workup. Most women can tell when you palpate their ovaries and can offer feedback.

25. The rectovaginal examination is the final step in the PVE. Insert your index finger in the vagina and your middle finger in the rectum and repeat the maneuvers of the bimanual examination.

Note: This approach allows assessment of the retroverted uterus and the region behind the cervix.

26. The examination is complete. Remind your patient to push back on the table before trying to sit up. Provide your patient with a towelette to remove any excess lubricant used during the examination.

SPECIAL CONSIDERATIONS

Pediatric genital examinations, when necessary, often can be performed using the "frog leg" position (Fig. 18-15). Special attention must be given to semantics and patient education when examining children. Keep in mind that most children have been taught not to allow anyone to touch their genitals.

In the geriatric population, frequency of PVE can often be decreased. Any posthysterectomy patient can receive less frequent examinations, varying from every 3 to 5 years. Some practitioners cease doing examinations altogether unless circumstance dictates. If the ovaries are still present, bimanual examination can still be important. Postmenopausal women often have dryer atrophic vaginas. This can make the PVE uncomfortable or painful. Care should be taken to use the smallest possible speculum and not tear the thin tissue.

Figure 18-15.   Pediatric "frog leg" position.

FOLLOW-UP CARE AND INSTRUCTIONS

- Inform the patient of the results of the examination, taking care not to imply that everything is completely normal until all test results are received.

- Educate her about when to return for her next screening examination. If anything was noted on examination, explain the possibilities and what follow-up may be necessary.

- Let her know what correspondence to expect from your office and the time period within which to expect it. Specifically tell her how she will receive her Pap smear results (e.g., letter, phone call, report).

- Ask her to call the office requesting her results if she has not heard anything within the specified period.

- Patient education handouts explaining Pap smear results are helpful and should be sent home with the patient. These handouts may increase the patient's understanding of Pap smears and increase compliance with the recommendations made based on the Pap smear results.

The PVE and the Pap smear are important parts of providing comprehensive well-woman care. Patient education and examiner sensitivity and competence increase compliance of the female patient in regard to this life-saving examination. For all examiners, competence and sensitivity toward the patient help make this examination repeatable for the patient and the next provider.

INTERPRETATION OF THE PAP SMEAR

Prior to the development of the Bethesda system, pap smears were divided and reported in 5 classes (see Table 18-2). The utilization of pap smear classes is now antiquated because:

- Do not reflect current understanding of pathology

- Classes not transferable to histology terms

- No classes for non-cancerous entities

- No longer uniform

- Years of experience have demonstrated a lack of reproducibility

The Bethesda system developed in 2001 incorporates important changes over older systems:

- Pap smear analysis considered a medical consult

- Pathologist responsible for diagnosis

- Referring physician provides history

- Must have a statement of adequacy

Recommendations regarding follow-up should be made by a pathologist.
   The Bethesda system is now used to interpret Pap smear findings. This system includes information on the following:

- Whether the Pap smear is an adequate sample

- Incidental findings such as evidence of infection

- Evidence of lesions: low-grade squamous intraepithelial lesion (SIL), high-grade SIL, or cancer

Providers performing the PVE and obtaining Pap smears must understand how to interpret the results to avoid errors in interpretation from failure of

Table 18.2	**Previous Systems and the Bethesda System**	
PAP CLASS	DESCRIPTION	BETHESDA 2001
I	Normal	Normal and variants
II	Reactive changes	Reactive changes
	Atypia	ASC, ASG
	Koilocytosis	Low-grade SIL
III CIN I	Mild dysplasia	Low-grade SIL
III CIN II	Moderate dysplasia	High-grade SIL
III CIN III	Severe dysplasia	High-grade SIL
IV	Carcinoma in situ, suspicious	High-grade SIL
V	Invasive	Microinvasion (<3mm)
		Frankly invasive (>3mm)

ASC, atypical squamous cells; ASG, atypical glandular cells; CIN, cervical intraepithelial neoplasia; SIL, squamous intraepithelial lesion.

Table 18.3 **New Bethesda System Classification Terms**

LOW-GRADE SQUAMOUS INTRAEPITHELIAL LESION
Cellular change associated with HPV
Mild (slight) dysplasia/CIN I

HIGH-GRADE SQUAMOUS INTRAEPITHELIAL LESION (HSIL)
Moderate dysplasia/CIN II
Severe dysplasia/CIN III
Carcinoma in situ/CIN III

ATYPICAL SQUAMOUS CELLS (ASC)
Unspecified (ASC-US)—includes unspecified and favor benign/inflammation
Cannot exclude HSIL (ASC-H)

ATYPICAL GLANDULAR CELLS OF UNCERTAIN SIGNIFICANCE (AGC-US)
AGC is broken down into favoring endocervical, endometrial, or not otherwise specified origin
  or endocervical adenocarcinoma in situ
Unspecified (AGC-US) (ASC-US)
Atypical glandular cells, favor neoplastic (AGC-H)

CIN, cervical intraepithelial neoplasia.

the clinician to understand or respond appropriately to Pap smear results (Tables 18-2 and 18-3). In October of 2005, the Institute for Clinical Systems Improvement provided a summary of changes for management of the abnormal pap smear. Algorithms delineate proper management for abnormal results and include management for benign endomatrial cells (BEC), ASC-US, and new LSIL management in special populations. These may be reviewed at the National Guidelines Clearing house web site (www.guideline.gov/summary/summary.ASPX?doc_ID=8327; Accessed 7/17/06).

REFERENCES

Saslow D, Runowicz CD, Solomon D, et al: American Cancer Society guidelines for the early detection of cervical neoplasia and cancer. CA Cancer J Clin 52:342-362, 2002.

U.S. Preventive Services Task Force: Screening for cervical cancer: Recommendations and rationale. AHRQ Publication No 03-515A. Rockville, Md, Agency for Healthcare Research and Quality, 2003.

BIBLIOGRAPHY

Agency for Health Care Policy and Research: Evidence Report/Technology Assessment. Rockville, Md, U.S. Department of Health and Human Services, Agency for Health Care Policy and Research, Jan 1, 1999.

Anderson JE: Grant's Atlas of Anatomy, 7th ed. Baltimore, Md, Williams & Wilkins, 1978.

Curtis P, Skinner B, Varenholt JJ, et al: Papanicolaou smear quality assurance: Providing feedback to physicians. J Fam Pract 36:309, 1993.

Eddy DM: Screening for cervical cancer. Ann Intern Med 113:214, 1990.

Goroll AH: Primary Care Medicine, 3rd ed. Philadelphia, Lippincott-Raven, 1995.

Lundber GD: The 1988 Bethesda system for reporting cervical/vaginal cytological diagnoses. JAMA 262:931, l989.

Optimizing the Papanicolaou Smear; accessed August 28, 2005. Available at: http://www.sh.lsuhsc.edu/fammed/OutpatientManual/PapSmear.htm

National Guideline Clearing house: Management of initial abnormal pap smear; accessed July 17, 2006. Available at: http://www.guideline.gov/summary/summary,aspx?doc_id=8327

Pfenninger JL, Fowler GC: Procedures for Primary Care Physicians. St. Louis, Mosby–Year Book, 1994.

Richart RM, Wright TC Jr: Controversies in the management of low-grade cervical intraepithelial neoplasia. Cancer 71:1413, 1993.

Ryan KJ, Berkowitz RS: Kistner's Gynecology and Women's Health, 7th ed. St. Louis, CV Mosby, 1999.

Wingo PA, Tong T, Bolden S: Cancer statistics, 1995. CA Cancer J Clin 45:8, 1995.

Chapter 19

Examination of the Male Genitalia

Richard Dehn

PROCEDURE GOALS AND OBJECTIVES

Goal: To perform a thorough examination of the male genitalia in a manner that preserves the patient's modesty while maximizing the likelihood of identifying abnormal findings.

Objectives: The student will be able to …

- Describe the indications, contraindications, and rationale for performing an examination of the male genitalia.

- Describe the essential anatomy and physiology associated with the performance of the examination of the male genitalia.

- Describe the logical order of the steps used to perform the examination of the male genitalia.

- Describe normal and abnormal findings associated with the examination of the male genitalia.

BACKGROUND AND HISTORY

Examination of the male genitalia is taught to practitioners as part of the physical examination and should be performed on all patients for whom information derived from the examination would be helpful. Although this examination has long been performed for diagnostic purposes, it has gained increasing importance as a screening examination for testicular cancer, prostatic cancer, and colon cancer.

The examination of the male genitalia typically is understood to include the physical examination of the external genitalia, which includes the perineum, penis, and scrotum, as well as a rectal examination in which the prostate is palpated. In addition, the examination often includes an assessment of the presence of an inguinal hernia.

The examination of the penis and scrotum also can have value for early disease detection, particularly if performed by the patient regularly as a self-examination regimen. Self-examination of the penis and urethra can be useful for the early detection of sexually transmitted diseases, and testicular self-examination can lead to early detection of testicular tumors. In young men, testicular tumors are often malignant and aggressive; thus, early detection is a significant factor in increasing survival rates, because testicular cancer is the most common malignancy in men 20 to 40 years of age (Kelly, 1998).

The rectal examination and associated prostate examination have also been used for screening directed at the early detection of cancer. A sample of stool is easily obtained during the rectal examination, and the presence of occult blood is correlated with colon cancers. Screening for stool occult blood has been demonstrated to reduce colon cancer mortality, especially in individuals older than 50 years of age, at which time the incidence of colon cancer greatly increases (Walsh, 2003). The incidence of prostate cancer also increases beginning at age 50. Prostate cancer is often discovered by digital rectal examination, although the value of digital rectal examination for detecting cancer before it has spread beyond the prostatic capsule is questionable (Woolf, 1995). Additionally, most examiners can palpate only part of the posterior prostatic surface when performing digital rectal examination; thus, this process does not detect all prostatic lesions.

INDICATIONS

The examination of the male genitalia is indicated in the following circumstances:

- For routine preventive screening for testicular cancer

- For routine preventive screening for prostate cancer

- For routine preventive screening for colon cancer

- To derive information concerning the male genital system

- To derive information concerning the male reproductive system

CONTRAINDICATIONS

There is no contraindication to performing an examination of the external genitalia. Palpation of the prostate is relatively contraindicated in patients suspected of having acute bacterial prostatitis, because this maneuver can result in septicemia (Dehn, 2001).

POTENTIAL COMPLICATIONS

Complications of the male genital examination include the following:
- Temporary discomfort from palpation of the penis and contents of the scrotum
- Rectal abrasions and fissures from the following:
  - Inadequate digit lubrication
  - Failure to allow the anal sphincter to relax adequately
  - Rectal masses or strictures
- Septicemia from prostatic manipulation if the patient has acute bacterial prostatitis

REVIEW OF ESSENTIAL ANATOMY AND PHYSIOLOGY

Examination of the male genitalia involves structures of the male reproductive system, the lower urinary tract, and the lower gastrointestinal tract (Fig. 19-1).

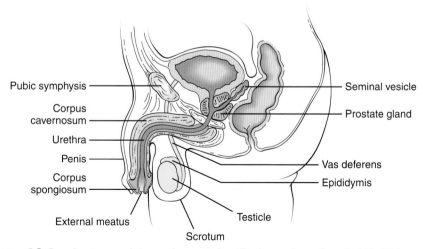

FIGURE 19-1.   Anatomy of the male genitalia. (Redrawn from Swartz MS: Male genitalia and hernias. In Swartz MS: Textbook of Physical Diagnosis, 3rd ed. Philadelphia, WB Saunders, 1998, p 391.)

The structures that are accessible by examination include the penis and internal penile structures, the scrotum, and the contents of the scrotal sac. The posterior surface of the prostate is palpable during a digital rectal examination. The anatomy of the rectum is illustrated in Figure 30-1.

The penis includes structures of both the reproductive system and the lower urinary system. The distal opening of the urethra is located at the glans penis. The urethra travels the corpus spongiosum the length of the penis, passing through the prostate gland to the bladder. The urethra serves as the conduit for both urination and ejaculation from the junction with the ejaculatory duct in the prostate distally. The two corpus cavernosa are located on the dorsum and sides of the penis and expand to produce penile erections when engorged with blood. The skin of the penis is thin and loose to accommodate the changes in size.

The scrotal sac contains the testicles, the epididymis, and the vas deferens. The testicles produce testosterone. Spermatozoa, also produced by the testicles, are transported by the vas deferens to the seminal vesicle at the point where it forms the ejaculatory duct, which then traverses the prostate. The vas deferens, testicular arteries, testicular veins, and associated nerves form the spermatic cord, which traverses the inguinal canal.

Examination of the male genitalia also identifies the presence of inguinal hernias. The inguinal canal, the remnants of where the scrotal sac contents passed through the abdominal wall at about the twelfth week of gestation, can present a point of weakness in the abdominal wall. Points of weakness of the abdominal wall include the internal and external rings of the inguinal canal. Occasionally, abdominal contents enter the inguinal canal and can present a strangulation risk. An indirect hernia traverses the inguinal canal from the internal ring to the external ring, sometimes resulting in abdominal contents in the scrotum. A direct hernia traverses the abdominal wall directly through the external ring.

PATIENT PREPARATION

- Because the examination of the male genitalia can be embarrassing to the patient, be sure to have the examination take place in an environment where privacy is established and maintained.

- Plan so that enough time can be taken not to rush the examination.

- Take the time to explain carefully to the patient what the examination involves and make sure the patient understands.

- Ask the patient to remove all clothing, at least from the waist down.

- Provide a hospital gown to ensure protection of the patient's modesty.

Materials Utilized for Performing an Examination of the Male Genitalia

The following materials should be assembled before initiating an examination of the male genitalia:

- Draping sheet and hospital gown (as noted in "Patient Preparation")

- An examination table for the patient to support himself during the rectal examination

- Unsterile gloves

- Water-soluble lubricant

- Sample collection apparatus and Hemoccult (diagnostic aid for occult blood) collection cards if needed

- A flashlight or penlight for transillumination

- Facial tissues

Note: Depending on the patient's presenting symptoms and clinical circumstances, samples may be needed for laboratory analysis. The urethra may be sampled with a urethral brush, and the skin and rectal mucosa may be swabbed with cotton applicators. Prostatic secretions may be collected on a microscope slide for cell analysis or collected for culture. Materials for appropriately collecting and transporting the necessary samples should be assembled before starting the examination, if possible.

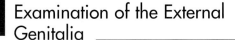

Performing the Procedure of Examining the Male Genitalia

Examination of the External Genitalia

1. Ask the patient to stand. If support is necessary, have the patient stand next to the examining table and use it for support.

2. Sit on an examination stool in front of the patient at approximate eye level with the patient's genitalia.

Note: If the patient is unable to stand, the examination can be performed with the patient in the supine position.

3. Put on unsterile examination gloves.

4. Expose the patient's genitalia fully.

5. Inspect the external genitalia, including the surrounding skin, penis, and scrotum. Note the hair distribution, the quality of the skin, the structures of the penis, and the structures of the scrotum. Also note any urethral discharge, lesions of the skin and hair, and structural deviations of the penis and scrotum, which should be investigated.

Note: If the patient is uncircumcised, the foreskin should be carefully pulled back for inspection and then returned to its original position when inspection is completed.

continued

Figure 19-2. Palpation of the internal structures of the scrotal sac. (Redrawn from Seidel HM, Benedict GW, Ball JW, et al: Male genitalia. In Mosby's Guide to Physical Examination, 4th ed. St. Louis, Mosby, 1999, p 654.)

Some patients prefer to do the foreskin manipulation themselves.

6. Palpate the meatus, penile shaft, and scrotum for abnormal structures and tenderness.

7. Palpate the internal structures of each side of the scrotal sac for masses and tenderness (Fig. 19-2).

8. Palpate symmetrical structures such as the testicles, epididymis, and vas deferens.

9. Insert the index finger into each external inguinal ring, then ask the patient to turn his head to the side and cough (turning the head avoids coughing on the examiner). If a hernia is present, it should be felt at this time.

10. Cover the patient's external genitalia area with the gown or drape.

Examination of the Rectum and Prostate

1. Ask the patient to flex forward at the waist, supporting his upper body with the examination table. Instruct the patient to spread his legs shoulder width apart and to place most of his weight on his upper extremities, which are supported by leaning on the examination table.

2. Sit on a stool facing the patient's rectal area.

Note: If the patient is unable to stand, the examination can be performed in the knee-to-chest position or the left lateral decubitus position with the hips and knees flexed.

3. Put on unsterile examination gloves if the gloves that were used for the first part of the examination were removed.

4. Inspect the area of the anus and surrounding structures. Note hair distribution and skin characteristics in the perineum and perianal region, and any lesions and areas of abnormal coloration.

5. Inspect the anus for lesions, fissures, hemorrhoids, and deviations from normal structure. Spread the patient's buttocks apart to facilitate the inspection process.

Note: Clock numbers define the geography of the anus, with the sacral surface located at 12 o'clock. Findings from the examination should use this convention in descriptions and documentation.

6. Liberally lubricate the gloved index finger of the dominant hand.

7. Gently press the lubricated gloved index finger into the anal opening.

8. Instruct the patient to bear down in a manner similar to having a bowel movement to facilitate the relaxation of the rectal sphincter.

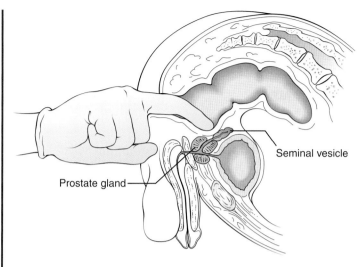

Prostate gland

Seminal vesicle

FIGURE 19-3. Palpation of the anterior rectum and examination of the surface of the prostate. (Redrawn from Seidel HM, Benedict GW, Ball JW, et al: Anus, rectum, and prostate. In Mosby's Guide to Physical Examination, 4th ed. St. Louis, CV Mosby, 1999, p 678.)

9. When the anal sphincter feels relaxed, gently advance your index finger into the anal canal.

10. Ask the patient to tighten the sphincter around the index finger; the muscle tone should be evaluated in this manner.

11. Rotate your finger using 360-degree motions, and use the pad of the distal finger to palpate for defects in the mucosa. Palpate the entire surface of the anal canal in this fashion by repeating the rotation at progressively deeper finger depths.

12. Advance the examining digit as far as is comfortably possible and palpate the anterior rectum to examine the posterior surface of the prostate (Fig. 19-3).

Note: Firm but gentle palpation should allow determination of the size, shape, consistency, mobility, and tenderness of the prostate.

   Note: Palpation of the prostate may cause prostatic secretions to exit the urethra. If clinically indicated, these should be collected for laboratory analysis.

13. Slowly and carefully withdraw your finger.

14. Transfer residual stool on the examination glove to testing medium for occult blood if indicated.

15. Wipe the external anal area clean of lubricating jelly.

16. Provide the patient with toilet paper or tissue to clean the lubricating jelly from his anal area, redrape the patient, and give him privacy to clean up and get dressed.

SPECIAL CONSIDERATIONS

■ Patients presenting with anatomy that deviates from normal because of past trauma, congenital defects, or past disease may be difficult to examine.

- Examination of young children requires patience and gentle technique.

- Rectal examinations and hernia examinations in children should be performed with the examiner's smallest digit.

FOLLOW-UP CARE AND INSTRUCTIONS

- Inform the patient before and during the examination that self-examination of the scrotal sac is useful for the early detection of testicular cancer.

- Instruct the patient in the technique for self-examination during the examination in a way that the patient would be able to perform self-examination in the future. The patient should be encouraged to establish a self-examination routine on a monthly basis.

- It is uncommon for the examination of the male genitalia to cause adverse effects. However, after the examination, instruct the patient to report any rectal tenderness, rectal bleeding, back pain, scrotal masses or tenderness, dysuria, pyuria, hematuria, hematospermia, fever, penile discomfort, or penile lesions.

REFERENCES

Dehn R: Prostatitis. In Moser RL (ed): Primary Care for Physician Assistants, 2nd ed. New York, McGraw-Hill, 2001, pp 712-713.
Kelly P: Testicular cancer. In Moser RL (ed): Primary Care for Physician Assistants, 2nd ed. New York, McGraw-Hill, 2001, pp 523-525.
Walsh JM, Terdiman JP: Colorectal cancer screening: Scientific review. JAMA 289:1288-1296, 2003.
Woolf SH: Screening for prostatic cancer with prostate-specific antigen. N Engl J Med 333:1401-1405, 1995.

BIBLIOGRAPHY

Seidel HM, Ball JW, Dains JE, Benedict GW: Male genitalia; Anus, rectum, and prostate. In Mosby's Guide to Physical Examination, 5th ed. St. Louis, Mosby, 2003, pp 648-693.
Swartz MS: Male genitalia and hernias. In Swartz MS: Textbook of Physical Diagnosis: History and Examination, 5th ed. Philadelphia, WB Saunders, 2006, pp 520-556.

Chapter 20

Joint and Bursal Aspiration

M. F. Winegardner

PROCEDURE GOALS AND OBJECTIVES

Goal: The goal of this procedure is to aspirate a knee joint or olecranon bursa successfully while observing standard precautions and with the minimal degree of risk to the patient.

Objectives: The student will be able to …

- Describe the indications, contraindications, and rationale for performing knee joint or olecranon bursa aspiration.

- Identify and describe common complications associated with knee joint or olecranon bursa aspiration.

- Describe the essential anatomy and physiology associated with the performance of a knee joint or olecranon bursa aspiration.

- Identify the materials necessary for performing a knee joint or olecranon bursa aspiration and their proper use.

- Identify the important aspects of post-procedure care after a knee joint or olecranon bursa aspiration.

BACKGROUND AND HISTORY

Joint aspiration offers both diagnostic and therapeutic benefits when managing joint effusion or inflammation. Diagnostically, the procedure permits acquisition of synovial fluid for analysis. Therapeutically, joint aspiration in the face of painful effusion relieves the patient's discomfort and may facilitate a more accurate joint examination. The same technique can be used for the administration of intra-articular medications. Aspiration of bursal distention relieves discomfort and restriction of motion and decreases the risk of chronicity, spontaneous drainage, or infection within the stagnant bursal fluid (Greene, 2001).

Despite the benefits, joint aspiration is an invasive procedure with the potential for grave injury if not carried out under strict sterile conditions. The procedure always necessitates careful, sterile preparation and sterile technique.

Each joint has specific anatomic landmarks by which the joint space is outlined and the needle can be placed for aspiration. In addition to reliance on anatomic landmarks, musculoskeletal ultrasound increasingly is used to guide needle placement (Grassi, 2004). The general steps in a joint aspiration procedure are the same, regardless of the joint. For the purposes of this chapter, knee joint aspiration is described.

Both traumatic and rheumatic processes affect the knee joint, although relatively more aspirations are performed at the knee for traumatic effusion than at other joints, where inflammation and effusion are more likely to be rheumatic in nature. A significant volume of joint effusion can collect within the knee joint. When assembling equipment for a therapeutic knee tap, it is important to recognize that there may be a significant volume of fluid to be aspirated and to plan accordingly.

INDICATIONS

Joint aspiration is indicated in the following situations:
- When there is a painful effusion of a joint, a monoarticular inflammation of a joint, or suspicion of a systemic rheumatic disorder of uncertain cause. In the mature patient, trauma can result in painful joint effusion, which can be remedied easily by joint aspiration.

- In the case of articular inflammation of unknown cause, the synovial fluid analysis—including viscosity, crystal examination, cell count, bacterial culture, Gram stain, and polymerase chain reaction studies—may be the most accurate diagnostic tool (Schumacher, 2001).

Bursal aspiration is indicated in the following situations:
- When painful bursal swelling persists despite conservative treatment or when questions arise about cause.

- When olecranon bursitis is perpetually aggravated by normal activities.

Like joint aspiration, strict sterile technique is indicated for bursal aspiration.

CONTRAINDICATIONS

■ Joint aspiration is contraindicated whenever circumstances exist by which entering the joint facilitates the seeding of bacteria into the joint. Introduction of a needle into the joint space through burns, infected skin, or infected subcutaneous tissue is contraindicated. Aspiration increases the risk of introducing bacteria into the joint when there is concern for overlying soft tissue cellulitis or impetigo, and joint aspiration should not be performed in this situation.

■ Aspiration of a bursa is likewise contraindicated when risks for introducing bacteria outweigh the benefits of aspiration.

■ Joint aspiration by the generalist is contraindicated after total joint arthroplasty except under the supervision of an orthopedic specialist. Should effusion or inflammation occur any time after joint replacement, the patient must be returned to the care of an orthopedist.

■ In the rare circumstance in which aspiration of a hemarthrosis is undertaken in a hemophiliac patient, the hemarthrosis will reaccumulate if bleeding has not been controlled before the procedure. Similarly, aspiration is relatively contraindicated in the patient who has undergone anticoagulation and has a significantly prolonged bleeding time.

POTENTIAL COMPLICATIONS

JOINT ASPIRATION

■ The most common complications of joint aspiration include bleeding, infection, pain, intra-articular injury, and reaccumulation of fluid. When providing patients with adequate information for informed consent, these complications should be outlined.

■ Inadvertent injury to vascular or neural structures near joint spaces can occur, as can a scoring injury of the intra-articular joint surface from the needle. Awareness of the proximity of nerves, arteries, or veins is necessary, as is caution when introducing a needle or infiltrating medications. As with any injection procedure, drawing back on the syringe plunger before administering medication is recommended to confirm that the needle is not within the lumen of a blood vessel.

■ Careful history taking concerning topical and systemic allergic reactions, with specific focus on iodine and anesthetic drug sensitivities, further minimizes complications associated with the procedure. With any parenterally administered medication, there must be prompt access to epinephrine 1:1000 for subcutaneous administration, and resuscitation equipment must be available in the event of a severe adverse reaction. Using a minimal volume of anesthetic is reasonable, and some authors recommend injecting no more than 5 mL of anesthetic solution within 30 minutes (Steinberg, 1999). When adequately anesthetizing the needle track for a joint aspiration, it is not difficult to exceed 5 mL of administered anesthetic. By respecting the landmarks and anatomy unique to each joint, one can minimize complications associated with an aspiration procedure.

BURSAL ASPIRATION

- The most common complications of bursal aspiration are infection, pain, chronic recurrence, chronic drainage via a sinus tract, and acute recurrent swelling. For bursal aspirations, keep in mind that some bursae communicate directly with the joint space.

- Baker's cysts, or popliteal bursae, are actually herniations of the joint capsule.

- Communication between the olecranon bursa and elbow joint may develop in rheumatoid arthritis. When aspirating the olecranon bursa, a lateral aspiration approach is recommended to prevent subsequent development of a chronic sinus tract that can result from introducing a needle directly into the tip of the elbow bursa (Steinberg, 1999). Despite the best technique, recurrence of olecranon bursitis with chronic painful inflammatory changes may necessitate definitive orthopedic resection of the bursa (Greene, 2001).

REVIEW OF ESSENTIAL ANATOMY AND PATHOPHYSIOLOGY: JOINT ASPIRATION

PATHOPHYSIOLOGY

The knee is representative of diarthrodial joints, with a synovial lining containing secretory cells and a fine capillary system from which synovial fluid is derived. Plasma transudation and mucin production within the joint combine to give synovial fluid its viscous, lubricating quality that reduces joint surface friction. Synovial fluid diffusion is an important factor in providing nutrition to the intra-articular structures (Weiner, 2004). Noninfectious effusions do not generally develop in fibrocartilaginous joints, such as the sacroiliac joint, because of the absence of synovial lining, but effusions do develop within bursae, which are cavities lined with secretory cells that function much like synovial cells (Sledge, 2001).

When trauma, inflammation, or infection occurs within the joint, the synovial fluid is characteristically altered, and sampling of the synovial fluid can be diagnostic. In the case of inflammatory reaction, the synovium produces increased synovial volume as a response to mechanical trauma or crystalline precipitants within the joint. Traumatically induced bleeding within the synovial fluid directly damages the synovial cartilage through the release of destructive proteolytic enzymes from blood cells. Hemarthrosis management should include aspiration to eliminate biochemical injury to the joint in addition to decreasing discomfort from mechanical distention.

Aspiration of a bloody synovial effusion is best attempted within the first couple of days after swelling develops. The clotting process makes aspiration nearly impossible between 3 and 7 days after injury, but aspiration becomes possible again 7 days after injury because of the breakdown of intra-articular clot. However, some cartilaginous damage is likely to have occurred by the time there is liquefaction of the intra-articular clot.

The synovial surface can also be transformed by chronic inflammatory changes that lead to proliferative changes on the synovial surface (Steinberg, 1999). This tissue proliferation can make aspiration techniques difficult or ineffective when the proliferative tissues obstruct the intra-articular needle and prevent aspiration of the joint fluid. Proper placement of the needle can reduce the likelihood of obstruction by avoiding areas commonly affected by synovial proliferation (Fig. 20-1).

ANATOMY AND PATHOMECHANICS

The knee joint is formed between the distal femur and proximal tibia, with the synovium covering the femur in a saddle configuration and reflecting anteriorly and superiorly on the femur behind the patella and draping inferiorly and posteriorly on the caudad surface of the femur, medially and inferiorly

Lateral anterior oblique   Posterior

FIGURE 20-1. Synovial surfaces of the knee joint.

Quadriceps

Suprapatellar fat

Femur

Patella

Synovium

Infrapatellar fat pad

Tibia

Fibula

Intracondylar space

Space narrowing with flexion

FIGURE 20-2. Anatomy of the knee joint.

over the lateral surfaces of the cruciate ligaments, and down to the tibial articular surfaces. A small synovial draping also occurs over the proximal fibula. The pommel of the synovial saddle lies on the anterior distal femur behind the patella, reflecting at the upper margin anteriorly toward the patella. The space medially between the femoral condyles and behind the patella generally permits better synovial aspiration because the probability of encountering synovial proliferation or abutting a bony surface is less, particularly when the knee is extended (Fig. 20-2).

PATIENT PREPARATION: JOINT ASPIRATION

■ Informed consent is appropriate for any invasive procedure. Whether using a formal written consent form or simply documenting the risks and benefits discussed, patients should be apprised of the risks for infection, bleeding, adverse reactions to anesthesia, joint surface injury, ongoing pain, and reaccumulation of fluid.

■ For some patients whose effusion has stabilized the knee, the removal of the fluid may uncover previously unnoticed knee instability. It is helpful to prepare patients for this by discussing the possibility before tapping the joint.

■ Let patients know that additional management after aspiration may include immobilization of the joint, antibiotic or anti-inflammatory therapy, hospitalization, or referral to a specialist, depending on the findings on aspiration.

■ Inform the patient that the procedure takes about 5 to 10 minutes after a 10-minute scrub of the joint area to ensure asepsis.

■ Patients must be reminded that once the preparation has begun, it is essential that the patient refrain from touching, pointing, or reaching over the area being prepared. Patients do well with this when told not to touch anywhere within the "covered area," when drapes are used, or where the "soap" was applied until the procedure is completed.

■ Patients should be prepared for a brief episode of stinging discomfort when the lidocaine anesthetic is administered subcutaneously. The "bee-sting" sensation lasts less than 30 seconds for most patients.

■ Considering overall safety for the patient as well as the position for optimal access of the effusion, it is preferable to have the patient in a supine position with the knee extended as much as the effusion permits. Knee flexion allows the patella to ride more closely to the femur, narrowing the retropatellar space. The widest patellofemoral space is afforded by placing the knee at the fullest extension allowable. Because the tension on the anterior cruciate ligament is greatest when the knee is in full extension or deep flexion, the patient may prefer to maintain a 30- to 70-degree flexion to maintain laxity of the anterior cruciate ligament and allow for comfort. Likewise, effusive distention of the joint may prevent full extension.

Table 20.1	**Synovial Fluid Testing**		
TEST	COLLECTION TUBE/ CONTAINER	AMOUNT OF FLUID NEEDED	SPECIAL CONSIDERATIONS*
Crystals	Red- or green-top tube (sodium heparin)	0.5 mL	Caution with other tubes containing EDTA—may be mistaken for joint fluid crystals
RA latex	Red-top tube	0.5 mL min	
Total protein	Red-top tube	0.5 mL min	
Glucose	Red- or gray-top* (sodium heparin)	0.5 mL min	
Mucin clot	Red-top tube	0.5 mL min	
Cell count	Purple-top tube (EDTA)	1.0 mL min	
Routine culture	Sterile syringe* Yellow top (ACD)*	0.5 mL min	Send to laboratory in syringe
Gram stain	Sterile syringe* Yellow top (ACD)*	0.5 mL min	Send to laboratory in syringe
TB culture	Sterile syringe* Yellow top (ACD)*	0.5 mL min	Send to laboratory in syringe
Fungal culture	Sterile syringe* Yellow top (ACD)*	0.5 mL min	Send to laboratory in syringe

*Individual microbiology and chemistry laboratories may have specific criteria for tests; confirm the laboratory's preference for the tests you are running.

ACD, anticoagulant citrate dextrose; EDTA, ethylenediaminetetra-acetic acid; min, minimum; RA, rheumatoid arthritis; TB, tuberculosis.

Materials Utilized for Performing Joint and Bursal Aspiration

- Tray table

- Sterile drapes

- Sterile gloves

- Povidone-iodine solution (or other topical antiseptic if iodine allergic)

- 1% lidocaine (unless contraindicated by allergy)

- Sterile 1-inch, 25-gauge needles; sterile 1½-inch, 19-gauge needles

- Three sterile 20- or 30-mL syringes, sterile 5- or 10-mL syringe

- Sterile hemostat

- Green-top sodium heparin tube or other Vacutainer tubes as indicated (Table 20-1).

Procedure for Performing Joint Aspiration

1. Determine the position that will allow the patient to be most comfortable and the effusion to be most easily accessed.

2. Perform a 10-minute scrub of the knee with povidone-iodine solution. The preparation must encircle the knee and extend 2 to 3 inches above and below the knee.

3. Draping of the knee is not essential but it reduces the risk of infection. If performed, the draping should allow adequate visualization of the joint space for the ballottement of fluid and determination of landmarks.

4. Prepare a sterile field on which to assemble all needed sterile equipment including syringes, needles, hemostat, and sterile cup.

5. Once prepared, don sterile gloves, drape if desired, and define the superior pole of the patella. Identify the joint spaces lateral to the patella by ballottement of fluid beneath the patella (Fig. 20-3).

6. Draw up 1% lidocaine in a 5- or 10-mL syringe.

7. Identify the landmarks to determine the location for needle placement.

Note: The needle may be introduced into the joint space either anteromedially or anterolaterally.

8. Draw a visual line along either lateral margin of the patella to intersect with the line of the superior patellar margin and, entering the skin at that point or slightly more laterally and superiorly, administer a small amount of the anesthetic subcutaneously. Angle 45 degrees off the sagittal plane and 30 degrees off the frontal plane, directing the needle caudally.

9. Advance the needle as deep as anesthesia is desired, aspirating for blood.

Note: When advancing to the joint capsule, resistance is encountered at the level of the joint capsule.

10. While withdrawing the needle, administer the anesthetic along the track from the joint capsule out to the skin (Fig. 20-4).

11. Remove the smaller gauge needle and syringe and assemble the 18-gauge needle on a 20- or 30-mL syringe. Hold the needle-syringe like a pencil and align to advance medially and caudally into the joint space behind the patella.

12. Introduce the 18-gauge needle into the anesthetized track angled 45 degrees laterally and directed 30 degrees caudally. Place gentle pressure on the syringe plunger while advancing and aspirate the synovial fluid on entering the joint space as the needle is directed medially and downward behind the patella (Fig. 20-5).

Note: Entering the joint space is painful briefly for the patient.

13. When the syringe is full, place the hemostat on the needle hub, remove the syringe, and replace it with an empty syringe or discharge the synovial fluid into a sterile cup. Repeat this step until the knee joint is no longer visibly distended or fluid can no longer be aspirated.

Note: Pressure applied above the knee joint can "milk" additional fluid centrally for aspiration. Caution must be exercised not to compromise sterile conditions.

continued

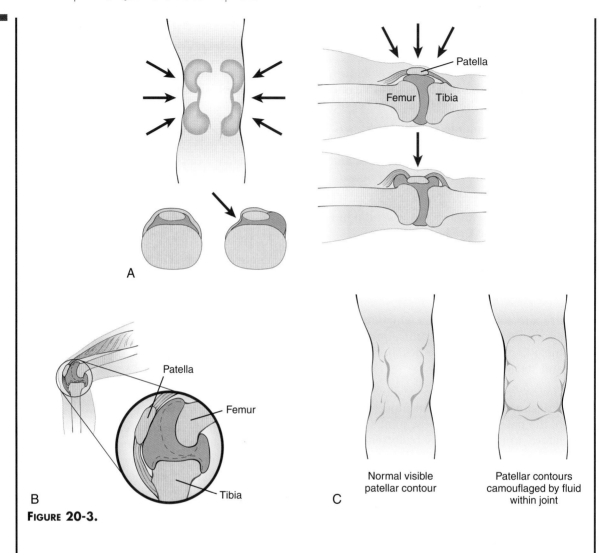

Femur Tibia

Patella

Patella

Femur

Tibia

Normal visible
patellar contour

Patellar contours
camouflaged by fluid
within joint

A

B

C

FIGURE 20-3.

14. Intra-articular medication can be administered after the aspiration if indicated.

15. Withdraw the needle from the joint space and apply direct pressure with sterile dressing over the puncture site for several minutes.

16. Confirm that the wound site is dry and active bleeding has stopped and then dress with sterile adhesive dressing.

17. Maintaining sterile conditions, observe the synovial fluid for evidence of a cloudy appearance and obtain Gram stain, cell counts, and cultures if there is suspicion of infection.

Note: Gram stain and cultures are usually collected in sterile syringes and transported promptly to the laboratory. Rapid transport and inoculation on special medium are essential for growth of fastidious bacteria

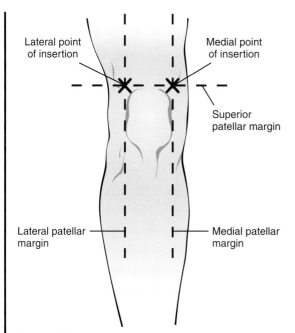

FIGURE 20-4. Landmarks for needle placement.

such as *Neisseria gonorrhoeae.* Specimens sent for crystal analysis should not be drawn into an ethylenediaminetetra-acetic acid (EDTA) tube because the EDTA crystals can be confused with intra-articular crystals. See Table 20-1 for guidelines on acquiring samples for the laboratory.

FIGURE 20-5. Positioning the needle for joint aspiration.

FOLLOW-UP CARE AND INSTRUCTIONS: JOINT ASPIRATION

- Advise patients to avoid use of the joint for at least 1 day. If traumatic injury preceded the effusion, longer immobilization or avoidance of weight bearing may be indicated. When aspiration eliminates internal splinting, the instability of the joint may become apparent and should be managed as would otherwise be indicated.

- Instruct the patient to call the office in the event of sudden reaccumulation of fluid, increased heat at the joint, fever, chills, or a severe increase in pain, which would necessitate the patient's prompt return for further evaluation.

- Evidence or strong suspicion of infection at the time of tapping necessitates an immediate referral to an orthopedist.

REVIEW OF ESSENTIAL ANATOMY AND PHYSIOLOGY: BURSAL ASPIRATION

Numerous bursae are found around the joints, many of which may accumulate excessive fluid as part of an inflammatory process. The olecranon bursa is one that can become visibly distended because of inflammation. This easily accessible bursa may swell slowly over time or accumulate suddenly from trauma or infection. Because of the relatively exposed and superficial anatomy of the bursa, external mechanical irritation plays a significant role in the initiation and perpetuation of olecranon bursitis. Other differential considerations include ulnar fracture, gout, acute rheumatoid arthritis, or a synovial cyst of the elbow joint (Greene, 2001).

Intrabursal scar tissue, which feels like small nodules within the bursa, can develop rather early as a sequela to olecranon bursitis. These "nodules" may result in chronic pain and tenderness when the elbow is mechanically aggravated.

The general approach to aspirating an olecranon bursitis can be applied to other bursae. Few others have such easily accessible anatomy. Some, such as the trochanteric bursae, are difficult to isolate anatomically because of overlying structures (Fig. 20-6). Others, such as the prepatellar bursae, are nearly as accessible as the olecranon bursae (Fig. 20-7).

PATIENT PREPARATION: BURSAL ASPIRATION

- Apprise the patient of the risks of infection, bleeding, adverse reactions to anesthesia, ongoing pain, and reaccumulation of fluid.

Trochanteric bursa

FIGURE 20-6. Trochanteric bursae are difficult to isolate because of overlying structures.

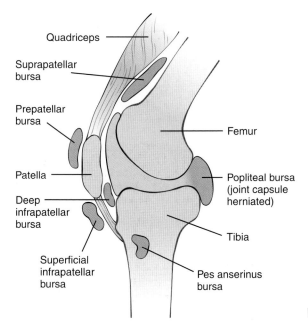

Quadriceps

Suprapatellar bursa

Prepatellar bursa

Patella

Deep infrapatellar bursa

Superficial infrapatellar bursa

Femur

Popliteal bursa (joint capsule herniated)

Tibia

Pes anserinus bursa

FIGURE 20-7. Knee bursae.

- Let the patient know that additional management after aspiration includes resting and protecting the elbow, antibiotic or anti-inflammatory therapy if indicated, or hospitalization or referral to a specialist, depending on the findings.

- Inform the patient that the procedure takes about 5 to 10 minutes after a 10-minute scrub of the joint area to ensure asepsis. Patients must be reminded that once the preparation has begun, it is essential that the patient refrain from touching, pointing, or reaching over the area being prepared.

- Warn the patient to be prepared for a brief episode of stinging discomfort when the lidocaine is administered subcutaneously. The "bee-sting" sensation lasts less than 30 seconds for most patients.

Procedure for Performing Bursal Aspiration

1. Have the patient sit well supported or lying down prone for the procedure. If sitting, the arm must be supported on a Mayo stand flexed at the elbow to 90 degrees. If lying down prone, have the patient rest the arm on the examination table with elbow flexed and shoulder comfortably abducted to allow access to the lateral olecranon bursa.

2. Prepare a sterile field on which to assemble all needed sterile equipment, including syringes, needles, hemostat, and sterile cup.

3. Perform a 10-minute scrub with povidone-iodine solution. Cover the entire olecranon process as well as the lateral elbow surface.

4. Once the patient is prepared, don sterile gloves and drape the area so that the bursa is easily accessible but sterility is maintained.

5. Draw up 1 mL of 1% lidocaine in a syringe. Identify the landmarks to determine the location for needle placement.

Note: The olecranon bursa is usually readily visible and distended beyond the typical elbow contour. Anesthesia to the skin and subcutaneous tissues may be administered as desired using a 25- to 27-gauge needle.

6. Administer the anesthetic under the skin of the elbow, centering the needle over the lateral surface of the distended bursa (Fig. 20-8).

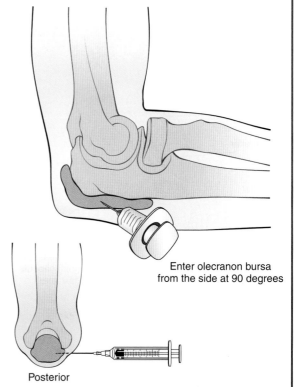

Enter olecranon bursa from the side at 90 degrees

Posterior

FIGURE 20-8. Positioning the needle for bursal aspiration.

7. With the elbow flexed to 90 degrees and resting comfortably, switch to an 18-gauge needle and syringe. Enter into the distended olecranon bursa at 90 degrees to the plane of the arm. Aspirate the fluid slowly until the bursal sac is flat.

8. Apply direct pressure over the puncture site. Dress with an adhesive bandage and wrap the elbow with an elastic compression bandage to retard the reaccumulation of fluid.

9. Observe the synovial fluid for evidence of a cloudy appearance and obtain a Gram stain, cell counts, and cultures if there is suspicion of infection. Tests for crystals or other rheumatoid parameters should proceed as was described in the joint aspiration section (see Table 20-1).

FOLLOW-UP CARE AND INSTRUCTIONS: BURSAL ASPIRATION

■ Advise the patient to avoid general use of the joint for at least 2 days. Recurrence of bursal effusion is more likely with persistent mechanical irritation of the bursa. Avoiding resting the elbow on tables, automobile arm rests, and chair arms decreases irritation. For some patients, these activities are so habitual that the elbow is inevitably chronically irritated and an elbow protector may be indicated. Another option is the placement of a posterior plaster splint after aspiration to limit elbow motion for the first week after the procedure. For those who go on to develop chronic bursitis, surgical excision may become necessary.

■ Instruct the patient to call the office in the event of the development of a warm elbow, fever, chills, or severe increase in pain, which would necessitate prompt return for further evaluation (Greene, 2001). Recurrence of olecranon bursitis more than three times probably indicates a need for surgical bursal excision, as does the development of a draining sinus tract.

REFERENCES

Grassi W, Filipucci E, Busilacchi P: Musculoskeletal ultrasound. Best Pract Res Clin Rheumatol 18::813-826, 2004.

Greene WB (ed): Essentials of Musculoskeletal Care. Rosemont, Ill, American Academy of Orthopaedic Surgeons, 2001.

Schumacher HR: Synovial fluid analysis and synovial biopsy. In Ruddy S, Harris ED, Sledge CB (eds): Kelley's Textbook of Rheumatology, 6th ed. Philadelphia, WB Saunders, 2001, pp 605-617.

Sledge CB, Reddi AH, Walsh DA, Blake DR: Biology of the normal joint. In Ruddy S, Harris ED, Sledge CB (eds): Kelley's Textbook of Rheumatology, 6th ed. Philadelphia, WB Saunders, 2001, pp 1-25.

Steinberg G, Akins C, Baran D (eds): Orthopaedics in Primary Care, 3rd ed. Philadelphia, Lippincott Williams & Wilkins, 1999.

Weiner DS (ed): Pediatric Orthopedics for Primary Care, 2nd ed. Cambridge, UK, Cambridge University Press, 2004.

BIBLIOGRAPHY

Carr AJ, Hamilton W (eds): Orthopedics in Primary Care, 2nd ed. Edinburgh, Elsevier/Butterworth-Heinemann, 2005.

McMahon PJ, Skinner HB: Sports medicine. In Skinner H (ed): Current Diagnosis and Treatment in Orthopedics. Norwalk, Conn, Lange Medical Books/McGraw-Hill, 2003.

Owens DS: Aspiration and injection of joints and soft tissues. In Ruddy S, Harris ED, Sledge CB (eds): Kelley's Textbook of Rheumatology, 6th ed. Philadelphia, WB Saunders, 2001, pp 583-603.

Ruddy S, Harris ED, Sledge CB (eds): Kelley's Textbook of Rheumatology, 6th ed. Philadelphia, WB Saunders, 2001.

Schumacher HR: Aspiration and injection therapies for joints. Arthritis Rheum 49:413-420, 2003.

Chapter 21

Casting and Splinting

Donald Frosch and Patrick Knott

PROCEDURE GOALS AND OBJECTIVES

Goal: To apply comfortable and well-fitting casts and splints that effectively immobilize an injured extremity in the appropriate position and minimize potential complications to the patient.

Objectives: The student will be able to …

- Compare and contrast the indications and contraindications of utilizing plaster and fiberglass materials for casts and splints.

- Distinguish the various types of splints and casts used to immobilize upper and lower extremity injuries.

- Describe the proper procedure for selecting and applying a short-arm cast, short-leg cast, short-arm gutter splint, short-leg posterior mold, and lower-leg sugar tong splint.

- Identify and describe potential complications associated with casting and splinting extremities.

- Describe how to perform a proper post-cast or post-splint assessment to determine if the device fits well, properly immobilizes the injured extremity, and is comfortable.

- Identify the important aspects of patient education and cast care following a casting and splinting application.

- Explain how to properly utilize an oscillating cast saw to remove a cast without causing injury to the patient.

FIGURE 21-1. Short-arm cast.

BACKGROUND AND HISTORY

Immobilization of the extremities in casts and splints is a practice that dates back to nearly 3000 BC, when tree bark was used to splint injured forearms. In the 1920s, plaster of Paris was commercially introduced to medicine as a powder that was impregnated into rolls of cloth. Since the 1970s, synthetic materials like fiberglass and plastic have been used to make casts and splints, but the principles of immobilization have remained remarkably constant throughout time.

There are numerous types of casts and splints used to treat an even greater number of specific fractures and soft tissue injuries. Some devices immobilize only the distal half of an extremity ("short-arm" or "short-leg" casts or splints), whereas others immobilize the entire extremity ("long-arm" or "long-leg" casts or splints) or only the upper arm. Describing the many special types of immobilization is beyond the scope of this chapter, and the use of many of these specialized types of casts and splints may be inappropriate in the primary care setting. What follows is an explanation of the basic principles of casting and splinting, and instructions for constructing several commonly used casts and splints.

A cast is an immobilization device that completely encases the circumference of an extremity. It consists of a rigid material (usually plaster or fiberglass), placed over several layers of padding and a cloth stockinette that together cover and protect the skin. Because a cast is circumferential, it must not be employed until the acute swelling phase of the injury has subsided. Two types of casts are discussed in this chapter, the short-arm cast (Fig. 21-1) and the short-leg cast (Fig. 21-2).

A splint is similar to a cast except that its rigid material encases only part of an extremity's circumference and must therefore be secured with a self-adherent and elastic wrap, such as an ACE bandage or Coban wrap. Although a splint provides less mechanical support and protection than a circumferential cast, its main advantage is that it allows for soft tissue swelling

FIGURE 21-2.   Short-leg cast.

FIGURE 21-3.   Gutter splint.

during the acute phase of an injury. It is typically employed as a temporary immobilization measure and is replaced with a cast after the acute swelling subsides. The stockinette is excluded from splint constructions because it is potentially constricting in the setting of acute swelling. A splint can be easily constructed from strips of fiberglass or plaster that are sandwiched between an upper and lower row of cast padding. Prefabricated splints, however, are commercially available in a variety of precut sizes or in cut-to-size rolls, and typically consist of an outer paper shell overlying fiberglass strips with foam padding on one side. Three general types of splints are discussed in this chapter: the "gutter," the "posterior mold," and the "sugar tong." The gutter splint (Fig. 21-3) is appropriately named for its gutter-like shape in supporting the extremity. The forearm gutter splint is an example of this type. The

FIGURE 21-4. Posterior mold splint.

FIGURE 21-5. Sugar tong splint for the lower leg.

posterior mold splint (Fig. 21-4) is so named because it is molded to the posterior aspect of the splinted extremity. Posterior mold splints of the short-leg, short-arm, or long-arm variety are commonly employed. The sugar tong splint (Figs. 21-5 and 21-6) forms a U-shaped strap around an extremity, resembling the kitchen accessory after which it is named. The sugar tong splint can be used to initially immobilize the lower leg, lower arm, or upper arm.

Plaster and fiberglass are the two primary materials used to make casts and splints today, although several other synthetic materials are gaining in popularity. Each material has inherent benefits and drawbacks that determine which is the best choice for the situation. Plaster is easier to mold to an extremity than is fiberglass, giving it an advantage when a snug and form-fitting cast is needed on an area with challenging contours, such as the chubby, cone-shaped arm or legs of a toddler. Despite this significant advantage, plaster has a number of drawbacks. It is much heavier than fiberglass, yet not as durable. It is also messy to apply and it emits quite a bit of heat as it cures. Because of the exothermic reaction generated, it is sometimes uncomfortable for the acutely injured patient and poses a potential burn risk in patients with sensory deficits. Fiberglass is an extremely popular casting material because of its strength, light weight, ease of application, and excellent durability. Unlike plaster, fiberglass cures rapidly and is water-resistant

FIGURE 21-6.   Sugar tong splint for the lower arm.

(although the underlying padding must still be kept dry). For these reasons, fiberglass is clearly the material of choice for the majority of cast and splint applications, and especially for weight bearing ("walking") casts. The drawback to fiberglass is that it is several times more expensive than plaster. Its higher initial cost can be justified because it lasts longer and requires fewer repairs and replacements during the period of immobilization.

INDICATIONS

Casts and splints are used in the primary care setting as follows:
■ To treat simple, acute, nondisplaced fractures

■ To immobilize a dislocation after it has been reduced

■ To treat soft tissue injuries, such as severe ligament sprains and muscle strains

Immobilization is necessary for comfort and healing after a bone fracture, and it is also beneficial in the short term following a soft tissue injury. Because long periods of immobilization cause disuse atrophy and stiffness in the affected limb, the benefits of immobilization must be weighed against these predictable side effects when deciding upon the optimal duration of immobilization.

CONTRAINDICATIONS

Cast (circumferential) immobilization should be avoided in the following situations:

■ During the acute injury phase (usually 3 to 4 days), when immediate swelling of the extremity is expected

■ When the cast would cover or conceal a known skin or soft tissue infection

■ When the cast would cover or conceal an open wound, where infection may occur

In these situations, a splint (noncircumferential) is much safer than a cast, because it allows the extremity to expand with swelling and provides access to the skin so that it can be periodically checked for wound healing and signs of infection.

POTENTIAL COMPLICATIONS

A circumferential cast on an injured extremity can be a potentially dangerous form of treatment, and the primary care provider must be vigilant to signs and symptoms of potential complications. These include compartment syndrome, cast dermatitis, pressure sores, nerve injuries, and deep venous thrombosis.

COMPARTMENT SYNDROME

The most serious complication after the application of a cast is the development of a compartment syndrome. This refers to a buildup of pressure within the soft tissues that can impede or cut off the blood supply to an injured extremity, causing permanent damage to muscles and nerves. A compartment syndrome typically follows an injury to a large bone in an area where there is a closed compartment formed by fascial layers (e.g., the forearm or lower leg). It is also more likely after a crush injury or arterial laceration. However, a compartment syndrome can occur without any of these predisposing factors. The classic example of a compartment syndrome in an upper extremity is Volkmann's ischemic contracture, a complication that results in muscle necrosis and loss of function of the affected arm and hand. The most predictive symptom of a compartment syndrome is pain that increases over time and is out of proportion to the severity of the injury. The pain is much worse with passive motion of the distal extremity and usually prevents active motion altogether. Less reliable signs and symptoms in the involved limb include paresthesias, decreased two-point discrimination, decreased capillary refill, pallor, and, ultimately, pulselessness. Normal soft tissue compartment resting pressures are in the range of 5 to 10 mm Hg. As these pressures rise above 30 mm Hg and begin to approach diastolic pressures, irreversible damage to the soft tissues can result. If suspected, one should look for compartment syndrome by directly measuring compartment pressure, rather than waiting for the later signs of decreased capillary refill or changes in the arterial pulse amplitude. Today, compartment pressure is most commonly measured with a special electronic hand-held device, although it can also be measured using a needle, three-way stopcock, intravenous tubing, and a mercury manometer (Whiteside's technique), or with a specially prepared catheter and pressure transducer (wick catheter technique). Treatment for a suspected compartment syndrome requires immediate loosening of the cast. This is accomplished by cutting and splitting the cast, padding, and stockinette down both sides of the extremity, and then separating the two halves to relieve pressure. Adequate relief of pressure may not be achieved unless the underlying padding and stockinette layers are cut all the way down to the skin. If symptoms do not resolve within a few minutes of this "bivalving" procedure, compartment pressures should be measured and surgical decompression undertaken, if necessary.

Cast Dermatitis

Cast dermatitis is a complication that occurs when air circulation is insufficient to clear residual moisture and ongoing limb perspiration from inside the cast. Patients often try to relieve the associated pruritus by scratching with coat hangers, pencils, or other long objects that they are able to insert into their cast. Such objects may cause skin abrasions or lacerations that become secondarily infected.

Cast Pressure Sores

Cast pressure sores result from inadequate cast padding over bony prominences or from finger indentations in the cast that result from poor technique during cast application. If not detected early, pressure sores may progress to pressure ulcers, and may require surgical debridement and skin grafting.

Nerve Injuries

Pressure over superficial nerves, especially the ulnar nerve at the elbow and the common fibular (common peroneal) nerve at the fibular head, can cause a temporary nerve palsy or permanent paralysis if left untreated. The causes are the same as for cast pressure sores.

DEEP VENOUS THROMBOSIS

In addition to lack of ambulation, long periods of immobilization of the lower extremities can lead to formation of deep venous thrombi or pulmonary emboli.

REVIEW OF ESSENTIAL ANATOMY AND PHYSIOLOGY

A rule of thumb when casting an injured extremity is that the immobilization should include the joints proximal *and* distal to the injured area. This rule is frequently broken, however, if the length of the limb proximal to the injury is sufficient to allow for proper immobilization and fixation of the fracture. For example, for a wrist fracture, the cast may not have to include the elbow if the length of cast along the forearm allows for adequate wrist joint immobilization. One should recognize that a short-arm cast never completely immobilizes the wrist joint because it does not prevent forearm pronation and supination. When uncertain about the length of cast required, an orthopedic specialist should be consulted.

Standard Precautions   Practitioners should use standard precautions at all times when interacting with patients. Determining the appropriate level of precaution requires the practitioner to exercise clinical judgment based on the patient's history and the potential for exposure to body fluids or aerosol-borne pathogens (for further discussion, see Chapter 2).

PATIENT PREPARATION

- Inform the patient about the procedure and answer any questions.

- Place the extremity in the position of function:

  - *For a short-arm cast, short-arm ulnar gutter splint, or short-arm sugar tong splint*: The elbow should be flexed to 90 degrees and the forearm maintained in neutral pronation-supination (with the thumb pointing upward). The wrist should be held in slight extension, with the fingers slightly curled as if holding a can of soda.

  - *For a short-leg cast, short-leg posterior mold splint, or short-leg sugar tong splint:* The ankle must be strictly maintained at 90 degrees of flexion. Allowing an ankle to drift into plantar flexion during cast application will result in a cast that is difficult to walk on. If uncorrected, a plantar-flexed cast will result in contraction of the Achilles tendon and stiffening of the calf and hamstring musculature. It is easiest to maintain proper ankle position during casting or splinting by applying the cast with the patient lying prone with the knee flexed to 90 degrees. If applying the cast with the patient sitting, it is helpful to have an assistant hold the patient by the toes to maintain proper ankle position. Whether performed in the prone or sitting position, casting the leg with the knee bent helps avoid the mistake of casting too high into the knee area and restricting knee flexion.

Materials Utilized for Applying Casts

■ Stockinette

Note: Stockinette is a stretchable socklike material that is available in 2-, 2½-, 3-, 4-, 5-, and 6-inch widths. It comes on a large roll that is cut to the desired length. The most appropriate width is selected based upon the limb involved, the size of the patient, and the degree of swelling of the limb. Stockinette serves two purposes. First, it acts as a barrier between the skin and the sometimes itchy cast padding. Second, after the cast padding and first layer of fiberglass are placed, the stockinette and cast padding are pulled over the rough edges of the cast to provide comfortable cast borders.

■ Cast padding

Note: Cast padding is available in 2-, 3-, 4-, and 5-inch widths and is packaged in individual small rolls. Depending on the size of the injured extremity, 2- or 3-inch padding is usually used on the arm, 3- or 4-inch padding on the lower leg, and 4- or 5-inch padding on the upper leg. Two types of padding are available, cotton and synthetic. Cotton was the type of cast padding originally used when plaster was the only type of casting material available. When fiberglass casting materials became available, synthetic cast padding was developed. An advantage of synthetic padding is that it absorbs less water than cotton if it gets wet. For these reasons, cotton padding is typically used with plaster, and synthetic padding with fiberglass. Two layers of padding are usually sufficient, with additional padding added to cast edges and over bony prominences. Too much padding may lead to a loose cast as the padding flattens over time.

■ Cast material

Note: Cast material (i.e., plaster, fiberglass) is available in 2-, 3-, 4-, and 6-inch widths and is usually packaged in individual rolls or various length strips. Smaller widths are used on the narrow, distal parts of the extremities (i.e., wrists, hands, ankles, feet), whereas larger widths are used on the wider and longer areas. The width of cast material selected is usually similar to that of the cast padding. Fiberglass cast material must be kept in its airtight foil package until it is ready to be applied, because the moisture in the air will initiate the curing process. This is not a concern with plaster.

■ Large basin or bucket

Note: This is filled with water and used to fully immerse the casting material.

■ Apron and gloves

Note: These are used to protect the clinician's skin and clothing from the sticky and permanently staining resin contained in fiberglass casting material, and from the messy splatter that occurs when using plaster casting material.

- Bandage scissors

Note: These are used to cut or trim the padding and casting materials, if needed.

- Cast saw and additional blades

Note: Specialized cast saws are used to remove or reshape casts after they harden. A cast saw has an oscillating blade that vibrates (instead of spinning like a conventional saw blade), thereby preventing the saw from inadvertently cutting the skin during cast removal.

General Procedure for Applying Casts

1. Select the appropriate size of stockinette.

2. Cut the stockinette to an appropriate length so that there will be about 3 to 4 inches of excess stockinette on each end of the cast (Fig. 21-7). Try to smooth out all wrinkles from the stockinette. If necessary, remove overlapping wrinkles with your scissors.

3. Select the appropriate size of cast padding. Roll the padding on smoothly, overlapping each time by about 50% (Fig. 21-8). It is easier to apply cast padding by starting at the narrow end of an extremity and rolling toward the wider part. Extend the padding about 1 to 2 inches *beyond* each border of where the cast material will be. One to two layers of foundation padding usually suffice.

FIGURE 21-8. Cast padding.

4. Add an additional layer or two of cast padding at the intended top and bottom borders of the cast. Add additional padding over bony prominences and in areas of potential cast friction by tearing small sections of padding from the roll and placing them where needed.

5. Put on your protective apron and gloves.

6. Immerse the casting material in a bucket of water. For *plaster*, immerse the roll in *cool* water until it is "sloppy wet." The excess cool water helps disperse the

FIGURE 21-7. Stockinette.

Figure 21-9. Casting material.

heat generated from the plaster's exothermic curing process. For *fiberglass*, immerse the roll in a bucket of water for about 10 seconds, and then squeeze it once gently to remove the bulk of the water.

7. Roll the casting material on smoothly, overlapping each time by about 50%. Start and finish each roll of casting material about 1 to 2 inches inside the border of the cast padding so that there will be sufficient padding to roll over the edge of the cast (Fig. 21-9). It is easier to apply cast material by starting at the narrow end of an extremity and rolling toward the wider part. Try to traverse the entire length of the planned cast with each roll. Avoid bunching or wrinkling the casting material by folding or tucking the roll when needed. Also, avoid stretching or pulling the casting material when applying. This is especially important when applying the first roll or two. The average cast may require 4 to 6 layers of plaster or 3 to 4 layers of fiberglass, with additional reinforcement at the foot for weight-bearing casts. Be sure to maintain the extremity in the position of function while rolling the casting material, and gently reposition it if needed.

8. Mold *each layer* to the contour of the extremity by gently, but firmly, rubbing the cast between the palms of your gloved hands. Proper molding is necessary to allow for a comfortable fit and appropriate immobilization of the extremity. With the proper amount of cast padding, molding can be accomplished with minimal discomfort to the patient. While molding, continue to ensure that the extremity is in the proper position of function. Be especially careful not to indent the cast with your fingertips when supporting the extremity!

9. Prior to rolling the final layer of cast material, pull the stockinette and cast padding over each cast edge and secure them with the final layer of cast material. This creates a nicely padded and rolled-edge border.

10. Perform a post-application assessment of the position of function, fit, extent of immobilization, and comfort of the cast.

Materials Utilized for Applying a Short-Arm Cast

- 2-, 2½-, or 3-inch stockinette (depending on arm size)
- One roll of 2- or 3-inch cast padding
- Two rolls of 2- or 3-inch fiberglass casting material

Procedure for Applying a Short-Arm Cast

Note: A short-arm cast should extend from about two fingerbreadths distal to the olecranon fossa to just proximal to the metacarpal-phalangeal (MCP) joints of all fingers. If properly applied, it should immobilize the hand, wrist, and distal forearm, yet allow for full flexion at the elbow, full range of motion of all the MCP joints (including the thumb), and an unobstructed thumb-index pinch. A short-arm cast is often used for hand, distal radius, and distal forearm fractures.

FIGURE 21-10.

1. Place (and maintain) the extremity in the proper position of function, as previously described.

2. Apply stockinette, as previously described. Be sure to extend the stockinette well beyond the anticipated cast borders. You will also need to cut an extra (distal) hole in the stockinette for the thumb when the stockinette is pulled down before the final layer of cast material is applied (see Fig. 21-7).

FIGURE 21-11.

3. Apply cast padding, as previously described. Be sure to extend the cast padding beyond the anticipated cast borders so that it (and the excess stockinette) can later be folded over the rough cast edges. Also apply extra padding over the radial and ulnar styloid processes.

4. Roll on the fiberglass casting material, starting in the narrow wrist area, then do a couple of figure eights around the hand before proceeding up the arm (Fig. 21-10). When rolling fiberglass through the narrow thumb-index web space, pinch or twist the tape so that it forms a small bridge that allows for thumb-finger opposition (Fig. 21-11).

FIGURE 21-12. Molding the cast.

5. After each roll of fiberglass is applied, mold the cast to the arm (and hand) using your palms, as previously described (Fig. 21-12).

6. Prior to rolling the final layer of cast material, pull the stockinette and cast padding over each cast edge and secure them with the final layer of cast material. This creates a nicely padded and rolled-edge border.

7. Perform a post-application assessment, evaluating each feature illustrated in Figure 21-13.

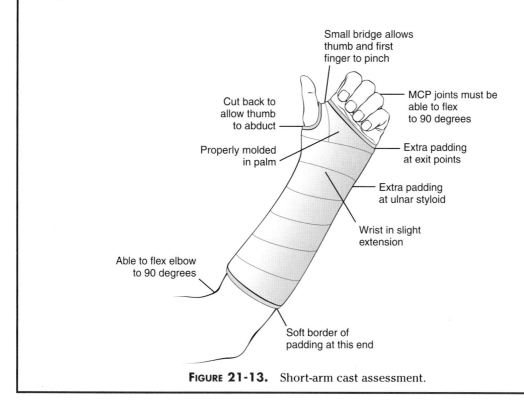

Small bridge allows thumb and first finger to pinch

Cut back to allow thumb to abduct

Properly molded in palm

MCP joints must be able to flex to 90 degrees

Extra padding at exit points

Extra padding at ulnar styloid

Wrist in slight extension

Able to flex elbow to 90 degrees

Soft border of padding at this end

FIGURE 21-13. Short-arm cast assessment.

Materials Utilized for Applying a Short-Leg Cast _____

- 3- or 4-inch stockinette (depending on leg size)
- Three rolls of 3- or 4-inch padding
- Three rolls of 4-inch fiberglass casting material

Procedure for Applying a Short-Leg Cast

Note: A short-leg cast should extend from the tibial tubercle to just proximal to the metatarsal-phalangeal (MTP) joints of all toes. If properly applied, it should immobilize the foot, ankle, and lower leg, yet allow full flexion at the knee and full range of motion of all the MTP joints, including the little toe. It is most often used for ankle fractures or severe ankle sprains.

1. Place (and maintain) the extremity in the proper position of function, as previously described.

2. Apply stockinette, as previously described. Be sure to extend the stockinette well beyond the anticipated cast borders.

3. Apply cast padding, as previously described. Be sure to extend the cast padding beyond the anticipated cast borders so that it (and the excess stockinette) can later be folded over the rough cast edges. Apply additional padding at the proximal end of the cast (at the tibial tubercle), over the metatarsal pad area, over the head of the fifth metatarsal, and especially over the heel.

Caution: **Do not pad the heel by wrapping circumferentially because cast padding will bulk up at the dorsal ankle area. To apply heavy padding to the heel, tear strips of cast padding and lay them over the heel.**

4. Roll on the fiberglass casting material, beginning at the ankle and proceeding proximally up the lower leg.

5. After each roll of fiberglass is applied, mold the cast to the leg (and foot) using your palms, as previously described.

6. Prior to rolling the final layer of cast material, pull the stockinette and cast padding over each cast edge and secure them with the final layer of cast material. This creates a nicely padded and rolled-edge border.

7. If the cast is to be used for walking, apply extra layers of reinforcement to the bottom surface and heel area for increased strength and durability, and strap a cast boot to the finished cast.

Note: Weight bearing must be restricted until the cast material has fully cured and hardened (1 to 2 hours for fiberglass casts; 4 to 6 hours for plaster casts). Premature weight bearing will cause cracking and denting of the cast.

8. Perform a post-application assessment, evaluating each feature illustrated in Figure 21-14.

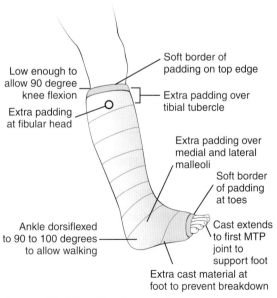

Low enough to allow 90 degree knee flexion

Extra padding at fibular head

Soft border of padding on top edge

Extra padding over tibial tubercle

Extra padding over medial and lateral malleoli

Soft border of padding at toes

Ankle dorsiflexed to 90 to 100 degrees to allow walking

Cast extends to first MTP joint to support foot

Extra cast material at foot to prevent breakdown

FIGURE 21-14. Short-leg cast assessment.

Materials Utilized for Applying a Short-Arm Ulnar Gutter Splint

- 3- × 12-inch prefabricated splint
- Bucket of cool water
- Dry towel
- 2- or 3-inch ACE bandage or Coban wrap

Procedure for Applying a Short-Arm Ulnar Gutter Splint

Note: A short-arm ulnar gutter splint extends from the tip of the little finger to just below the elbow and like a U-shaped gutter. It runs along the ulnar border of the hand and forearm. If properly applied, it immobilizes the fourth to fifth digits, the ulnar border of the hand, the wrist, and the distal forearm. It is used to treat fractures of the fifth metacarpal.

1. Although prefabricated splints contain a layer of padding, additional padding can be added over the ulnar styloid process for additional comfort.

Note: No stockinette is used with splints because of the risk of constriction from acute swelling.

2. Immerse the splint in a bucket of cool water.

3. Remove excess water from the splint by rolling it up tightly, or by rolling it like a jellyroll in a dry towel.

4. With the help of an assistant, maintain the patient's arm in the position of function while properly positioning the splint on the patient's bare arm. If the splint is too long, simply fold it away from the arm at the proximal end. Carefully avoid making fingerprint indentations in the splint.

Caution: **When using a prefabricated splint, remember to place the padded side of the splint against the patient's skin.**

5. Secure the splint using an ACE bandage or Coban wrap, beginning distally and proceeding proximally.

6. Gently mold the splint around the ulnar aspect of the arm and hand.

7. After the splint sufficiently hardens, remove the wrap and neatly rewrap it. In order to permit mobility of the thumb, index, and middle fingers, exclude them from the final elastic wrapping.

8. Perform a post-application splint assessment.

Materials Utilized for Applying a Short-Leg Posterior Mold Splint

- 5- × 30-inch prefabricated splint

- Bucket of cool water

- Dry towel

- 3- or 4-inch ACE bandage or Coban wrap

Procedure for Applying a Short-Leg Posterior Mold Splint

Note: A short-leg posterior mold splint extends along the posterior aspect of the lower leg, from two fingerbreadths distal to the popliteal fossa to the distal ends of the toes. If properly applied, it should immobilize the foot and ankle yet allow full flexion at the knee. This type of splint is commonly used for initial immobilization of ankle sprains and fractures.

1. Although prefabricated splints contain a layer of padding, additional padding is frequently used over the medial and lateral malleoli, metatarsal pad area, head of the fifth metatarsal, and heel.

Note: No stockinette is used with splints because of the risk of constriction from acute swelling.

2. Immerse the splint in a bucket of cool water.

3. Remove excess water from the splint by rolling it up tightly, or by rolling it like a jellyroll in a dry towel. It is important to remove as much water from the splint as possible in order to prevent water from pooling at the heel of the splint and causing skin breakdown.

4. With the help of an assistant, maintain the patient's foot and ankle in the position of function. Properly position the splint on the patient's lower leg, starting behind the knee and progressing to the foot. If the splint is too long, simply fold it back on itself, away from the body, at the distal end. Carefully avoid making fingerprint indentations in the splint.

Caution: **When using a prefabricated splint, remember to place the padded side of the splint against the patient's skin.**

5. Secure the splint using an ACE bandage or Coban wrap, starting just below the knee and working to the foot. To prevent pressure sores, be sure that the folds in the splint at the ankle area are directed outward and are not pointing in toward the skin.

6. Gently mold the splint around the posterior aspect of the lower leg, ankle, and foot.

7. Perform a post-application splint assessment.

Note: A *long-leg* posterior mold splint is constructed in a similar fashion, except that it includes the entire lower extremity with the knee in full extension. It is constructed using 2 to 3 rolls of 4-inch padding, a 5- × 45-inch splint, and additional padding over the medial and lateral malleoli, metatarsal pad area, head of the fifth metatarsal, and heel. It is often used for initial stabilization of tibia fractures.

Note: A *long-arm* posterior mold is constructed in a similar fashion, except that the entire upper extremity is splinted with 90 degrees of elbow flexion and neutral forearm pronation/supination. It is constructed using three rolls of 3-inch padding, a 4- × 30-inch splint, and additional padding over olecranon, medial and lateral epicondyles, and ulnar styloid process. It is often used for initial stabilization of mid- or proximal forearm fractures, or fractures of the distal humerus.

Materials Utilized for Applying a Lower Leg Sugar Tong Splint

- 3- × 45-inch prefabricated splint
- Bucket of cool water
- Dry towel
- 3- or 4-inch ACE bandage or Coban wrap

Procedure for Applying a Lower Leg Sugar Tong Splint

Note: A lower leg sugar tong (or "stirrup") splint is a U-shaped splint that starts at the medial aspect of the knee, passes under the foot, and extends to the lateral aspect of the knee. If properly applied, it provides great mediolateral support to the ankle, while allowing full range of motion of toes and knee. The sugar tong splint is an alternative to the posterior mold when splinting the lower leg.

1. Although prefabricated splints contain a layer of padding, additional padding is frequently used over the bony prominences, especially at the medial and lateral malleoli.

Note: No stockinette is used with splints because of the risk of constriction from acute swelling.

2. Immerse the splint in a bucket of cool water.

3. Remove excess water from the splint by rolling it up tightly, or by rolling it like a jellyroll in a dry towel.

4. With the help of an assistant, maintain the patient's foot and ankle in the position of function while properly positioning the splint. Start by positioning the splint just inferior to the knee on the medial side of the leg, pass it under the heel, and then up along the lateral side of the leg in a symmetrical fashion. If the splint is too long, simply fold it back on itself, away from the leg, at its lateral end. Carefully avoid making fingerprint indentations in the splint.

Caution: **When using a prefabricated splint, remember to place the padded side of the splint against the patient's skin.**

5. Secure the splint using an ACE bandage or Coban wrap, starting at the foot and working to the knee.

continued

6. Gently mold the splint around the medial and lateral aspects of the lower leg, ankle, and foot.

7. Perform a post-application splint assessment.

Note: An *upper arm* sugar tong splint is constructed in a similar manner, but it starts at the proximal medial upper arm, passes under the elbow, and extends to the distal lateral aspect of the upper arm. It requires a 3- × 30-inch splint and additional padding over the medial and lateral epicondyles. If properly applied, it provides good stabilization (and some traction) of the upper arm while allowing for some pronation/supination and full range of motion of the wrist and hand. It is often used for initial stabilization of humeral fractures.

Note: A *lower arm (forearm, short-arm)* sugar tong splint is constructed in a similar manner, but it starts at the volar wrist, passes around the elbow, and extends to the volar wrist. It requires two or three rolls of 2- or 3-inch cast padding, a 3- × 30-inch splint, and additional padding over the bony prominences, especially at the medial and lateral epicondyles. If properly applied, it provides good stabilization of the forearm while allowing full range of motion of the fingers and shoulder. It is often used for initial stabilization of mid- or proximal forearm fractures.

FOLLOW-UP CARE AND INSTRUCTIONS

EVALUATION AFTER CASTING

- Perform a careful assessment of the cast or splint before sending the patient out of the casting area.

- Make sure that the cast or splint extends to the proper boundaries, yet does not interfere with the range of motion of necessary joints.

- Check for finger indentations and sharp edges. Using the cast saw or bandage scissors, trim back the cast and repad or recast if necessary.

- Be sure to ask the patient how the cast feels, allowing a few minutes so he or she can determine whether there are areas of increased pressure or sharp edges. If this step is neglected, an unhappy patient will return hours later for cast modification.

CAST AFTERCARE

- For upper extremity casts and splints, a sling provides elevation (to reduce swelling) and support (for comfort). When issued a sling, the patient should be instructed to briefly remove it three to four times each day to perform shoulder and elbow range-of-motion exercises to help prevent excessive stiffness and loss of function.

- A cast boot is usually applied to protect a short-leg cast. Most lower extremity casts initially are non–weight bearing until healing progresses over the following days or weeks.

- Provide the patient with crutches, a walker, or another assistive device, if needed, along with complete instructions.

- Advise the patient to avoid getting the cast wet. A wet cast leads to cast breakdown and skin maceration. Before showering, a towel should be wrapped around the top of the cast, followed by a plastic bag that is tightly secured over the cast with tape. Tell the patient that a hairdryer may be used to dry a fiberglass cast and its padding, if needed. If minimally damaged, a plaster cast can be reinforced with additional casting material. More extensive damage may necessitate cast removal and reapplication.

- Instruct the patient not to insert any objects under the cast in an attempt to relieve itching.

- Instruct the patient to return for a cast or splint check in 3 to 7 days. A splint may be replaced with a cast at this time.

- Instruct patient to notify you promptly of any numbness, tingling, weakness, skin lesions or discolorations, or, most important, increasing pain in the immobilized extremity.

Cast Removal

- Inform the patient that an oscillating cast saw (Fig. 21-15) is designed to cut rigid cast material, but not padding, stockinette, or underlying skin. The clinician may demonstrate to the patient that the saw does not cut skin by gently touching the oscillating saw to the fleshy part of his or her hand.

- Sawing over bony prominences, however, should be avoided because skin injuries can potentially occur in these locations. A long strip of rigid plastic is sometimes used to slip inside the cast to form a barrier between the saw blade and the patient's skin. This is especially useful

Figure 21-15. Oscillating cast saw.

when removing a cast from an especially anxious patient. If this device is not available, a wooden tongue depressor can be used to protect the skin at either end of the cast.

- When sawing, the saw blade should be firmly pressed against the cast at a 90-degree angle until it can be felt to completely pass through the cast shell. It should then be lifted out, moved to an adjacent spot, and the process repeated. This vertical "in-and-out" sawing motion minimizes the heat generated by the cast saw and minimizes the potential for skin burns or abrasions that frequently occur when the saw is improperly angled and dragged or pulled along the cast.

- If the cast saw becomes too hot, turn it off until it sufficiently cools. Don't risk burning the patient.

- The cast should be cut down both sides. A special instrument known as a cast spreader is then used to further widen the cut until the two cast shells can be separated and removed. A bandage scissors is then used to carefully cut off the underlying cast padding and stockinette.

Cast Window

Occasionally a window-like opening must be cut into an existing cast, or incorporated into a new cast, to provide access for wound care or for removal of a foreign object. The cast window must be large enough to accomplish its purpose, yet not so large that it leads to window edema, compromises the structural integrity of the cast, or compromises fracture immobilization. Generally, a cast window for wound care should be no more than $\frac{1}{2}$ to 1 inch larger than the underlying wound.

Bibliography

Bucholtz RW, Kasser JR, Heckman JD, Beaty JH (eds): Rockwood, Green, and Wilkins' Fractures, 5th ed. Philadelphia, Lippincott Williams & Wilkins, 2001.

Hart J: Cast window. Body Cast. Accessed July 28, 2005. Available at: http://www.pappin.com/csot/summer_2004a.html

Hutchinson MR, Ireland ML: Chronic exertional compartment syndrome: Gauging pressure. Phys Sportsmed 27:101-102, 1999.

Mercier LR: Practical Orthopedics, 5th ed. St. Louis, Mosby, 2000.

Swain R, Ross D: Lower extremity compartment syndrome. When to suspect acute or chronic pressure buildup. Postgrad Med 105:159-162, 165, 168, 1999.

Chapter 22

Local Anesthesia

Michelle DiBaise

PROCEDURE GOALS AND OBJECTIVES

Goal: To perform local anesthesia successfully while observing standard precautions and with the minimal degree of risk to the patient.

Objectives: The student will be able to ...

- Describe the essential anatomy and physiology associated with administering local anesthesia.

- Describe the indications, contraindications, and rationale for administering local anesthesia.

- Identify and describe common complications associated with administering local anesthesia.

- Identify the materials necessary for the administration of local anesthesia and their proper use.

- Identify the important aspects of care after administration of local anesthesia.

BACKGROUND AND HISTORY

Local anesthesia provides reversible blockade of nerves, leading to loss of sensation of pain. Topical application and direct infiltration anesthetizes the immediate area. Regional blocks are designed to anesthetize larger areas via a nerve or field block. Local anesthesia is used for a variety of reasons, including but not limited to elimination of pain so that the following can be carried out: repair of lacerations, skin surgery, treatment of painful oral or genital lesions, and the removal of superficial lesions by chemical or physical means.

Nearly painless anesthesia may be achieved in wound repair or skin surgery when the location, surface area involved, and estimated length of time for the procedure are considered. A patient's emotional response is also critical in ensuring nearly painless anesthesia, as most patients fear that the injection will be painful. Throughout this chapter, a combination of certain anesthetics and procedural techniques are discussed that can help lessen the patient's pain and anxiety.

REVIEW OF ESSENTIAL ANATOMY AND PHYSIOLOGY

Local anesthetics act to block the conduction of nerve impulses by selectively binding to voltage-dependent sodium channels. The vast majority of local anesthetics may be divided into two main categories: esters and amides. Local anesthetics contain a hydrophobic and a hydrophilic end joined together by an ester or amide linkage (Strichartz, 1998; Page, 1997). The hydrophilic portion allows the anesthetic to be water soluble so that it can be injected in solution and diffuse to the nerves requiring blockade. The hydrophobic portion allows the anesthetic to be lipid soluble and enter the neuronal membrane. It is the hydrophilic end that subsequently binds to the voltage-dependent sodium channel. The ester anesthetics include benzocaine (e.g., Anbesol), cocaine, procaine (Novocain), and tetracaine (Cetacaine, Pontocaine). The amide anesthetics include lidocaine (e.g., ELA-Max, Xylocaine), mepivacaine (Carbocaine), bupivacaine (Marcaine), dibucaine (Nupercaine), and prilocaine (EMLA, Citanest) (Table 22-1).

When proper concentrations of anesthetic are used, the conduction of action potentials is blocked. This effect is reversible and nonspecific. Once anesthetics are absorbed by the local circulation and metabolized or excreted, nerve function returns to normal. Because local anesthetics are nonspecific, they can act on all sensory nerves, depending on the dose administered. A number of factors affect the rate of onset, intensity, and duration of sensory nerve anesthesia. After reading this section and reviewing the multiple variables that affect the quality of local anesthesia, it can be understood that sensory nerve impulses are lost in the order of temperature sensation, pain, touch, deep pressure, and, finally, motor.

Table 22.1	**Drugs for Local Anesthesia**						
	DRUG CLASS	TRADE NAME	CONCENTRATION AVAILABLE (%)	ONSET OF LOCAL	ONSET OF NERVE BLOCK	DURATION	MAXIMAL DOSE	MAXIMAL DOSE WITH EPINEPHRINE
TOPICAL AGENTS								
Benzocaine	Ester	Anbesol		Rapid		Short		
Cocaine	Ester		2-11.8	2-10 min		45-180 min	3 mg/kg	
Tetracaine	Ester	Cetacaine	0.25, 0.5, 1.0	Rapid		Short		
Proparacaine	Ester	Ophthaine		Rapid		Short		
Dibucaine	Amide	Nupercaine		Rapid		Short		
Lidocaine	Amide	ELA-Max/ LAT/TLE	4.0-5.0	5-30 min		20-60 min	2-5 mL of mixture	
Prilocaine + lidocaine	Amide	EMLA	50/50	30-120 min		20-60 min	2-5 mL of mixture	
INJECTABLE AGENTS								
Lidocaine	Amide	Xylocaine	0.5, 1, 2	Rapid	4-10 min	20-120 min*	4.5 mg/kg of 1%	7 mg/kg of 1%
Mepivacaine	Amide	Carbocaine	1, 2	1-3 min	6-10 min	30-180 min	4.5 mg/kg of 1%	5.5 mg/kg of 1%
Prilocaine	Amide	Citanest	1, 2, 3	2-6 min		90-240 min	5.5 mg/kg of 1%	8.5 mg/kg of 1%
Bupivacaine	Amide	Marcaine	0.25, 0.5, 0.75	3-10 min	8-12 min	120-480 min	2 mg/kg of 0.25%	3.5 mg/kg of 0.25%
Procaine	Ester	Novocain	0.5, 1, 2	5 min		60-90 min	7 mg/kg	7 mg/kg
Tetracaine	Ester	Pontocaine	0.1, 0.25	7 min		120-180 min	0.3-1.4 mg/kg	8.5 mg/kg

*Epinephrine added to lidocaine doubles the duration of action.

Rate of Conduction

Local anesthetics are much more likely to bind to sodium channels that have rapid action potentials (such as those that carry pain impulses) than those with slower action potentials.

Presence of Myelin

Unmyelinated nerve fibers (such as C-type pain and temperature fibers) are more easily blocked by local anesthetics because they are smaller in diameter and lack the lipid barrier of the myelin sheath. Pressure, touch, and motor conduction are transmitted by larger diameter, A-type myelinated fibers. The lipophilic local anesthetics become bound by the highly lipid myelin sheath, which slows the amount of drug at the node, leading to slower onset but longer duration.

Nerve Fiber Diameter

Larger doses of drug are needed to anesthetize larger nerve trunks, such as digital nerves, and the onset of action is slower.

Vascularity of the Location Anesthetized

In highly vascular areas, drug is rapidly removed from the area that requires anesthesia, leading to the need for more drug or a vasoconstricting agent. A shorter duration of action also results. All the local anesthetics are vasodilatory in nature, except cocaine, which is a vasoconstrictor.

Use of Epinephrine

Adding a vasoconstricting agent such as epinephrine decreases blood flow, reduces systemic absorption, shortens onset, and extends duration of action. Epinephrine tends to be more effective with the less lipid-soluble agents (lidocaine and mepivacaine) than with the more lipid-soluble agents (bupivacaine) (Strichartz, 1998; Gage, 1997). As a general rule, the use of epinephrine doubles the duration of anesthesia achieved with lidocaine (Gonzalez del Rey, 1997). Caution must be exercised in using vasoconstrictive agents in regions of the body supplied by a single vascular source, because tissue necrosis may result.

ANESTHETIC SOLUTION AND TISSUE pH

Most anesthetic solutions are acidic in order to maintain their stability or shelf life. Once injected, however, they equilibrate to the pH of normal tissues. This leads to the sensation of burning on injection. Buffering the anesthetic solution with sodium bicarbonate can effectively eliminate this undesirable side effect. Although buffering decreases the onset of action and increases the effectiveness of the blockade, it decreases the shelf life. Plain lidocaine buffered with bicarbonate has a shelf life of approximately 7 days (Usatine, 1998; Gonzalez del Rey, 1997). In addition, buffering can degrade epinephrine if it is kept in a container exposed to light (Gonzalez del Rey, 1997). It is unknown what the shelf lives of buffered mepivacaine and bupivacaine are because studies have not been performed.

Because anesthetic solutions work best at physiologic pH, they are less effective in infected tissues than in normal tissues because of the resultant metabolic acidosis, which decreases pH (Strichartz, 1998).

METHOD AND TECHNIQUE OF INJECTION

The nerve fibers are present at the junction of the dermis and the subcutaneous fat. Direct infiltration of an open wound at this level provides immediate blockade (Gonzalez del Rey, 1997). Direct infiltration of intact skin, if started at the junction of the dermis and the subcutaneous fat, also provides immediate and nearly painless anesthesia. If the injection is started higher in the epidermis or at the dermal-epidermal junction, the blockade is slightly slower and more painful. Digital nerve block is slower in onset because of the larger nerve fibers. Technique is important because placement of anesthetic immediately adjacent to a digital nerve can lead to blockade within minutes, whereas delivery that is further from the nerve trunk can delay onset and can lead to inadequate blockade and the possible need for repeat injections.

CONCENTRATION OF SOLUTION

Solutions of higher concentration may lead to a slightly shorter onset of action when compared with solutions of lower concentration, but this difference is not markedly significant. For example, adding epinephrine to 1% lidocaine achieves the same effect as using 2% lidocaine (Gonzalez del Rey, 1997).

TOTAL DOSE PROVIDED

Increasing the dose leads to more effective blockade; however, too much can lead to side effects. Maximal doses of anesthetic solutions are provided in Table 22-1.

RATE OF METABOLISM

The ester anesthetics undergo metabolism first by being hydrolyzed by plasma cholinesterases and liver esterases and then being excreted by the kidneys (Hruza, 1999; Strichartz, 1998). They tend to have a shorter half-life than the amide anesthetics (Strichartz, 1998). Amide anesthetics are metabolized by first being *N*-dealkylated and then being hydrolyzed by the liver's endoplasmic reticulum. Because bupivacaine is highly bound to plasma proteins and tissue at the injection site, it is more likely to cause side effects in patients with severe liver disease (Strichartz, 1998). This is because of reduced liver metabolism and a decreased concentration of plasma proteins, which are made in the liver.

INDICATIONS

Local anesthesia in any procedure can be confined to one area of the body in which pain or discomfort associated with the procedure can be anticipated. The most common indication is in minor surgical procedures, including repair of lacerations, incision and drainage of abscesses, removal of lesions, biopsies, and nail removal.

CONTRAINDICATIONS

TOPICAL ANESTHETICS

- Cocaine-containing products are occasionally used to anesthetize adult nasal mucosa; however, contact with these agents should be avoided in infants and neonates. Unless used by a provider skilled in the use of cocaine-containing products on the nasal mucosa, these products should not be administered on the conjunctiva or nasal or oral mucosa. There is a case report of an infant death associated with the use of a cocaine-containing solution that accidentally came into contact with the nasal and oral mucosa (Dailey, 1988). Cocaine-containing products should also not be administered on the fingers, toes, penis, nose, and pinna of the ear because of their vasoconstricting properties.

- There are a few relative contraindications to the use of non–cocaine-containing topical anesthetics in premature infants. Studies are mixed concerning the possibility of the development of methemoglobinemia in premature infants who were given a topical eutectic mixture of lidocaine anesthetics (EMLA), but overall EMLA appears to be safe and effective in most infants and children (Frey, 1999; Essink-Tjebbes, 1999).

LOCAL ANESTHETICS

Listed contraindications to the use of local anesthetics include the following:
- Severely unstable blood pressure

- True allergy

- Severe liver disease when amide anesthetics are being considered

- Severe renal disease when ester anesthetics are being considered (esters are renally excreted) and mental instability (which might mask the symptoms of adverse effects of lidocaine) (Hruza, 1999; Gonzalez del Rey, 1997).

EPINEPHRINE

Absolute contraindications to the use of epinephrine include the following:
- Untreated hyperthyroidism or untreated pheochromocytoma

- Administration to locations of the body that have a single, dependent blood supply—such as the fingers, toes, penis, nose, and pinna of the ear—or for use in a digital block

Relative contraindications to the use of epinephrine include the following:
- Untreated hypertension

- Severe coronary artery or peripheral vascular disease

- Pregnancy

- Narrow-angle glaucoma

- Use in patients taking β-blockers, phenothiazines, monoamine oxidase (MAO) inhibitors, or tricyclic antidepressants

Epinephrine should be used cautiously in patients with relative contraindications by diluting the epinephrine in half or using it sparingly, or determining not to use it at all.

POTENTIAL COMPLICATIONS

The most common complication seen with injection of anesthesia follows:
- Development of anxiety over the impending injection and a subsequent vasovagal reaction demonstrated by hypotension, bradycardia, and syncope (Hruza, 1999; Gonzalez del Rey, 1997)

Local complications of injection are not as common and include the following:
- Bruising

- Edema

- Infection

■ Prolonged or permanent nerve damage

■ Temporary motor nerve paralysis (Hruza, 1999; Gonzalez del Rey, 1997)

Systemic complications are uncommon; when they occur it is usually because anesthetic is inadvertently injected into a vessel. This complication can be avoided by making sure that blood cannot be aspirated before injecting the anesthetic. Systemic reactions include the following:

■ Hypotension

■ Bradycardia

■ Central nervous system depression or stimulation, leading to slurred speech, drowsiness, disorientation, tremor, restlessness, weakness, seizures, paralysis, coma, respiratory failure, and cardiac dysrhythmias

This last complication is more common with bupivacaine than with the other anesthetics. Prilocaine in large doses can lead to methemoglobinemia (Hruza, 1999).

Epinephrine can lead to a number of side effects such as the following:

■ Cardiac dysrhythmias

■ Increased blood pressure

■ Anxiety

■ Cardiac arrest

■ Cerebral hemorrhage

■ Ischemia if used in areas of end artery flow such as the digits, penis, nose, and pinna of the ear, leading to skin necrosis, especially in patients with poor circulation

Treatment of complications tends to be supportive. The patient should be placed in the Trendelenburg position, which usually reverses hypotension and bradycardia (Hruza, 1999; Gonzalez del Rey, 1997). If hypotension continues, an intravenous infusion of normal saline can be started, an airway maintained, supplemental oxygen administered, and cardiac monitoring with frequent vital signs begun (Gonzalez del Rey, 1997). Seizures are generally controlled by administration of intravenous diazepam (Valium).

Benzocaine is a para-aminobenzoic acid (PABA) derivative that has a tendency to cause allergic contact dermatitis. The literature cites that patients sensitive to benzocaine may also be sensitive to thiazide diuretics, sulfonylureas, sulfonamides, paraphenylenediamine, and para-aminobenzoic acid–based preparations. Because benzocaine is an ester anesthetic, patients hypersensitive to this agent may also be sensitive to other ester anesthetics such as procaine (Novocain), which is rarely used because of the rate of true allergic reactions, and tetracaine, but they will not be sensitive to the amide anesthetics.

True allergic reactions are rare among amide anesthetics but are more frequent with the older ester anesthetics. Allergic reactions may be caused by the preservative methylparaben or bisulfites, which are used in multiple-dose vials. True allergy is characterized by a skin rash, localized or general urticaria, angioedema, and, rarely, anaphylaxis with hypotension and bradycardia. Only 1% of all patients receiving local anesthesia demonstrate a true allergic response (Gonzalez del Rey, 1997).

Allergic reactions are managed with airway management and administration of supplemental oxygen, intravenous access, and administration of epinephrine, diphenhydramine, and corticosteroids as needed (Hruza, 1999, Gonzalez del Rey, 1997).

Assessment of patients with a reported allergy to local anesthetics should include determining the offending anesthetic and substituting it with a different class (i.e., if allergic to an ester, use an amide, and vice versa) or skin test the patient with a preservative-free anesthetic. If the patient has a true anesthetic allergy, Benadryl, normal saline, no anesthetic, or conscious sedation are all accepted alternatives.

Standard Precautions   Practitioners should use standard precautions at all times when interacting with patients. Determining the level of precaution necessary requires the practitioner to exercise clinical judgment based on the patient's history and the potential for exposure to body fluids or aerosol-borne pathogens (for further discussion, see Chapter 2).

PATIENT PREPARATION

Several techniques have been offered to decrease the pain and anxiety that can accompany an injection of anesthetic.

- Because of the way local anesthesia affects the sensory nerve impulses (see "Review of Essential Anatomy and Physiology"), an anxious patient may perceive touch as if it were pain. Therefore, reassuring the patient and explaining the expectations of the procedure are key to ensuring nearly painless anesthesia.

- Because the most common reaction to local anesthesia is a vasovagal response or syncope, the patient needs to be in the supine position, placed so that he or she cannot see the injection being administered.

- Engaging in conversation should distract the patient.

- Inform the patient what is being done at each step.

- Encourage the patient to take deep, slow breaths to avoid hyperventilation.

- Continue to reassure the patient throughout the procedure of injection.

- For anxious patients or children, conscious sedation with a benzodiazepine may be necessary; however, detailing its use is beyond the scope of this chapter.

- Use cryoanesthetic, such as ice, ethyl chloride, tetrafluoroethane (Medi-Frig), fluoroethyl (25% ethyl chloride, 75% dichlorotetrafluoroethane), or liquid nitrogen before an injection. This technique can also be used for anesthesia before curettage of superficial lesions as described in Chapter 24. Cryoanesthetics provide short periods of decreased pain sensation. For purposes of anesthesia before injection, liquid nitrogen is not preferred because it can be painful and may lead to unwanted tissue destruction.

■ Warming the local anesthetic has not been known to reduce the pain of anesthetic injection significantly and requires time and effort to warm the vial or syringe to 37° C to 40° C and then rapidly inject the anesthetic before it cools (Gonzalez del Rey, 1997).

Materials Utilized for Administering Anesthetics

Topical Anesthesia

Note: There are a number of benefits to topical anesthesia compared with injection and include lack of injection (therefore, no discomfort), ease of administration, decreased need for physical restraints, and no distortion of the anatomy. Topical anesthesia tends to work better on the highly vascular face and scalp than on the trunk or proximal extremities (Gonzalez del Rey, 1997; Trott, 1997). When using topical anesthesia for wound closure, it should be limited to lacerations of 5 cm or less in order to avoid the complication of systemic absorption (Gonzalez del Rey, 1997; Trott, 1997).

Note: Topical anesthetics are divided into amides (lidocaine, prilocaine), esters (benzocaine, tetracaine), and nonamides, nonesters (dimethisoquin, dyclonine, pramoxine). Each specialty tends to have one topical anesthetic that is preferred over others. Anesthesia of the conjunctiva can be accomplished by the use of proparacaine or tetracaine eye drops (Hruza, 1999). Topical benzocaine is commonly added as an agent for sunburn relief. It is, however, a common contact sensitizer and should generally be avoided. Anesthetics available for use on the superficial mucous membranes include dyclonine (Dyclone), benzocaine (Anbesol and others), tetracaine (Cetacaine), viscous lidocaine, and lidocaine jelly. Deeper anesthesia of the mucous membranes can be accomplished with a 4% to 10% solution of cocaine. Cocaine-containing products increase the cost of the anesthetic and need to be stored and disposed of under strict protocols. Cocaine-containing products also may be used to anesthetize lacerations. Examples of cocaine-containing products include:

■ TAC: tetracaine 0.5%, epinephrine 1:2000, cocaine 11.8%

■ TAC, ½ strength: tetracaine 1%, epinephrine 1:2000, cocaine 4%

■ *or* tetracaine 0.25%, epinephrine 1:4000, cocaine 5.9%

Other topical agents without cocaine used for wound repair include:
■ LAT: lidocaine 4%, epinephrine 1:2000, tetracaine 1%

- TLE: lidocaine 5%, epinephrine 1:2000

Note: All these products can be prepared by a pharmacist as a liquid or gel; however, although gels decrease the risk of mucosal exposure, they may also decrease the amount of total dose delivered (Usatine, 1998; Gonzalez del Rey, 1997). Some authors have stated that TAC/LAT/TLE combinations provide inconsistent anesthesia for lacerations on the extremities, leading to the need for supplemental anesthetic injection (Gonzalez del Rey, 1997).

 Note: For intact skin, superficial anesthesia can be achieved with EMLA (eutectic mixture of lidocaine anesthetics) or ELA-Max (4% lidocaine). EMLA is 50% lidocaine and 50% prilocaine in an acid-mantle cream. Neither cream should be used on mucous membranes or conjunctiva because of the risk of greater absorption leading to potential systemic side effects.

- Other equipment

    - Cotton-tipped applicators or gauze pads

    - Materials to clean the wound or anesthesia site

Injection Anesthesia

The most commonly used agents follow:

- Lidocaine (Xylocaine 1% and 2%, with and without epinephrine)

    - Rapid onset of action

    - Readily penetrates nerve sheaths, leading to an almost immediate anesthesia with local infiltration

    - For direct wound infiltration, the duration of action is approximately 20 to 30 minutes and is approximately 60 to 120 minutes for nerve blocks

Caution: There is a subset of patients who metabolize lidocaine quickly and require repeat injections.

 Note: The use of epinephrine with lidocaine increases the duration of action and improves local hemostasis.

    - Method of buffering lidocaine: 1 mL of bicarbonate + 9 mL of 1% lidocaine

Note: Buffering of 2% solutions may cause precipitation.

 Note: The shelf-life of buffered lidocaine is 7 days.

- Mepivacaine (Carbocaine 1% and 2%)

    - Slightly longer onset of action with direct infiltration (6 to 10 minutes), but the duration of action is longer, approximately 30 to 60 minutes

    - Does not cause as much vasodilation as lidocaine; therefore, does not require epinephrine for hemostasis

    - Method of buffering mepivacaine: 0.5 to 1 mL of bicarbonate + 9 mL of mepivacaine

    - Shelf life unknown; therefore, do not use after 24 hours

■ Bupivacaine (Marcaine 0.25% and 0.5%)

■ Slow onset of action (8 to 12 minutes) with direct infiltration, but the duration of action is much longer than with either lidocaine or mepivacaine. It lasts approximately four times longer than lidocaine, offering significant postsurgical relief from pain.

■ Method of buffering bupivacaine: 0.1 mL of bicarbonate + 20 mL of bupivacaine

Note: The shelf life is unknown; therefore, do not use after 24 hours.

■ Diphenhydramine (Benadryl)

■ For allergic reaction to amide or ester anesthetics, or both, alternatives include Benadryl and normal saline or no anesthesia.

■ Provide adequate anesthesia for at least 30 minutes.

■ Benadryl should be diluted to 12.5 mg/mL with normal saline.

Note: The technique for direct infiltration with Benadryl is the same as with other anesthetics. Benadryl, however, is more painful to inject than lidocaine and is not reduced by buffering.

■ Other equipment

■ Materials to clean the site or wound

■ Materials to ensure sterile technique

■ 27- or 30-gauge needle $\frac{1}{2}$- to $\frac{1}{4}$-inch length

■ A syringe, size dependent on the quantity of anesthetic to be injected

■ The injectable anesthetic

Procedure for Using Topical Anesthesia

1. For intact skin, achieve superficial anesthesia with EMLA (50% lidocaine and 50% prilocaine in an acid-mantle cream) or ELA-Max (4% lidocaine).

Note: Neither cream should be used on mucous membranes or conjunctivae because of the risk of greater absorption leading to potential systemic side effects. Young children should be watched closely to avoid accidental ingestion.

2. When applying ELA-Max, do not keep on skin for more than 2 hours at a time.

Note: Anesthesia with EMLA and ELA-Max works best for removal of superficial skin lesions, for some laser procedures, and before injection of anesthetic. With both creams, the depth of anesthesia is directly proportional to the duration of application and lasts for several hours. ELA-Max appears to have a more rapid onset of action than does EMLA. Neither cream appears to cause irritating effects or hypersensitivity reactions with repeated or prolonged use.

3. Gently remove blood clots from the area.

4. For wound repair, saturate a gauze sponge or cotton swab with anesthetic.

5. Fold the anesthetic-saturated sponge into and around the wound and tape into place.

6. Have the parent or assistant (or yourself) apply constant, gentle pressure for 15 to 20 minutes.

Note: The person applying pressure should wear gloves in order to avoid absorption.

   Note: Anesthesia is complete when blanching is observed around the wound. One report stated that about 5% of wounds require supplemental injection of local anesthetic to achieve complete anesthesia. Studies have also shown that about 2 to 3 mL of topical anesthetic is sufficient to provide anesthesia for most wound repairs (Gonzalez del Rey, 1997).

7. If administering EMLA or ELA-Max, cover the area requiring treatment with a $\frac{1}{4}$-inch-thick layer of cream.

Note: EMLA is then occluded with a plastic adhesive dressing 1 hour before the procedure. ELA-Max does not require occlusion, although this may be performed.

8. Remove both creams before the start of the procedure.

Procedure for Administering Local Anesthetic by Injection

Note: Nearly painless anesthesia is more likely with the use of a 27- or 30-gauge needle. This occurs not only because the caliber of the needle is smaller but also because it decreases the speed with which anesthetic is injected. Rapid tissue expansion is more uncomfortable for the patient, so the provider should aim for a slow injection technique, which will be facilitated by selecting a 1- to 3-mL syringe.

   Note: Needle length varies from $\frac{1}{2}$ to $1\frac{1}{4}$ inch. The shorter length is adequate for small punch biopsies, whereas longer needles are better for larger excisions, wound infiltration, and field and digital blocks.

Direct Infiltration of Wounds

1. Initiate the injection on the side where sensory innervation originates and then proceed distally.

Note: Direct wound infiltration is recommended in most minimally contaminated wounds. The injection should be located between the dermis and the subcutaneous fat. Tissue resistance is less and the sensory nerves are rapidly affected by the anesthetic at this level.

2. Once the needle is inserted, aspirate to ensure that the needle is not in a vessel. If no blood is withdrawn, inject a small amount of anesthetic.

3. Reposition the needle adjacent to, but still within, the area where anesthetic was placed.

4. Aspirate and proceed to inject if no blood is withdrawn.

5. Continue to repeat the preceding steps until all edges of the wound are anesthetized.

6. If at any time bloody aspirate is obtained, withdraw the needle slightly and aspirate until clear. A 3- to 4-cm laceration should

continued

FIGURE 22-1.

require about 3 to 5 mL of anesthetic (Hruza, 1999; Gonzalez del Rey, 1997) (Fig. 22-1).

Local Infiltration of Intact Skin

1. Clean the intended procedure site with an alcohol wipe or alternative antiseptic.

2. Pinch the skin in the vicinity of the injection site. This decreases the sensation of pain from the injection.

3. Infiltrate at the junction of the dermis and subcutaneous fat and then reposition the needle to the level of the epidermis and inject a small amount of anesthetic.

Note: Always remember to aspirate before injection. For punch biopsies, only 1 to 2 mL of anesthetic is generally required.

Field Block

Note: Field block is an alternative to direct wound infiltration when a larger area requires treatment or, in wounds that are grossly contaminated, to avoid bacterial spread. It has the advantage of fewer injections than direct wound infiltration.

1. Start the injection in the same plane as described in local infiltration of intact skin; however, a larger bore (25- to 27-gauge), 1¼- to 2-inch needle is required.

2. Insert the needle into the skin and advance to the hub parallel to the dermis and subcutaneous fat. After aspiration, a slow injection of anesthetic is left as the needle is withdrawn to the insertion site.

3. Reinsert the needle at the end of the first track and repeat the procedure until a wall of anesthesia surrounds the area to be treated (Usatine, 1998; Gonzalez del Rey, 1997) (Fig. 22-2).

FIGURE 22-2. (Adapted from Pfenninger JL, Fowler JC: Procedures for Primary Care Physicians. St. Louis, Mosby–Year Book, 1994, p 147.)

Digital Block

Note: 1% lidocaine or 1% mepivacaine without epinephrine, with or without bicarbonate, and 2% lidocaine without epinephrine or bicarbonate are commonly used for digital blocks (Strichartz, 1998; Page, 1997; Gage, 1997). Lidocaine with bupivacaine is an alternative. Bupivacaine's onset of action is too slow to use alone. It does accord longer duration of action for extended procedures as well as significant postoperative relief of discomfort for the patient.

   Note: A digital block is generally recommended for procedures distal to the midproximal phalanx of the digit and is preferred for nail avulsion, paronychial drainage, and repair of lacerations of the digits.

1. A digital nerve block is accomplished by injecting anesthetic just distal to the web space in the middle of the digit.

2. After aspirating, inject 0.1 mL of anesthetic locally into the epidermis.

3. Advance the needle to the bone, withdraw slightly, and then move dorsally, where 0.5 mL of anesthetic is injected after aspiration.

4. Withdraw the needle again to the midline, advance to bone, and move ventrally where another 0.5 to 1 mL of anesthetic is injected after aspiration.

5. Withdraw the needle and repeat the whole procedure on the other side of the digit (Fig. 22-3).

Note: Larger volumes of anesthetic are not required if injected near the nerve. The needle should always be withdrawn between dorsal and ventral injections to avoid nerve and vessel damage. Anesthesia is reported to occur anywhere from 4 to 20 minutes after injection, depending on the anesthetic and technique used.

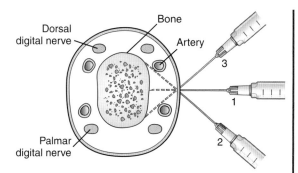

FIGURE 22-3. (Adapted from Pfenninger JL, Fowler JC: Procedures for Primary Care Physicians. St. Louis, Mosby–Year Book, 1994, p 149.)

   Note: There are alternatives to the method described for performing a digital block.

Alternatives to Performing a Digital Block

1. Since the second to fifth toes are small, one technique uses a dorsal midline injection. Anesthetic is then deposited on one side of the toe.

2. Withdraw the needle and move to the opposite side without completely withdrawing the needle from the skin (Gonzalez del Rey, 1997).

Caution: This technique is not recommended for the great toe.
   Note: For surgery on the distal nail unit, periungual administration may be performed. It is essentially a field block technique of the nail unit (see Chapter 28). It is more painful than a digital block but is more rapid in onset.

1. It is completed by injecting first along one lateral nail fold, then perpendicularly along the proximal nail fold, and then along the opposite lateral nail fold. Lastly, anesthetic is administered in the hyponychial area (Gonzalez del Rey, 1997).

continued

2. Another alternative is to inject at a 30-degree angle into the middle of the proximal nail fold, where the needle is then advanced distally under the nail matrix.

3. After aspiration, inject anesthetic as the needle pierces the nail plate, the nail matrix, and the nail bed.

Note: The nail matrix and nail bed will blanch with injection of anesthetic. It is painful, but anesthesia is immediate. This type of anesthesia can be used for most procedures performed on the proximal half of the nail unit, but not for removal of the nail matrix or complete nail avulsion (Gonzalez del Rey, 1997).

Note: Other digital blocks used include supraorbital, supratrochlear, infraorbital, mental, auricular, median, ulnar, radial, sural, and tibial. These are used for procedures or repair of lacerations covering a large surface area; however, their description is beyond the scope of this book.

FOLLOW-UP CARE AND INSTRUCTIONS

Complications from local anesthesia are uncommon. Occasionally a patient exhibits sensitivity to a component of the anesthetic, which may later present as a rash or inflammatory reaction.

■ Instruct the patient to notify the office if there is any unusual skin color, itching, or pain in the area where the anesthetic was injected, or if sensation does not return promptly after the anesthesia was to have worn off.

REFERENCES

Dailey RH: Fatality secondary to misuse of TAC solution. Ann Emerg Med 17:159-160, 1988.

Essink-Tjebbes CM, Hekster YA, Liem KD, et al: Topical use of local anesthetics in neonates. Pharm World Sci 21:173-176, 1999.

Frey B, Kehrer B: Toxic methaemoglobin concentrations in premature infants after application of a prilocaine-containing cream and peridural prilocaine. Eur J Pediatr 158:785-788, 1999.

Gage TW: Drugs in dentistry. In Page CP, Curtis MJ, Sutter MC, et al (eds): Integrated Pharmacology. St. Louis, CV Mosby, 1997, pp 383-398.

Gonzalez del Rey JA, DiGiulo GA: Wound care and the pediatric patient. In Trott AT (ed): Wounds and Lacerations: Emergency Care and Closure, 2nd ed. St. Louis, CV Mosby, 1997, pp 38-52.

Hruza GJ: Dermatologic surgery: Introduction and approach. In Fitzpatrick TB, Eisen AZ, Wolff K, et al (eds): Dermatology in General Medicine, 5th ed. New York, McGraw-Hill, 1999, pp 2923-2937.

Page CP, Curtis MJ, Sutter MC, et al: General principles of drug action. In Page CP, Curtis MJ, Sutter MC, et al (eds): Integrated Pharmacology. St. Louis, CV Mosby, 1997, pp 17-52.

Strichartz GR: Drugs affecting peripheral transmission: Local anesthetics. In Brody TM, Larner J, Minneman KP (eds): Human Pharmacology: Molecular to Clinical, 3rd ed. St. Louis, CV Mosby, 1998, pp 151-156.

Trott AT: Infiltration and nerve block anesthesia. In Trott AT (ed): Wounds and Lacerations, 2nd ed. St. Louis, CV Mosby, 1997, pp 53-89.

Usatine RP, Moy RL: Anesthesia. In Usatine RP, Moy RL, Tobinick EL, et al (eds): Skin Surgery: A Practical Guide. St Louis, CV Mosby, 1998, pp 20-30.

BIBLIOGRAPHY

Fine JD, Arndt KA: Medical dermatologic therapy. In Orkin M, Maibach HI, Dahl MV (eds): Dermatology. Norwalk, Conn, Appleton & Lange, 1991, pp 635-656.

Kechijian P: Nail surgery. In Fitzpatrick TB, Eisen AZ, Wolff K, et al (eds): Dermatology in General Medicine, 5th ed. New York, McGraw-Hill, 1999, pp 2992-3002.

Kongsiri AS, Ciesielski-Carlucci C, Stiller MJ: Topical nonglucocorticoid therapy. In Fitzpatrick TB, Eisen AZ, Wolff K, et al (eds): Dermatology in General Medicine, 5th ed. New York, McGraw-Hill, 1999, pp 2717-2726.

Ries CR, Sutter FM, Sutter MC: Drugs used in surgery. In Page CP, Curtis MJ, Sutter MC, et al (eds): Integrated Pharmacology. St. Louis, CV Mosby, 1997, pp 399-410.

Roenigk HH: Dermatologic surgery in dermatology. In Orkin M, Maibach HI, Dahl MV (eds): Dermatology. Norwalk, Conn, Appleton & Lange, 1991, pp 657-662.

Chapter 23

Wound Closure

Karen A. Newell

PROCEDURE GOALS AND OBJECTIVES

Goal: To reapproximate wound edges with sutures, staples, or skin adhesive successfully in order to facilitate wound healing and reduce the likelihood of infection.

Objectives: The student will be able to ...

- Describe the indications, contraindications, and rationale for performing wound closure.

- Identify and describe common complications associated with wound closure.

- Describe the essential anatomy and physiology of the skin associated with the performance of wound closure.

- Identify the materials and tools necessary for performing wound closure and their proper use.

- Identify the important aspects of post-procedure care after wound closure.

BACKGROUND AND HISTORY

Wound closure has been in existence for many years in the practice of medicine. Although wound closure typically is associated with suturing the wound, many materials have been used over time. The word *suture* describes any strand of material used to ligate (tie) blood vessels or approximate (sew) tissues. The first written description of sutures used in operative procedures is recorded in the Edwin Smith Papyrus, the oldest known surgical document. This document has Egyptian origins and dates back to the 16th century BC. Dating as far back as 2000 BC, written references have been found describing the use of strings and animal sinews for suturing.

Rhazes of Arabia was credited in 900 AD with first using kit gut to suture abdominal wounds. The Arabic word *kit* means a dancing master's fiddle. In those days the musical strings of fiddles, called *kit strings,* were made of sheep's intestines. It has been speculated that Rhazes used these to suture. The term *catgut* is thought to have evolved from these origins.

Through the centuries, a wide variety of materials—silk, linen, cotton, horsehair, animal tendons and intestines, and wire made of precious metals—has been used in operative procedures. Some of these materials are still in use today. The evolution of suturing material has brought us to a point of refinement that includes sutures designed for specific surgical procedures. They not only eliminate some of the difficulties the surgeon may have previously encountered during closure but decrease the potential for infection postoperatively. Despite the sophistication of today's suture materials and surgical techniques, closing a wound still involves the same basic procedure used by physicians to the Roman emperors (Ethicon, 1985).

INDICATIONS

Most superficial wounds heal without intervention. However, a superficial skin laceration extending into the subcutaneous tissues should be considered for closure in order to avoid undesirable outcomes. Suture, staple, or skin adhesive closure of wounds may be warranted for the following reasons:

- To decrease the time required for the wound to heal

- To reduce the likelihood of infection

- To decrease the amount of scar tissue likely to form

- To repair the loss of structure or function, or both, of the tissue

- To improve cosmetic appearance

CONTRAINDICATIONS

Before any wound or laceration repair is initiated, a thorough evaluation of the patient must be carried out. Remember that all wounds, no matter how minor they may appear, can be the result of serious injury to underlying structures. The basic history, general physical examination, and wound examination help define the repair strategy and help identify more serious problems that may necessitate specialized care.

Contraindications to suture closure of wounds relate largely to the risk of infection and disruption of underlying structures such as nerves, arteries, and tendons. Wounds that have the following characteristics should be left unclosed, or at least very careful consideration should be given (weighing the pros and cons of closure) before electing to suture the wound:

- Wounds that have a high likelihood of contamination should not be closed with sutures. Doing so may mask a developing underlying infection, thus delaying appropriate treatment. This delayed treatment may result in spread of infection to underlying and surrounding structures, which has the potential to cause considerable morbidity. Classification of the wound helps the clinician to make an informed decision about the appropriateness of closing the wound (see "Review of Essential Anatomy and Physiology").

- Wounds that require suturing to minimize infection and scar potential should be closed within 8 hours of the injury. Some wounds can be closed up to 24 hours after injury if the anatomic location is highly vascular (e.g., face, neck, and scalp) and the cosmetic appearance is an important consideration.

- The presence of foreign bodies in the underlying tissues is a consideration. Foreign bodies may remain a source of repeated infections if not thoroughly removed through irrigation, exploration, and extraction or debridement of devitalized and contaminated tissue.

- Extensive wounds involving tendons, nerves, or arteries should be carefully considered before closure.

POTENTIAL COMPLICATIONS

The primary complications associated with wound closure include the following:

- Infection

- Scarring, including keloid formation

- Loss of function and structure (an example might be scarring of an eyelid repair, resulting in incomplete closure of the eyelids)

- Loss of a cosmetically desirable appearance

- Wound dehiscence (wound margins separate and wound reopens)

- Tetanus

Stratum germinativum

Stratum corneum

Hair follicle

Duct of sweat gland

Body of sweat gland

Blood vessels and nerves

Epidermis

Dermis

Subcutaneous fat

Superficial fascia (subcutaneous fascia)

Deep fascia

Muscle group

Blood vessels

FIGURE 23-1. Anatomy of the skin, illustrating structures pertinent to wound repair. (Redrawn from Trott AT: Wounds and Lacerations: Emergency Care and Closure, 2nd ed. St. Louis, Mosby–Year Book, 1998, p 27.)

REVIEW OF ESSENTIAL ANATOMY AND PHYSIOLOGY

ANATOMY OF THE SKIN AND FASCIA

The epidermis is a thin layer of squamous epithelial cells located on the outermost surface of the skin. This layer is void of blood vessels or nerve endings. The epidermis provides an excellent protective barrier when healthy and intact. The stratum germinativum, or basal layer, is the parent layer for new cells. This layer provides the cells for new epidermis formation during wound healing (Fig. 23-1).

The dermis is much thicker than the epidermis. It is composed largely of connective tissue such as fibroblasts; macrophages, lymphocytes, and mast cells are also present. Some small blood vessels and nerve fiber endings are present at this level.

Deep to the dermis is a layer of loose connective tissue that composes the superficial fascia or subcutaneous tissue. Many blood vessels and nerve endings are located at this level. Subcutaneous fat is present here, and the quantity varies depending on the region of the body. Sensory nerve branches to the skin travel in the superficial fascia just deep to the dermis, which makes it ideal for injecting local anesthetic, because the anesthetic spreads easily along this plane and abolishes sensation in the overlying skin.

The deep fascia is a relatively thick, dense, and discrete fibrous tissue layer. It lies just above muscle, tendon, or bone. If disrupted by the injury, it should be repaired to re-establish the supportive function of this layer. Failure to do so may result in disfiguration of the surrounding area.

SKIN TENSION LINES (LANGER'S LINES)

Skin tension lines, also known as Langer's lines or lines of cleavage, are linear clefts in the skin that indicate the direction of orientation of the underlying collagen fibers. If the skin is disrupted parallel to the long axis of the fibers, the wound tends to reapproximate. However, if the wound crosses the long axis of the fibers perpendicularly, they are disrupted in a manner that causes the wound to gape open; therefore, greater tension is required to close the wound. Lacerations that run parallel to these lines naturally reapproximate the skin edges. Lacerations that run at right angles to the tension lines tend to gape apart. Figure 23-2 illustrates the typical orientation of Langer's lines throughout the body.

Wounds should be classified based on their degree of contamination with bacteria or foreign matter, or both. Timing of the closure is also important to consider. The chance of wound infection developing increases each hour that wound closure is delayed. There is general agreement that wounds less than 6 to 8 hours old that are considered clean are eligible for primary closure with sutures. Highly vascular areas such as the face and scalp can be considered for primary closure with sutures up to 24 hours after the injury. In each case, the clinician must consider the degree of contamination and evaluate each wound individually.

CLASSIFICATION OF WOUNDS

- Clean: incisions made during a surgical procedure in which aseptic techniques were followed, without involvement of the gastrointestinal, respiratory, or genitourinary tract; likelihood of infection is less than 2% and warrants routine primary closure

- Clean-contaminated: similar to clean wounds except that the gastrointestinal, respiratory, or genitourinary tract is involved

- Contaminated: similar to clean and clean-contaminated except there is gross spillage (e.g., bile, stool); traumatic wounds fall into this category

- Infected: established infection before wound is made (e.g., incision and drainage of an abscess) or heavily contaminated wounds (e.g., gross spillage of stool)

FIGURE 23-2. Skin tension lines of the body surface. (Adapted from Trott AT: Wounds and Lacerations: Emergency Care and Closure, 2nd ed. St. Louis, Mosby–Year Book, 1998, p 17.)

Wound Closure Classification

- Primary intention: All layers are closed.
  - Best chance for minimal scarring
  - Usually performed in clean and clean-contaminated wounds
- Secondary intention: The deep layers are closed, whereas superficial layers are left open to granulate on their own from the inside out.
  - Often leaves a wide scar and requires frequent wound care, consisting of irrigation and assorted types of packing and dressings

- Prolonged process

- Reasons for use include excessive tissue loss and infection

- Third intention or delayed primary intention: The deep layers may be closed primarily, whereas the superficial layers are left open until reassessment on day 4 or 5 after initial closure, at which time the wound is inspected for signs of infection.

  - If it looks clean and has begun to granulate, it is irrigated and closed.

  - If it looks as if it may be infected, it is left open to heal by secondary intention.

  - These wounds often arise initially from contaminated wounds.

Standard Precautions   Every practitioner should use standard precautions at all times when interacting with patients, especially when performing procedures. Determining the level of precaution necessary requires the practitioner to exercise clinical judgment based on the patient's history and the potential for exposure to body fluids or aerosol-borne pathogens (for further discussion, see Chapter 2).

PATIENT PREPARATION

- Take the patient's history to denote when, where, and how the injury occurred. Other pertinent information in the history may include handedness, tetanus status, other past or concurrent medical problems (e.g., diabetes mellitus, peripheral vascular diseases, immune status), smoking history, occupation, hobbies, family history, medications, and allergies.

- Begin the physical examination with a meticulous inspection detailing the type of wound, anatomic location, extent of injury, and level of contamination. Bleeding can usually be controlled with direct manual pressure applied to the site with a clean bandage. A careful sensory and motor examination should precede any wound exploration or anesthetic infiltration.

- Prepare the patient for the initial treatment of the wound. This involves irrigation of the wound, which is the major step in reducing the likelihood of infection. Some advocate cleansing the wound with 1% povidone-iodine and then, with the patient properly anesthetized, suturing the wound.

- Immunize the patient against tetanus, if necessary.

A discussion regarding tetanus status and potential risk is warranted in any patient with a wound. Tetanus is a preventable endotoxin-mediated disease caused by *Clostridium tetani*. When present, it may cause trismus, neck rigidity, dysphagia, and severe, uncontrolled reflex spasms. Populations at particular risk are the elderly and those who have immigrated to the United States and had inadequate immunization, those who are immunocompromised, and those who inject drugs regularly and have frequent skin abscesses, impaired immune status, and reluctance to seek health care.

It is therefore important to determine when the patient last received a tetanus immunization and to classify the wound as either tetanus prone or non–tetanus prone.

Tetanus-prone wounds have the following characteristics:

■ Greater than 6 hours old

■ Greater than 1 cm deep

■ Stellate or have an avulsion configuration

■ Associated with devitalized tissue

■ Contaminated with soil, feces, or saliva

■ From a missile (e.g., gunshot wound)

■ From a puncture or crush

■ Associated with a burn or frostbite

All other wounds can be considered non–tetanus prone. To determine the appropriate treatment, see Table 23-1 and the following guidelines:

■ A non–tetanus-prone wound in an adult patient with up-to-date immunization requires tetanus and diphtheria toxoid (Td) if it has been 10 years since the last immunization.

■ A tetanus-prone wound in a patient with up-to-date immunization requires Td if it has been more than 5 years since the last immunization.

■ A non–tetanus-prone wound in an adult patient with inadequate immunization requires Td.

Table 23.1 **Summary Guide to Tetanus Prophylaxis in Routine Wound Management, 1991**				
HISTORY OF ADSORBED TETANUS TOXOID (DOSES)	CLEAN, MINOR WOUNDS		ALL OTHER WOUNDS*	
	Td[†]	TIG (250 U)	Td[†]	TIG (250 U)
Unknown or <3	Yes	No	Yes	Yes
≥3[‡]	No[§]	No	No	No

TIG, tetanus immune globulin.

*Such as, but not limited to, wounds contaminated with dirt, feces, soil, and saliva; puncture wounds; avulsions; and wounds resulting from missiles, crushing, burns, and frostbite.

[†]For children <7 years old, DTP (DT, if pertussis vaccine is contraindicated) is preferred to tetanus toxoid alone. For persons ≥7 years of age, Td is preferred to tetanus toxoid alone.

[‡]If only three doses of *fluid* toxoid have been received, a fourth dose of toxoid, preferably an adsorbed toxoid, should be given.

[§]Yes, if >10 years since last dose.

[¶]Yes, if >5 years since last dose. (More frequent boosters are not needed and can accentuate side effects.)

Adapted from Diphtheria, tetanus, and pertussis: Recommendations for vaccine use and other preventive measures. Recommendations of the Immunization Practices Advisory Committee (ACIP). MMWR Recomm Rep 40(RR-10):1-28, 1991.

- Tetanus-prone wounds in adult patients with inadequate immunization require both passive immunity with tetanus immunoglobulin (TIG) and active immunity with Td. When giving both Td and TIG, place them in different syringes and deliver them at separate anatomic locations. Adults with an unknown history should receive the three-dose regimen and therefore will require follow-up. The initial dose of Td toxoid is given at the time of wound closure; 4 to 8 weeks later, a second dose of Td toxoid is administered. The last dose is given 6 to 12 weeks after the second dose. Booster doses of Td toxoid should then be given every 10 years to maintain an adequate tetanus status.

- Diphtheria, tetanus toxoid, and pertussis (DTP) or acellular pertussis (DTaP) is used instead of Td in children.

- TIG is considered safe in pregnancy, whereas Td toxoid can be safely given in the second trimester and later in those who have high-risk wounds.

Materials Utilized for Performing Irrigation, Cleansing, and Debridement

- Gloves and goggles

Irrigation
- 60-mL syringe

- 21-gauge plastic intravenous catheter or irrigation needle with "blunted" end for fluid irrigation

- Several liters of saline solution

Cleansing
- A cleansing agent (Table 23-2) may be considered, but due to tissue toxicity and lack of supportive evidence, it cannot be routinely recommended.

- Sterile, fenestrated drape

- Several sterile square or rectangular drapes

Debridement
- Scalpel or sharp tissue scissors

Table 23.2	**Summary of Wound Cleansing Agents**			
SKIN CLEANSER	ANTIBACTERIAL ACTIVITY	TISSUE TOXICITY	SYSTEMIC TOXICITY	POTENTIAL USES
Povidone-iodine surgical scrub	Strongly bactericidal against gram-positive and gram-negative bacteria	Detergent can be toxic to wound tissues	Painful to open wounds Other reactions extremely rare	Hand cleanser
Povidone-iodine solution	Strongly bactericidal against gram-positive and gram-negative bacteria	Minimally toxic to wound tissues	Extremely rare	Wound periphery cleanser
Chlorhexidine	Strongly bactericidal against gram-positive organisms, less strong against gram-negative bacteria	Detergent can be toxic to wound tissues	Extremely rare	Hand cleanser Alternative wound periphery cleanser
Poloxamer 188	No antibacterial activity	None known	None known	Wound cleanser (particularly useful on face)
Hexa-chlorophene	Bacteriostatic against gram-positive bacteria; poor activity against gram-negative bacteria	Detergent can be toxic to wound tissues	Teratogenic with repeated use	Alternative hand cleanser
Hydrogen peroxide	Very weak antibacterial agent	Toxic to red cells	Extremely rare	Wound cleanser adjunct

Adapted from Trott AT: Wounds and Lacerations:Emergency Care and Closure, 2nd ed. St. Louis, Mosby–Year Book, 1998, p 91.

Procedure for Irrigating and Cleansing the Wound

1. Put on gloves and goggles to avoid exposure to blood-borne pathogens.

2. Using a 60-mL syringe and a 21-gauge plastic intravenous catheter or blunt needle designed for irrigation, repeatedly squirt normal saline into the site in short bursts to dislodge remaining particulate matter. Minimally, 250 to 500 mL of irrigation solution should be used. Several liters may be necessary for large wounds that are heavily contaminated.

3. Apply a cleansing agent (see Table 23-2) to the wound edges and surrounding skin using a bull's-eye or circular motion from the inside moving outward and repeat three times. Avoid allowing the agent to enter the wound.

Note: One example of a cleansing agent might include three sterile diluted povidone-iodine (1%)-soaked 4 × 4 pads. Please be advised that standard povidone-iodine solution is 10% and the scrub is even more concentrated.

4. Place a sterile fenestrated drape over the wound site and several sterile square or rectangular drapes around the site to create a sterile field.

Note: If the wound is on a limb, a sterile drape should be placed under the extremity before the other drapes are applied. Drapes are often found in prepackaged suture kits or on a laceration tray and are placed after the clinician dons sterile gloves.

5. If debridement is necessary to remove dead or devitalized tissue, use a scalpel or sharp tissue scissors.

Note: Care should be taken to preserve tissue, yet conversion of a jagged laceration to a surgical one may be required for optimal closure to occur. Sometimes the subcutaneous tissue may need to be undermined to allow for adequate closure of tight wound edges.

Materials Utilized to Perform Suturing _____

■ Sterile gloves

Suture Selection

Note: Once it is determined that a wound should be closed primarily, suture selection begins. The first item to consider is whether to use absorbable or nonabsorbable suture based on anatomic location and healing potential.

■ Absorbable suture is used in mucosal areas such as the oral cavity and tongue and disintegrates by one of two methods: enzymatic breakdown of organic material (e.g., surgical gut—plain or chromic) or by hydrolysis of synthetic material (e.g., polyglactin 910 [Vicryl]).

■ Nonabsorbable suture (silk, stainless steel, nylon, polypropylene, polyester fiber) can be further classified into monofilament (single strand) or multifilament (several strands, which are often braided).

Note: One advantage of monofilament is that it passes through tissue more easily than does braided suture. However, a disadvantage is that it has less tensile strength than a multifilament. Advantages of a multifilament suture include better flexibility, whereas a disadvantage would be that it may harbor organisms more easily within the braid. It is also important to recognize that loss of tensile strength and absorption are separate processes (i.e., suture may lose tensile strength rapidly but absorb slowly or vice versa).

   Note: Suture size is denoted by the number of zeros, and increases in number as the diameter of suture decreases; for example, 7-0 is smaller than 1-0. Refer to Table 23-3 as a guide for suggested suture size based on anatomic location.

■ Needles

Note: The final consideration for proper suture selection is based on needle characteristics and includes the following:

   ■ The smallest-diameter needle to accomplish the task should be chosen to avoid unnecessary tissue trauma.

Table 23.3 Suggested Guidelines for Suture Material and Size for Body Region

BODY REGION	PERCUTANEOUS (SKIN)	DEEP (DERMAL)
Scalp	5-0/4-0 monofilament*	4-0 absorbable[†]
Ear	6-0 monofilament	—
Eyelid	7-0/6-0 monofilament	—
Eyebrow	6-0/5-0 monofilament	5-0 absorbable
Nose	6-0 monofilament	5-0 absorbable
Lip	6-0 monofilament	5-0 absorbable
Oral mucosa	—	5-0 absorbable[‡]
Other parts of face/forehead	6-0 monofilament	5-0 absorbable
Trunk	5-0/4-0 monofilament	3-0 absorbable
Extremities	5-0/4-0 monofilament	4-0 absorbable
Hand	5-0 monofilament	5-0 absorbable
Extensor tendon	4-0 monofilament	—
Foot/sole	4-0/3-0 monofilament	4-0 absorbable
Vagina	—	4-0 absorbable
Scrotum	—	5-0 absorbable[‡]
Penis	5-0 monofilament	—

*Nonabsorbable monofilaments include nylon (Ethilon, Dermalon), polypropylene (Prolene), and polybutester (Novafil).

[†]Absorbable materials for dermal and fascial closures include polyglycolic acid (Dexon, Dexon Plus), polyglactin 910 (Vicryl), polydioxanone (PDS [monofilament absorbable]), and polyglyconate (Maxon [monofilament absorbable]).

[‡]Absorbable materials for mucosal and scrotal closure include chromic gut and polyglactin 910 (Vicryl).

Adapted from Trott AT: Wounds and Lacerations: Emergency Care and Closure, 2nd ed. St. Louis, Mosby–Year Book, 1998, p 179.

■ The type and shape of needle should be considered:

■ A conventional cutting needle is often used for skin and has three cutting edges (two lateral and one on the *inner* concave curve).

■ A reverse cutting needle is often used for tough tissue such as ligament and also has three cutting edges (two lateral and one on the *outer* concave curve).

■ A taper needle is circumferentially rounded with a point and it is useful intraoperatively on delicate tissue such as peritoneum. Figure 23-3 illustrates the various parts of a needle.

Other Instruments

■ Needle driver or holder, appropriate for the size of needle and suturing material being used

■ Skin forceps

■ Suture scissors

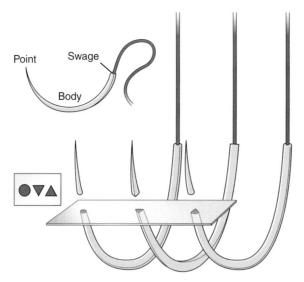

FIGURE 23-3. The parts of a taper and reverse cutting needle. (Redrawn from Trott AT: Wounds and Lacerations: Emergency Care and Closure, 2nd ed. St. Louis, Mosby–Year Book, 1998, p 31.)

Procedure for Performing Suture Techniques (General Information)

Caution: **Proper instrument technique is paramount.**

 ### Needle Driver-Holder

1. Using sterile gloves, hold the needle driver with the dominant hand while the nondominant hand holds the forceps.

Note: The tripod grip is an excellent method for use with both the needle driver and scissors as it maximizes hand control (Fig. 23-4). This may include the distal phalanx of the thumb and fourth digit inserted into the rings of the needle driver but never allowing the digits to move into rings more proximal than the distal interphalangeal joint.

2. Grasp the needle at the tip of the needle driver and load so that it is perpendicular to the needle driver, as shown in Figure 23-5.

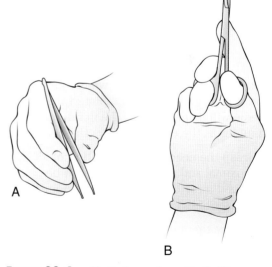

A

B

FIGURE 23-4. (**A**, Redrawn from Trott AT: Wounds and Lacerations: Emergency Care and Closure, 2nd ed. St. Louis, Mosby–Year Book, 1998, p 32.)

continued

A

B

Figure 23-5. (A, Redrawn from Trott AT: Wounds and Lacerations: Emergency Care and Closure, 2nd ed. St. Louis, Mosby–Year Book, 1998, p 33.)

Note: The needle concavity will be furthest from the clinician, and the point of the needle will be pointing to the nondominant shoulder as the clinician views the needle.

3. Grasp the needle at the junction of its proximal and middle third. It can be moved more distal (toward the point) for smaller bites.

Note: The tip of the needle should never be grasped because it can become dull. To minimize needle stick injuries, **needles should never be touched with the fingers**; they can be loaded easily from the packet they come in or from any flat surface.

Forceps

1. For maximal control, hold the forceps like a pencil, as shown in Figure 23-4.

Note: If the forceps have teeth, avoid a tight tissue grasp to eliminate skin trauma ("teeth marks").

2. One method lifts the tissue rather than grasping it by placing one tooth of the forceps into the wound edge and lifting gently without closing the other toothed face to the skin surface.

Scissors

1. Cut with the tips of the scissors using the tripod grip and with the screw of the scissors facing up and at a 45-degree angle to the suture as in Figure 23-4.

Note: Scissors are manufactured to cut most accurately with the tips.

Note: The technique of cutting at a 45-degree angle helps eliminate the possibility of accidentally cutting out the knots when no tail is left intraoperatively. One should never attempt to cut suture without full visualization of the distal scissor tips to avoid cutting tissue inadvertently.

Procedure for Suture Placement

1. Introduce the suture needle into the tissue at a 90-degree angle or less (toward the wound) (see Figure 23-5); try to approximate this angle as closely as possible. This can be maximized with full wrist pronation.

Note: This is to promote skin eversion or a slight tenting of the wound edge at closure to minimize the ultimate scar visibility. With time, a normal scar contracts and flattens and appears flush, casting no shadow. Conversely, a wound that initially is closed flush often later "sinks-in" and creates a shadow of light that highlights and draws attention to the scar.

Note: The depth of needle penetration is determined by the wound depth. Sometimes a bite can be completed by one pass through the tissue (skin surface, wound edge, wound edge, skin surface); other times the needle should be reloaded halfway through or after it passes from skin surface through the first wound edge. This allows for specific placement of the wound edge to the adjacent wound edge to ensure a side-to-side match and is necessary for larger bites in a deep wound. Typically, the total stitch length should be as wide as the wound is deep, as shown in Figure 23-6.

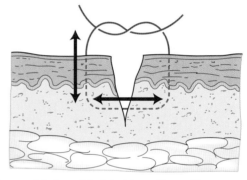

FIGURE 23-6. (Modified from Trott AT: Wounds and Lacerations: Emergency Care and Closure, 2nd ed. St. Louis, Mosby–Year Book, p 113.)

Note: If a needle begins to bend, excessive pressure has been placed on it by either poor technique or attempting too large a bite. Taking a bite deeper than the wound may cause important structures to be traumatized from blind needle placement. Conversely, taking too superficial a bite may leave dead space below the closure, inviting blood accumulation, bacterial growth, and infection.

2. Place the needle bite just superficial to the wound depth.

Note: This allows complete visualization of structures penetrated and adequately closes the wound.

Procedure for Performing the Instrument Tie

1. Place the needle driver between the suture ends and, with the nondominant hand, wrap the suture with the needle attached over the instrument twice on the first throw of the first knot only (surgeon's knot, used to prevent slippage) (Fig. 23-7A and B).

2. Grasp the short end of the suture with the needle driver, and the short and long suture ends switch sides (see Fig. 23-7C).

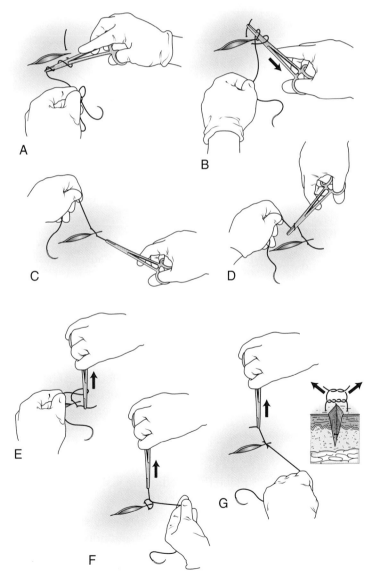

FIGURE 23-7. (Redrawn from Trott AT: Wounds and Lacerations: Emergency Care and Closure, 2nd ed. St. Louis, Mosby–Year Book, 1998, pp 98-102.)

Note: This is considered one throw. Two throws makes one knot. Next, the needle driver is placed between the two suture ends and one wrap of the long suture over the instrument is used (Fig. 23-7D).

3. Again, grasp the short suture end with the needle driver. The long and short suture ends again switch sides (see Fig. 23-7E).

Note: A circle should be seen as the suture comes down to the skin surface. This suture circle should be placed at 90 degrees to the wound length for simple interrupted and vertical mattress sutures (horizontal mattress sutures will be parallel with the wound) (see Fig. 23-7F).

4. Repeat these steps with only one wrap over the needle driver on every successive throw until the suture is cut.

Note: Remember the only throw that gets two wraps is the first throw of the first knot in a series. Therefore, an even number of throws ensures completion of all knots. Compare the diagrams of a typical knot (see Fig. 23-6) with a surgeon's knot (see Fig. 23-7G).
  Note: The number of knots depends on the anatomic location (below the skin

surface requires fewer knots; above the skin surface requires more knots) and suture material (those with "memory" often require more knots). Usually three or four knots on the skin surface are sufficient. The needle remains connected throughout these steps and usually poses no problem to the clinician or patient, as it remains stationary lying on the sterile field. There is no need to remember where you are in a sequence with this method, as in the "over-under technique."

5. After an adequate number of knots are secured, pull the suture knot to one side to avoid knot placement directly over the wound to minimize debris collection and potential infection.

Note: The suture is now ready for cutting. The "suture tail" or "suture tag" will be used during suture removal.
  Note: Two helpful rules can be used to estimate this length: (1) The tail length should be equal to the distance from the wound edge to the suture border. (2) The tail length should be slightly less than the distance between adjacent knots. Use the previously described scissor technique to cut the suture.

Procedure for Performing the Simple Interrupted Stitch

Note: It is important to estimate carefully the number and size of sutures necessary to close the wound adequately without placing too many and too small or too few and too large stitches. Most simple interrupted stitches should measure between 3 and 10 mm in length and should be about this same distance apart. The method described in the instrument tie section is consistent with the simple interrupted stitch, which is frequently used to close most lacerations.

1. One method of closure includes closure by halves. Place the first stitch at the halfway point along the length of the wound.

2. Place the next stitches at the halfway point between the first stitch and each end of the wound.

3. Place the next stitches between each of the previous stitches until the wound is approximated.

continued

Note: An alternate method involves beginning at one end of the wound and placing evenly spaced sutures along the length until you reach the opposite end of the wound. Be careful to place the sutures evenly on both sides of the wound; failure to do so may result in an asymmetric end to the wound known as a dog ear, in which one side of the wound appears to be longer than the other side, creating a redundant "ear" of tissue.

Procedure for Correcting Dog Ear Deformity

If a dog ear develops, the sutures should be removed and the closure reattempted. If it appears that correction cannot be achieved by reapproximation, the following method illustrates an acceptable procedure for correction.

1. Make an incision 45 degrees at the end of the redundant side.

Note: This tissue is undermined to create a small flap, which when gentle traction is applied can be excised as shown.

2. Close the wound in the usual fashion, creating a "hockey-stick" appearance (Fig. 23-8).

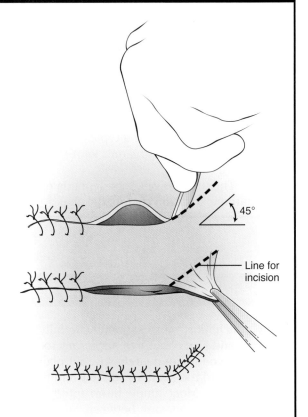

FIGURE 23-8. (Redrawn from Trott AT: Wounds and Lacerations: Emergency Care and Closure, 2nd ed. St. Louis, Mosby–Year Book, 1998, p 37.)

Procedure for Performing the Vertical Mattress ("Far-Far/Near-Near") Stitch

The next most commonly performed stitch is the vertical mattress stitch. This stitch is so named because the stitch lies in a plane perpendicular (vertical) to the skin. It is useful for closing deeper wounds (e.g., those of the scalp) in which the closure occurs at two levels (superficial and deep), eliminating dead space.

1. To perform the vertical mattress stitch, introduce the needle "far" and exit "far" from the wound edge, diving deep but just superficial to the wound depth (Fig. 23-9).

Note: Figure 23-9 illustrates a wound with first stitch traversing the lower wound margin. Most wounds will have the first stitch traverse within the lower portion of the wound margin, as illustrated in Figure 23-6.

2. Next, starting on the same side as the first exit point, load the needle backhand (needle points to dominant shoulder while all other criteria remain unchanged) and enter "near" the wound edge and exit on the original side "near" the wound edge, both at a level more superficial than the original deep first pass.

3. The remainder of the instrument tying steps is the same (see Fig. 23-7).

Note: Performing the second step first, or a "near-near/far-far" stitch, should be avoided to eliminate "blind" needle placement and creating inadvertent trauma to unseen structures.

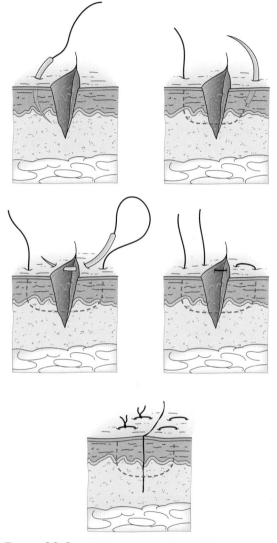

Figure 23-9. (Redrawn from Trott AT: Wounds and Lacerations: Emergency Care and Closure, 2nd ed. St. Louis, Mosby–Year Book, 1998, p 38.)

Procedure for Performing the Horizontal Mattress Stitch

The horizontal mattress stitch lies in a plane parallel to the skin. It is useful when there is a flap of tissue or when the tension of the stitch is to be predominantly on one side (the knotted side). For example, this method works well in a wound with a vascular side and a relatively avascular side, as the avascular area is pulled toward the vascular side, with most of the tension being on the vascular side. In other stitch types, the tension is shared equally by each side.

1. To perform the horizontal mattress stitch, start on the vascular side and exit on the relatively avascular side.

2. Re-enter backhanded on this avascular side parallel to the wound edge and adjacent to the original exit site; the final exit is on the original vascular side.

Note: The stitch should look like a box. All knot tying steps are performed as previously discussed except that the stitch is brought down parallel (not perpendicular) to the wound line (Fig. 23-10).

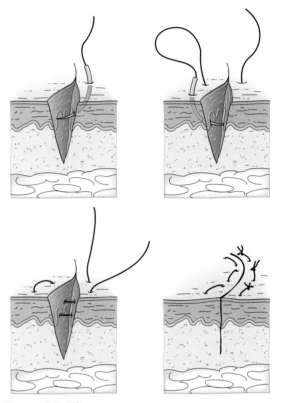

Figure 23-10. (Redrawn from Trott AT: Wounds and Lacerations: Emergency Care and Closure, 2nd ed. St. Louis, Mosby–Year Book, 1998, p 39.)

Procedure for Performing the Continuous-Running-Baseball Stitch

The advantages of the continuous stitch is that it can be performed quickly and can be applied tightly if "locked." The disadvantages are as follows:

- If one loop is broken, the entire wound may open.

- It cannot be partially removed as can other stitch types (e.g., every other or a wound segment) to allow for drainage when managing an early wound infection.

- It may leave a cosmetically suboptimal scar with a "railroad tracks" appearance.

The continuous suture is performed as follows:

1. Place a suture at the end of the wound in the same fashion as that outlined for a

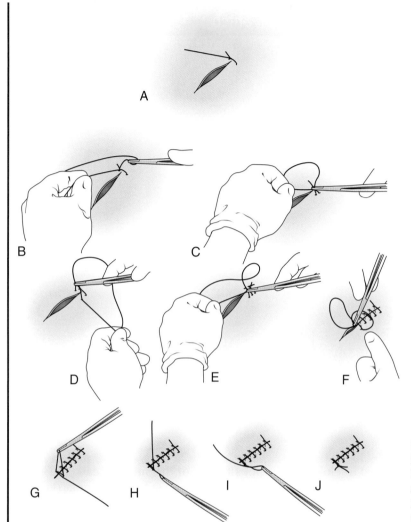

A

B

C

D

E

F

G

H

I

J

Figure 23-11. (Redrawn from Trott AT: Wounds and Lacerations: Emergency Care and Closure, 2nd ed. St. Louis, Mosby–Year Book, 1998, pp 123-128.)

simple interrupted suture (only cut suture on non-needle side after knot is tied).

2. Using the initial suture as an anchor, additional sutures are placed (throws) in a continuous fashion until the entire wound is reapproximated. Enter next to knot and exit on opposite side skin surface at a 45-degree angle to the wound and re-enter through skin surface directly across and repeat (Fig. 23-11).

3. When the end of the wound is reached, the final suture is tied in the same manner as that outlined for the simple interrupted suture, but the needle side is tied to the last loop before it has been pulled taut. When cut, it will yield three tails.

Note: The method illustrated demonstrates the "non-locking" method. To "lock" the suture, bring the needle up through the previous loop before it has been pulled taut creating a tight seal, which can be particularly useful intraoperatively.

Procedure for Performing the Subcuticular Stitch

FIGURE 23-12. (Redrawn from Trott AT: Wounds and Lacerations: Emergency Care and Closure, 2nd ed. St. Louis, Mosby–Year Book, 1998, p 41.)

The subcuticular stitch is often used to close a surgical incision or a very clean wound. Absorbable suture material must be used if the suture will not be removed at a later time.

1. Create an initial buried knot to anchor the suture (Fig. 23-12).

2. Begin making equal passes through the wound edges in the horizontal plane until you have traversed the length of the wound (entering and exiting the dermal layer from side to side).

Note: It is important to keep the bites equal and approximate the tissue so that it aligns properly.

3. A final buried knot is tied at the opposite wound end to complete and anchor the opposite end of the suture. Leave the needle side of the suture tail uncut (cut the loop side).

Note: The suture is secure because of the final buried anchor knot.

4. Bury the final tail by re-entering the closed wound with the needle and attached suture and exiting on the skin surface 1 cm away from the wound edge.

5. Cut it flush with the skin.

6. Apply skin tapes over the wound surface.

Note: No suture will be visible on the skin surface.

SPECIAL CONSIDERATIONS

Several important general concepts exist and are discussed based on anatomic location.

- Hair can be shaved to allow for better wound exploration, irrigation, and closure, but this is *not* routinely recommended. Often just trimming the surrounding hair is helpful without further traumatizing the skin by creating potential sites of infection from the minute lacerations and skin abrasions that often occur during the shaving process. Cutting the suture tails longer than usual and using an alternate suture color also facilitates removal in hairy anatomic locations and minimizes the need for shaving hair.

- Never shave an eyebrow, as the hair may not grow back at all or will grow back irregularly. It is also critical to line up the hair and skin borders exactly to avoid misalignment. If an eyebrow has been shaved and the wound is sutured closed, it is difficult to know where these borders exist. Therefore, the possibility of even slight misalignment of the hair to the skin border can occur, and if the hair grows back it will look very disfiguring. Usually these areas can be visualized well enough to suture them adequately without the need for hair removal.

- Following this same principle is the concept of aligning the vermilion border of the lips. The best method for doing this begins by placing the first stitch at the border of the skin and mucosal edges (use 6-0 nylon). The remaining wound can be closed using nonabsorbable suture for the skin and absorbable suture for the lip itself. It is critical that this border be aligned exactly.

- If an incision has to be made, it is important to recognize and follow the natural skin tension lines. Scar visibility is minimized when it runs parallel to these lines and is more prominent when placed perpendicular or oblique to them (see Fig. 23-2).

 ## Materials Utilized for Using Skin Staplers _____

- Stapler with staples—sterile disposable type
- Tissue forceps
- Skin tape

Procedure for Using Skin Staplers

Note: Skin staplers are sterile, disposable, cost-effective, and useful for long, linear lacerations of the scalp, trunk, and extremities because they can be applied quickly with the same ultimate cosmetic result as suture.

1. Place staples over the approximated wound and firmly squeeze the trigger to deliver each staple, everting the tissue edges.

Note: Staplers should not be used to close lacerations of the face or hands or those over a joint. They should also be avoided in areas that might later require computed tomography or magnetic resonance imaging (e.g., head injury).

2. To remove, use a special sterile, disposable device and squeeze this device at each staple. The staple legs are straightened. Then pull the staple from the tissue.

Note: Skin tapes are often placed after removal of the staples.

Materials Utilized for Applying Wound Adhesives

- Ampules or other delivery devices (ProPen) of wound adhesive
- Cotton-tipped applicator

Procedure for Applying Wound Adhesives

Note: Wound adhesives are another variation of wound closure that may be used; they can be applied quickly and painlessly for easily approximating skin edges of surgical incisions or lacerations of the face, trunk, and limbs. They are not recommended over skin creases, areas of movement, or long lacerations or for hand injuries. Other contraindications include wounds with active infection, those that involve mucosal surfaces or occur at mucocutaneous junctions, and areas exposed to body fluids. In addition, some clinicians avoid areas of dense hair such as the scalp. After the usual cleaning, debriding, and care to achieve hemostasis, the area is carefully dried.

1. Crush an ampule and invert it, soaking the cotton-tipped applicator with solution.

2. With the applicator, lightly paint over the approximated wound edge three times in succession with 30 seconds' drying time between.

Caution: **It is important to avoid applying the fluid into the wound and to avoid spillage to surrounding areas such as the eye.**

3. Because the adhesive is of low viscosity (runny), position the anatomic area in the horizontal plane to avoid runoff or protect surrounding skin with a barrier.

4. After full strength is reached at 2.5 minutes, a protective dressing can be applied at 5 minutes, but it is not required.

Note: Follow manufacturer's instructions for other application delivery devices, which deliver a high viscosity version skin adhesive.

FOLLOW-UP CARE AND INSTRUCTIONS FOR SUTURED OR STAPLED WOUNDS

- Advise the patient to keep the wound site clean and dry. Some clinicians advocate no contact with water at all for 48 hours, whereas others allow gentle bathing with soap and water or a quick shower with careful drying of the site afterward, but all emphasize no prolonged soaking of the site in water.

- If applicable, elevate the area.

- Instruct the patient verbally and in writing regarding the desired frequency of wound checking and dressing changing. It is suggested that the patient remove the dressing twice each day to visualize the site for signs of infection and to reapply antibiotic ointment. A clean, dry dressing should then be applied. Some sites may be left open to the air (face, neck, scalp).

- Instruct the patient to apply a cold compress for the first 48 hours after surgery in sites with significant associated soft tissue involvement, such as a contusion (20 minutes each time four to five times per day).

- Verbalize and write the signs of infection for the patient to watch for and instruct him or her to return if there is an increase in pain, redness beyond the wound margin, or red streaking; if the area becomes warm, swollen, and tender; if there is discharge or drainage from the wound; if there is tenderness under the arms or groin; or if he or she experiences fever or chills.

- Consider possible activity restriction or immobilization.

- Consider analgesics (acetaminophen, nonsteroidal anti-inflammatory drugs [NSAIDs]).

- Advise the patient about when he or she should return for a wound check and suture or staple removal.

- Educate the patient that scars take 1 year to fully mature and that after initial healing it is best to avoid strong sunlight and to apply sunscreen to the site.

- Administration of antibiotics is sometimes advised, although small, uncomplicated wounds and lacerations often do not require them. If the particular wound is high risk, a wound check in 24 to 48 hours may be necessary. It is always best to have the original provider assess the wound if possible, because he or she has a baseline for comparison. Antibiotics should be considered in the following high-risk wounds:

- Wounds that are more than 12 hours old at initial presentation, especially those of the hands

- Human or animal bites, including those caused by the patient's teeth (intraoral laceration)

- Crush wounds

- Heavily contaminated wounds

- Wounds involving relatively avascular areas, such as the cartilage of the ear

- Wounds involving joint spaces, tendon, or bone

- Severe paronychia and felons

- Wounds in patients with a history of valvular heart disease

- Wounds in patients with immunosuppression (diabetes, chronic steroid use, infection with human immunodeficiency virus [HIV])

SUTURE REMOVAL

Anatomic location dictates the length of time sutures should be left in place to ensure adequate healing. Table 23-4 may be useful as a general guide. It is important to remember that adults heal more slowly than do children and that other medical conditions may increase healing time.

- The wound should be inspected for signs of infection before the sutures are removed, including erythema beyond the wound margin, discharge, swelling, pain, or tenderness.

- Some practitioners advocate the use of povidone-iodine (Betadine) both before and after suture or staple removal.

Table 23.4 **Recommended Intervals for Removal of Percutaneous (Skin) Sutures**	
LOCATION	DAYS TO REMOVAL
Scalp	6-8
Face	4-5
Ear	4-5
Chest/abdomen	8-10
Back	12-14
Arm/leg*	8-10
Hand*	8-10
Fingertip	10-12
Foot	12-14

*Add 2 to 3 days for joint extensor surfaces.

From Trott AT: Wounds and Lacerations: Emergency Care and Closure, 2nd ed. St. Louis, Mosby–Year Book, 1998, p 366.

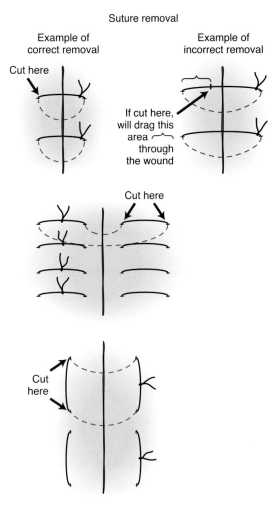

Suture removal

Example of correct removal

Example of incorrect removal

Cut here

If cut here, will drag this area through the wound

Cut here

Cut here

FIGURE 23-13.   Suture removal.

- Using sterile instruments, cut the suture to minimize dragging contaminated suture through the patient's body.

- If sutures are tight and difficult to cut, use of a No. 11 scalpel blade should be considered. Turn the sharp side away from the patient to sneak under the suture to avoid excessive pulling. Diagrams of correct and incorrect methods of various stitch removals are shown in Figure 23-13.

- It is important to ensure that all the nonabsorbable suture is removed and that none is left inside the wound to act as a foreign body.

- Often, minimal erythema surrounding the wound, secondary to local reaction to these materials, is alleviated 24 to 48 hours after the sutures are removed.

■ Some practitioners advocate the use of antibacterial ointment.

■ Most wounds should be left open to the air at this point and do not require a dressing.

STAPLE REMOVAL

■ Align the staple remover so that it is centered under the staple.

■ It is important to recognize that the staple removal device is squeezed and then the staple is lifted in two distinct motions; combining them is painful to the patient and traumatizes tissue.

■ Often, minimal erythema surrounding the wound, secondary to local reaction to the staples, is alleviated 24 to 48 hours after the staples are removed.

■ Some practitioners advocate the use of antibacterial ointment.

■ Most wounds should be left open to the air at this point and do not require a dressing.

FOLLOW-UP CARE AND INSTRUCTIONS FOR ADHESIVE-CLOSED WOUNDS

■ Notify the patient that the adhesive naturally starts to slough off 5 to 10 days after placement.

■ Caution the patient to avoid scratching, rubbing, or picking at the site.

■ Instruct the patient that the area should not be scrubbed, soaked, or exposed to prolonged wetness (the area should be kept dry; a quick shower can be taken, if necessary).

■ Advise the patient not to apply medication in liquid or ointment form to the site.

The cost of skin adhesives is comparable when costs for suture kits, suture materials, clinician time, and follow-up visits for suture removal are considered.

REFERENCE

Ethicon: Wound Closure Manual. New Brunswick, NJ, Ethicon, 1985.
   Available at: http://www.ethiconinc.com/

BIBLIOGRAPHY

Pfenninger JL, Fowler GC (eds): Procedures for Primary Care
Physicians, St. Louis, CV Mosby, 1994.
Principles of Primary Wound Management: A Guide to the
Fundamentals. Fairfax, Va, Mortiere, 1996.
Trott AT: Wounds and Lacerations: Emergency Care and Closure, 2nd
ed. St. Louis, Mosby–Year Book, 1998.
Wedmore IS: Wound care: Modern evidence in the treatment of man's
age-old injuries. Emerg Med Pract 7:1-24, 2005.

Chapter 24

Dermatologic Procedures

Michelle DiBaise

PROCEDURE GOALS AND OBJECTIVES

Goal: To perform biopsies, electrosurgery, and acne surgery successfully while observing standard precautions and with the minimal degree of risk to the patient.

Objectives: The student will be able to ...

- Describe the indications, contraindications, and rationale for performing biopsies, electrosurgery, and acne surgery.

- Identify and describe common complications associated with performing biopsies, electrosurgery, and acne surgery.

- Describe the essential anatomy and physiology associated with performing biopsies, electrosurgery, and acne surgery.

- Identify the materials necessary for performing biopsies, electrosurgery, and acne surgery and their proper use.

- Describe the steps in performing biopsies, electrosurgery, and acne surgery.

- Identify the important aspects of post-procedure care after biopsies, electrosurgery, and acne surgery.

FIGURE 24-1. Algorithm for biopsy technique based on clinical assessment.

Biopsies

BACKGROUND AND HISTORY

Skin biopsies are performed to determine the cause of a lesion or to remove a lesion, or both. The general categories of biopsies include shave, punch, and excision. A shave biopsy removes the epidermis and a portion of the upper dermis and is performed along the horizontal plane. Variations on the shave technique include snip excisions, as performed for skin tag removal, and curettage, as performed for many benign superficial lesions. A punch biopsy can be either incisional or excisional. An incisional biopsy removes only a portion of a lesion, whereas an excisional biopsy removes the entire lesion. Larger excisional biopsies can be completed using a No. 15 blade. Incisional and excisional biopsies extend to the subcutaneous fat. Determining the correct biopsy technique is based on the clinical diagnosis (Fig. 24-1) and the desired cosmetic outcome (Tobinick, 1998).

SHAVE BIOPSY

INDICATIONS

- Seborrheic keratoses
- Verrucous lesions
- Molluscum contagiosum
- Superficial basal cell carcinomas

Occasionally, a shave biopsy may be performed on benign nevi, particularly on the face, when a good cosmetic result is essential (Bennett, 1988a; Siegel and Usatine, 1998b; Tobinick, 1998).

Snip excisions may be performed for the following (Bennett, 1988a; Siegel and Usatine, 1998b):

- Acrochordons (skin tags)
- Pedunculated nevi

Care must be taken not to perform this technique on dermal nevi without anesthesia, because the patient will experience greater discomfort because of innervation of nevi.

Curettage may be performed on benign superficial lesions, such as the following (Ho, 1999):

- Molluscum contagiosum
- Verruca vulgaris
- Seborrheic keratoses, with or without cryotherapy

For superficial multicentric basal cell carcinomas and Bowen's disease, curettage and desiccation are alternatives to excision (Bennett, 1988a; Schwartz, 1999; Usatine, 1998a).

When curettage is used, histologic margins are impossible to determine. If tumor margins need to be determined, an alternative biopsy technique should be used.

CONTRAINDICATIONS

Contraindications for a shave biopsy include the following (Siegel and Usatine, 1998b):

- Most pigmented lesions, except in the case of benign nevi, as stated earlier
- For the diagnosis of infiltrative dermatoses
- In a suspected sclerosing basal cell carcinoma
- Any lesion with a dermal component

POTENTIAL COMPLICATIONS

The most common complications seen with shave biopsy include the following (Siegel and Usatine, 1998b):

■ Bleeding: Most bleeding is readily stopped with the use of 20% aluminum chloride (Drysol). If bleeding is more brisk, as occurs when patients are taking aspirin or warfarin, or if the shave is too deep into the dermis, hand-held cautery may be used. Monsel's solution (ferric subsulfate) and silver nitrate may be used, but tattooing can occur with their use. It is not recommended that Monsel's solution or silver nitrate be used on the face or highly visible areas (Siegel and Usatine, 1998b; Stasko, 1996; Usatine, 1998b).

■ Infection

■ Regrowth of the lesion: Lesions such as warts and incompletely removed nevi or seborrheic keratoses can regrow. An estimated 1 in 20 nevi regenerates (Siegel and Usatine, 1998b).

■ Scarring: Scarring, which usually has the appearance of an atrophic, lighter than normal area, may occur even when the procedure is performed correctly. It is more of a risk if the shave is too deep into the dermis.

■ Some discomfort may be experienced with the injection of anesthetic.

REVIEW OF ESSENTIAL ANATOMY AND PHYSIOLOGY

For simplicity, the skin structure consists of the epidermis or topmost layer of the skin, the dermal-epidermal junction, the dermis, and the subcutaneous fat. It is essential that the practitioner have knowledge of the vasculature and nerves of the biopsy site before performing any biopsy of the skin. In addition, adequate knowledge of the lines of skin tension is required to determine the orientation of punch and excisional biopsies. Suture lines are less likely to develop into a widened scar if placed parallel to the lines of tension (Fig. 24-2) (Moy and Usatine, 1998b; Zalla, 1996). In addition, placing suture lines parallel to wrinkles improves the cosmetic appearance of the end defect. Caution must be used when performing elliptical excisions on the face—particularly on the forehead or near the eye or lips—so that distortion does not occur. Large excisions in these areas may necessitate a graft or flap closure.

Standard Precautions   Every practitioner should use standard precautions at all times when interacting with patients, especially when performing procedures. Determining the level of precaution necessary requires the practitioner to exercise clinical judgment based on the patient's history and the potential for exposure to body fluids or aerosol-borne pathogens (for further discussion, see Chapter 2).

FIGURE 24-2.   Skin tension lines of the body surface. (Adapted from Trott AT: Wounds and Lacerations: Emergency Care and Closure, 2nd ed. St. Louis, Mosby–Year Book, 1998, p 17.)

PATIENT PREPARATION

- Explain the procedure to the patient or guardian, or both, and be prepared to answer any questions.

- The patient or patient's guardian must give informed consent before start of the procedure.

- A topical anesthetic can be provided, which must be applied 20 to 60 minutes before the procedure, depending on the topical agent used (see Chapter 22 for selection of topical anesthetics). If topical anesthesia is used, the occlusive tape, if any, is removed and cleaned with gauze.

Materials Utilized to Perform a Shave, Snip, or Curettage Biopsy

■ Topical anesthetic, if used

■ Sterile gloves

■ Sterile towels

■ Alcohol pads

■ No. 15 blade or a razor blade

■ Lidocaine with or without epinephrine, as indicated

■ 3-mL syringe and 30-gauge needle for local anesthesia

■ 4 × 4-inch gauze

■ Forceps

■ Cotton-tipped applicator and 20% aluminum chloride for hemostasis (for more vascular lesions, hand-held cautery may be needed)

■ Specimen container

Note: Most biopsy specimens may be sent in formalin containers. The exceptions to this are specimens sent for culture or immunofluorescent studies and specimens in which formalin breaks down the tissue, such as in xanthomatous lesions (Fitzpatrick, 1999; Schultz, 1996). In these instances, specimens should be sent fresh. This is accomplished by placing the specimen on sterile 4 × 4-inch gauze moistened with sterile water or normal saline in a sterile urine cup. All fresh specimens need to be transported immediately to the pathology department for examination.

■ Polymyxin B sulfate-bacitracin zinc (Polysporin) and an adhesive bandage

If skin tags (acrochordons) are to be removed, the following equipment is needed:

■ Alcohol pads

■ Forceps

■ Tonometry scissors

■ 4 × 4-inch gauze

■ 20% aluminum chloride

■ Cotton-tipped applicator

■ Polymyxin B sulfate-bacitracin zinc (Polysporin) and an adhesive bandage

For curettage the following equipment is needed:
- Alcohol pads
- 4 × 4-inch gauze
- 20% aluminum chloride
- Cotton-tipped applicator
- Polymyxin B sulfate-bacitracin zinc (Polysporin) and an adhesive bandage
- Hand-held cautery and cryogun (optional)

Procedure for Performing a Shave, Snip, or Curettage Biopsy

Shave Biopsy

1. Place a sterile towel around the biopsy site.

2. Lightly clean the area with an alcohol pad unless cautery use is anticipated.

Note: Because alcohol is flammable, use nonflammable povidone-iodine and water to prepare the skin if cautery may be used.

3. If the lesion has the potential to blanch with an injection of lidocaine with epinephrine, such as in basal cell carcinomas, mark the margins of the lesion with a sterile surgical marker before the anesthetic is injected (Bennett, 1988a; Siegel and Usatine, 1998b).

4. Inject the lesion with anesthetic so that a wheal is raised.

5. Hold the No. 15 blade flat and parallel with the skin surface.

6. If a razor blade is used, snap it in half lengthwise and bow the ends so that the middle of the blade is flat and parallel with the skin surface.

7. Use a gentle sawing motion to shave through the lesion (Fig. 24-3).

Figure 24-3.   Shave biopsy. (Redrawn from Pfenninger JL, Fowler GC: Procedures for Primary Care Physicians. St. Louis, Mosby–Year Book, 1994, p 22.)

8. The lesion may be elevated with the use of forceps or by spearing the lesion with a needle.

Note: Care must be taken not to crush the lesion with the forceps, which will distort the histologic specimen (referred to as crush artifact).

9. Attempt to shave the base of the lesion completely by shaving into the uppermost portion of the dermis.

Note: If the specimen is too thin (just epidermis), a good histologic diagnosis may not be made.

10. To complete the shave, it is sometimes useful to stabilize the far end of the lesion with a cotton-tipped applicator to cut against.

continued

11. Once the lesion is removed, most light bleeding can be stopped with direct pressure and 20% aluminum chloride on a cotton-tipped applicator.

Note: If bleeding is more brisk or is not stopped with the preceding procedure, hand-held cautery should be used.

12. Place an antibiotic ointment such as mupirocin (Bactroban) or polymyxin B sulfate-bacitracin zinc on an adhesive bandage to dress the wound.

Snip Excision

1. Clean the area lightly with an alcohol pad.

Note: There is usually no need to anesthetize the area. The exception is larger skin tags because they may actually be dermal nevi.

2. Pick up the skin tag with forceps and cut at the base with tonometry scissors.

3. If there is any bleeding, stop with 20% aluminum chloride on a cotton-tipped applicator.

4. Place antibiotic ointment on an adhesive bandage to dress the wound.

Curettage

Note: For seborrheic keratoses, verrucous lesions, or molluscum contagiosum, cryotherapy (see Chapter 27) applied first and followed quickly by curettage requires no local injection because liquid nitrogen acts as a partial anesthetic (Graham, 1999).

1. If the patient is apprehensive, a topical anesthetic can be applied before the procedure.

2. For superficial basal cell carcinomas or any other lesion in which the use of cautery is anticipated, the lesion should be injected with anesthetic.

3. Hold the curette like a pencil with the sharp side down.

4. Stabilize the skin and use quick scraping motions.

Note: When the lesion has been removed, the skin feels different under the curette. Differentiating this change develops with the experience of the provider.

5. Once the lesion is completely removed, obtain hemostasis with 20% aluminum chloride on a cotton-tipped applicator or with hand-held cautery.

Note: Curettage and desiccation for basal cell carcinomas and Bowen's disease requires the following procedure: Curette the lesion until all visible signs of tumor are gone (generally 1 to 2 mm onto normal skin), desiccate the whole base of the lesion with hand-held cautery, and then repeat both steps for three full cycles of curettage and desiccation (Schwartz, 1999; Usatine, 1998a).

6. Place antibiotic ointment on an adhesive bandage to dress the wound.

FOLLOW-UP CARE AND INSTRUCTIONS

■ Written instructions on wound care can be provided.

■ Instruct the patient to keep the area clean and dry for 24 hours (Siegel, 1998; Zalla, 1996).

- After that time, instruct the patient to remove the adhesive bandage and to clean the wound site with soap and water as usual.

- Instruct the patient that if an adhesive bandage is applied, more antibiotic ointment should be placed on the biopsy site. For most small shave biopsy sites, however, the adhesive bandage does not need to be reapplied after the first 24 hours.

- Caution the patient that infection is a rare complication, as antibiotic ointment is applied under the dressing after the procedure is complete.

- Instruct the patient to call the office if the following signs appear: erythematous, tender, warm skin with purulent drainage. When this occurs, antibiotic treatment should be initiated. A broad-spectrum oral antibiotic that covers *Staphylococcus* and *Streptococcus* species should be used, such as cephalexin, dicloxacillin, or erythromycin (Moy and Usatine, 1998a).

- Barring infection, it is not necessary to schedule a return appointment, but the patient should be informed of the results of the pathologic examination.

PUNCH BIOPSY

INDICATIONS

When there is a lesion or dermatosis that covers a large surface area and diagnosis needs to be confirmed before treatment is started, taking just a portion of the lesion is indicated (Siegel and Usatine, 1998a).
- It is important to take the most representative area of the lesion for the highest diagnostic yield.

- In the case of pruritic dermatoses, it is best to biopsy a lesion that has not been excoriated.

- For vesicular lesions, an intact vesicle or bulla may provide the best diagnostic yield for general histology. If an autoimmune bullous disorder is suspected, an additional punch biopsy should be obtained within 1 cm but not on the vesicle or bulla. This specimen would be sent to pathology for direct immunofluorescence staining. In suspected melanoma that is too large to excise at that time, the biopsy should be obtained from the darkest or thickest area of the lesion.

CONTRAINDICATIONS

Contraindications for an incisional biopsy would be any lesion with highly suspected malignant potential, such as melanoma, that could be easily excised at the initial visit (Siegel and Usatine, 1998a). Any lesion smaller than

8 to 10 mm, regardless of malignant potential, can easily be removed completely with a punch biopsy.

POTENTIAL COMPLICATIONS

The risks for a punch biopsy are similar to those of shave biopsies:

- There is discomfort with the injection of anesthetic.

- The risk for bleeding is higher than in shave biopsies because the skin is incised to the subcutaneous fat, increasing the risk of severing small vessels. Hand-held cautery is the method of choice to stop brisk bleeding.

- In any punch biopsy of 8 mm or larger, subcutaneous sutures also decrease the bleeding and improve wound healing.

- The infection rate is higher because the procedure is slightly more invasive. As with a shave biopsy, secondary infection can be easily treated with a 5- to 7-day course of a broad-spectrum antibiotic.

- Scarring will occur, but the extent depends on the patient's ability to heal versus the size of the end defect. In punch biopsies of 1 cm or larger, it is more cosmetically appealing to perform an excision with a No. 15 blade (Moy and Usatine, 1998b; Siegel and Usatine, 1998a), which avoids the potential problem of dog-eared closures.

Standard Precautions   Every practitioner should use standard precautions at all times when interacting with patients, especially when performing procedures. Determining the level of precaution necessary requires the practitioner to exercise clinical judgment based on the patient's history and the potential for exposure to body fluids or aerosol-borne pathogens (for further discussion, see Chapter 2).

PATIENT PREPARATION

- Explain the procedure to the patient or guardian, or both, and be prepared to answer any questions.

- The patient or guardian must give informed consent before start of the procedure.

- A topical anesthetic can be provided, which must be applied 20 to 60 minutes before the procedure, depending on the topical agent used (see Chapter 22 for selection of topical anesthetics). If topical anesthesia is used, the occlusive tape, if any, is removed and cleaned with gauze.

Materials Utilized to Perform a Punch Biopsy _____

- Topical anesthetic, if used
- Metric ruler to determine the size of the lesion
- Sterile gloves
- Sterile towels
- Alcohol pads
- Lidocaine with or without epinephrine, as indicated
- 3-mL syringe and 30-gauge needle for local anesthesia (for larger lesions use a 27-gauge, 1½-inch needle)
- 4 × 4-inch gauze
- Forceps
- Curved scissors
- Needle driver
- Appropriate suture to close skin (see Chapter 23)
- Specimen container
- Polymyxin B sulfate-bacitracin zinc (Polysporin) and an adhesive bandage
- Appropriately sized punch (A punch is selected that is the appropriate size to completely excise the lesion with minimal surrounding normal skin.)

Note: Disposable punches are available in the following sizes: 2, 3, 4, 6, and 8 mm. Nondisposable punches are available in 10, 12, and 15 mm sizes. In the case of incisional biopsies, a 3- or 4-mm punch should be sufficient to make the diagnosis. If enough tissue is needed to send a portion for histologic examination and another portion for culture or immunofluorescent studies, two 3- or 4-mm biopsy specimens may be taken. Alternatively, one 6-mm specimen may be sent with a request to the pathology department to split the specimen and explicit directions on what is to be done with each half.

Procedure for Performing a Punch Biopsy

1. With punch biopsy specimens smaller than 1 cm, place a sterile towel around the biopsy site.

2. Use an alcohol pad to lightly clean the area.

3. If the punch biopsy specimen is to be 1 cm or larger, scrub the area first for 3 minutes with chlorhexidine or povidone-iodine (Hruza, 1999; Moy and Usatine, 1998b).

4. Drape the area with sterile towels.

5. If the lesion has the potential to blanch with the injection of lidocaine with epinephrine, such as in basal cell carcinomas, the margins of the lesion should be marked with a sterile surgical marker before the anesthetic is injected.

6. Inject the lesion with the anesthetic so that the area where the punch will be placed and the surrounding tissue will be sutured is anesthetized.

Note: It is also important to ensure that the full depth of where the punch will extend is anesthetized. Local anesthetic works rapidly, within a minute; however, in highly vascular areas such as the scalp it is prudent to wait 10 minutes to allow the epinephrine to work (Siegel and Usatine, 1998a).

7. After selecting the appropriate size punch, hold the skin taut perpendicular to the lines of tension, wrinkle, or skin fold.

8. Hold the punch perpendicular to the skin and place it so that the lesion is centered within the punch area (Fig. 24-4A).

9. Apply downward pressure while rotating the punch.

Note: It is useful to get into the habit of rotating the punch in one direction, as it is necessary for the biopsy of vesicular or bullous lesions. Rotating back and forth in these cases distorts the plane of cleavage (Bennett, 1988c).

10. The punch should extend to the subcutaneous fat.

Note: When performing a punch biopsy over large vessels or nerves and in areas of thin skin, it is sometimes helpful to pinch the skin upward to avoid damaging underlying structures.

11. Once complete, remove the punch, and the specimen will remain attached to the subcutaneous fat by a pedicle (see Fig. 24-4B).

12. Gently lift the specimen with a pair of forceps and cut at the base with a pair of scissors (Fig. 24-4C).

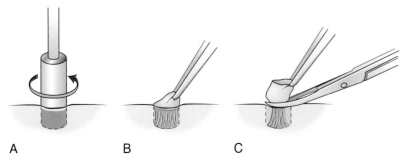

A   B   C

FIGURE 24-4. A-C, Punch biopsy. (Redrawn from Pfenninger JL, Fowler GC: Procedures for Primary Care Physicians. St. Louis, Mosby–Year Book, 1994, p 23.)

Note: Care must be taken not to crush the lesion with the forceps, which could distort the histologic specimen.

  Note: If the punch is removed and the pedicle is missing, it may be found in one of two places. Most commonly it is inside the punch. Removal can be accomplished by spearing it with a needle and pulling it out. It may also be under the skin. Gently explore under the skin through the defect to look for the specimen.

13. Once the specimen is removed completely, place it in the specimen container.

14. Suture the wound, placing half as many sutures as the size of the punch (see Chapter 23). For instance, a 6-mm punch requires three evenly spaced sutures.

15. Apply an antibiotic ointment on an adhesive bandage to dress the wound.

FOLLOW-UP CARE AND INSTRUCTIONS

- Written instructions on wound care should be provided.

- Instruct the patient to keep the area clean and dry for 24 hours. After that time, the adhesive bandage may be removed and the site cleaned with soap and water as usual.

- If a new adhesive bandage is applied, instruct the patient to place more antibiotic ointment on the biopsy site. For most punch biopsy sites, however, the adhesive bandage does not need to be reapplied after the first 24 hours. The exception to this is in areas of friction or if drainage will get on the patient's clothing.

- Schedule a return appointment in 5 to 21 days, depending on the area biopsied. The head tends to heal faster, whereas areas of tension such as the anterior tibia require longer healing times. A basic time schedule for suture removal is as follows (Hruza, 1999; Moy, 1998):

  - Face and ears: 5 to 7 days

  - Neck: 7 days

  - Scalp: 7 to 10 days

  - Trunk and extremities: 7 to 14 days

  - Distal lower extremities: 10 to 21 days

- Advise the patient to not do any heavy lifting or exercising that might cause the sutures to break or lead to a widened scar.

- The patient should be informed of the results of the pathologic examination, either when the results are provided to the practitioner or when the patient returns for suture removal.

EXCISIONAL BIOPSY

INDICATIONS

Any lesion that is smaller than 8 to 10 mm can be completely excised as stated earlier with a punch biopsy. Most lesions larger than 1 cm have a better cosmetic appearance if the excision is performed using a No. 15 blade. Lesions that are excised routinely are as follows (Moy and Usatine, 1998b; Schultz, 1996; Zalla, 1996):

■ Suspected melanomas

■ Epidermal inclusion cysts

■ Lipomas

■ Larger basal cell and squamous cell carcinomas

■ Dermal lesions larger than 1 cm

Mohs micrographic surgical procedures are beyond the scope of most primary care providers, as they require special training to perform. However, they bear mentioning with respect to removal of malignant lesions. Mohs procedures are preferred in sclerosing and morpheaform basal cell carcinomas, recurrent tumors, and any malignant tumor around the eyes, nose, or lips, and on the ears. They use a special technique of excising and color-coding the specimen before histologic examination. This method has a higher overall cure rate and lower recurrence rate than do standard excisions (Randle, 1996; Russell, 1999; Zalla, 1996). Patients who meet the preceding criteria and in whom surgery is being considered should be referred to a dermatologist trained in the Mohs technique.

POTENTIAL COMPLICATIONS

The complications are similar to those of punch biopsies.

■ There is discomfort with the injection of anesthetic.

■ The risk for bleeding is higher because a larger area of skin is incised to the subcutaneous fat, increasing the risk of severing small vessels.

■ Hand-held cautery is the method of choice to stop brisk bleeding in addition to subcutaneous sutures.

■ The infection rate is also higher because the procedure is more invasive. Secondary infection can be easily treated with a 5- to 7-day course of a broad-spectrum antibiotic covering *Staphylococcus* and *Streptococcus* species.

■ Scarring will occur, but the extent depends on the patient's ability to heal versus the size and placement of the end defect.

■ More than with any other biopsy technique, adequate knowledge of the lines of skin tension is required to determine orientation of excisional biopsies (see Fig. 24-2).

Caution must be used when performing elliptic excisions on the face—particularly on the forehead or near the eyes or lips—so that distortion does not occur (Moy and Usatine, 1998b). Large excisions in these areas may necessitate a graft or flap closure.

Standard Precautions   Every practitioner should use standard precautions at all times when interacting with patients, especially when performing procedures. Determining the level of precaution necessary requires the practitioner to exercise clinical judgment based on the patient's history and the potential for exposure to body fluids or aerosol-borne pathogens (for further discussion, see Chapter 2).

PATIENT PREPARATION

■ Explain the procedure to the patient or the patient's guardian, or both, and be prepared to answer any questions.

■ The patient or guardian must give informed consent before the start of the procedure.

■ A topical anesthetic can be provided, which must be applied 20 to 60 minutes before the procedure, depending on the topical agent used (see Chapter 22 for selection of topical anesthetics).

■ If topical anesthesia is used, the occlusive tape, if any, is removed and cleaned with gauze.

Materials Utilized to Perform an Excisional Biopsy

■ Topical anesthesia, if used

■ Chlorhexidine or povidone-iodine

■ Sterile surgical marker

■ Sterile gloves

■ Sterile towels

■ Alcohol pads

■ Lidocaine with or without epinephrine, as indicated

■ 3-mL syringe and 27-gauge, 1-inch needle for local anesthesia

■ 4 × 4-inch gauze

- Forceps

- Curved scissors

- Needle driver

- Appropriate suture to close subcutaneous tissue and skin (see Chapter 23)

- Hand-held cautery

- Specimen container

- Polymyxin B sulfate-bacitracin zinc (Polysporin) and a dressing of 4 × 4-inch gauze and paper tape or a large adhesive bandage

- Metric ruler to determine the size of the end defect

Procedure for Performing an Excisional Biopsy

Note: Proper anesthetic technique is determined by the size of the area being excised and may warrant direct infiltration of the biopsy site, digital block, or a field block (see Chapter 22).

Note: It is also important to ensure that anesthesia is adequate for the full depth and width of the excision and placement of sutures. Local anesthesia works rapidly, within a minute; however, in highly vascular areas such as the scalp it is prudent to wait 10 minutes to allow the epinephrine, when used, to work.

1. Scrub the area for 5 minutes with chlorhexidine or povidone-iodine.

2. Drape the area with sterile towels.

3. If the lesion has the potential to blanch with the injection of lidocaine with epinephrine, such as in basal cell carcinomas, the margins of the lesion should be marked with a sterile surgical marker before the anesthetic is injected.

4. Use a sterile surgical marker to mark the intended incision line, taking into account the lines of tension, wrinkles, or skin folds (see Fig. 24-2).

5. Hold the No. 15 blade like a pencil, perpendicular to the skin.

6. Use the tip of the blade to incise the corner of the ellipse, but use the belly for the rest of the incision (Moy and Usatine, 1998b; Zalla, 1996).

7. Continue the incision through the dermis to the subcutaneous fat (Fig. 24-5).

FIGURE 24-5. Excisional biopsy. (Redrawn from Pfenninger JL, Fowler GC: Procedures for Primary Care Physicians. St. Louis, Mosby–Year Book, 1994, p 24.)

8. Use the forceps to lift the specimen gently, taking care not to crush it.

9. Use the No. 15 blade to cut the specimen at the base or subcutaneous fat.

Note: In the case of potentially malignant lesions, it is useful to place a tag suture on one corner of the specimen, indicating where the tag was placed on the form sent to pathology (e.g., tag is placed on medial corner).

10. Once the specimen is completely removed, place it in the specimen container.

11. In larger excisions, push the skin edges of the defect together or pull them together with skin hooks to see how much tension will be placed on the sutures.

Note: If there is tension, undermining is needed. Undermining is performed by blunt dissection to mobilize adequate tissue for closure.

12. Stop any bleeding with hand-held cautery.

13. Begin wound closure of the excision with the placement of subcutaneous vertical mattress sutures to approximate the wound edges, decrease wound tension, and reduce the risk of wound dehiscence. This is performed with an absorbable suture material.

14. Place nonabsorbable sutures to close the skin.

Note: This can be performed with running or simple interrupted sutures for most wounds. In areas of greater tension, mattress sutures may need to be placed for strength.

15. Leave the skin edges everted at the end closure for the best outcome.

16. Apply an antibiotic ointment on a dressing over the wound.

SPECIAL CONSIDERATIONS

With any invasive procedure, a good history and review of systems should be taken to determine if there are any contraindications to surgery. In addition, the patient's ability to heal, history of allergies, need for subbacterial endocarditis (SBE) prophylaxis and use of anticoagulants should be assessed. If possible, the patient should discontinue warfarin and nonsteroidal antiinflammatory agents approximately 2 to 4 days before any invasive procedure, and aspirin should be discontinued for approximately 10 days (Hruza, 1999; Moy and Usatine, 1998a; Stasko, 1996; Zalla, 1996).

It is difficult to perform biopsies on small children, particularly those between the ages of 1 and 5. The provider needs to discuss the absolute need for biopsy with the parents or guardian before deciding to perform the procedure. Once it is determined that the biopsy is necessary, the child may need to be sedated. However, with the use of topical anesthetics, many children experience little discomfort.

FOLLOW-UP CARE AND INSTRUCTIONS

- Written instructions on wound care should be provided.

- Instruct the patient to keep the area clean and dry for 24 hours.

- After that time, the dressing may be removed and the site cleaned with soap and water as usual.

- If a new dressing is applied, instruct the patient to place more antibiotic ointment on the biopsy site. For most biopsy sites, however, the dressing does not need to be reapplied after the first 24 hours. The exception to this is in areas of friction or if drainage will get on the patient's clothing.

- Schedule a return appointment in 5 to 21 days, depending on the area biopsied. (Refer to the time schedule for suture removal given in "Follow-up Care and Instructions" under "Punch Biopsy.")

- Inform the patient that care should be taken to not do any heavy lifting or exercising that might cause the sutures to break or lead to a widened scar.

- Inform the patient of the results of the pathologic examination either when the results are provided to the practitioner or when the patient returns for suture removal.

Electrosurgery

BACKGROUND AND HISTORY

Electrosurgery encompasses electrodesiccation, electrocoagulation, electrofulguration, electrosection, electrolysis, and electrocautery. The focus of this section is electrodesiccation. This is a high-voltage, low-amperage damped current, which generates heat in the tissue, causing coagulation and dehydration (Hruza, 1999; Pollack, 1997). There is no current channeling along blood vessels and nerves with electrodesiccation, so it is relatively safe in patients with cardiac pacemakers. Despite this, it should not be used immediately near the pacemaker (Bennett, 1988b; Hruza, 1999; Pollack, 1997; Usatine, 1998a). Lesions larger than 3 to 4 mm do better with cryosurgery, whereas smaller, 1- to 2-mm lesions may respond better to electrodesiccation (Graham, 1999).

INDICATIONS

Lesions commonly treated with electrodesiccation include the following:
- Acrochordons

- Pyogenic granulomas and other vascular lesions

- Verruca vulgaris

- Condyloma acuminata

- Actinic keratoses

- Superficial multicentric basal cell carcinomas, in combination with curettage

CONTRAINDICATIONS

- The procedure should not be performed near a pacemaker.

- It also should not be performed if flammable material or gases are present in the immediate surgical field.

POTENTIAL COMPLICATIONS

Common complications of electrodesiccation include the following:
- Pain

- Scarring

- Delayed bleeding

- Risk of burns

- Pigment alterations: A crust will form within 24 hours. Within 5 to 7 days, the crust sloughs off. Once this occurs, there may be a hypopigmented area remaining, which is generally temporary. Occasionally, an area of hyperpigmentation may develop that could require further treatment with keratolytic (e.g., topical retinoids) or bleaching agents (e.g., 4% hydroquinone) to lighten the skin (Stasko, 1996). Scarring may be hypertrophic, atrophic, or a keloid on rare occasions.

- The use of alcohol to prepare the skin could lead to fire during electrosurgery. A nonflammable alternative preparation such as povidone-iodine is preferred. Care must also be taken when electrosurgery is performed in the perianal area. Bowel gas, which is composed of methane and hydrogen gas, can ignite. This can be prevented with adequate bowel preparation before the procedure or the placement of cotton in the rectum (Bennett, 1998b).

- Viral particles can be aerosolized in cautery and laser smoke, particularly human papillomavirus (HPV) and human immunodeficiency virus (HIV). There are no case reports of HIV transmission through cautery and laser smoke. There are, however, reports of laryngeal papillomatosis in health care providers from cautery and laser ablation of warts (Lowry, 1999; Seabury-Stone, 1996; Usatine, 1998a).

Standard Precautions   Every practitioner should use standard precautions at all times when interacting with patients, especially when performing procedures. Determining the level of precaution necessary requires the practitioner to exercise clinical judgment based on the patient's history and the potential for exposure to body fluids or aerosol-borne pathogens (for further discussion, see Chapter 2).

PATIENT PREPARATION

- Explain the procedure to the patient or the patient's guardian, or both, and be prepared to answer any questions.

- The patient or guardian must give informed consent before start of the procedure.

- A topical anesthetic can be provided, which must be applied 20 to 60 minutes before the procedure, depending on the topical agent used (see Chapter 22 for selection of topical anesthetics).

- If topical anesthesia is used, the occlusive tape, if any, is removed and cleaned with gauze.

- Electrodesiccation does not induce partial anesthesia; therefore, the procedure is better tolerated if a topical anesthetic is applied before starting the procedure or local anesthesia infiltration is used. After the procedure, patients rarely need any analgesia, but acetaminophen may be required.

 Materials Utilized to Perform Electrosurgery _____

- Topical anesthetic, if used

- Hyfrecator and desiccation electrode needle

- Face mask (for protection from smoke generated during the procedure)

- 4 × 4-inch gauze

- Antibiotic ointment and an adhesive bandage

- 5- or 7-mm curette and 4 × 4-inch gauze, if curettage of a lesion will follow the electrosurgery

Procedure for Performing Electrosurgery

1. Clean the area with povidone-iodine and water only for electrodesiccation. Alcohol is flammable, and therefore should not be used.

2. For electrodesiccation, remove the occlusive tape from the topical anesthetic.

3. Use the hyfrecator with desiccation electrode needle.

Note: Set the hyfrecator to a low setting to begin and turn it up as needed. Lightly touch the lesion to determine if the power setting is adequate.

4. Once the correct power setting is found, ablate the lesion.

Note: Small lesions usually are ablated immediately, whereas larger lesions require gentle passes with the electrode.

5. Gently wipe the charred lesion with 4 × 4-inch gauze or curette. No bleeding should occur.

6. Apply an antibiotic ointment and an adhesive bandage.

FOLLOW-UP CARE AND INSTRUCTIONS

■ Written instructions on wound care should be provided.

■ For areas of electrodesiccation, instruct the patient to keep the area clean and dry for 24 hours.

■ After that time, the dressing may be removed and the site cleaned with soap and water as usual.

■ If a new dressing is applied, instruct the patient to place more antibiotic ointment on the biopsy site. For most biopsy sites, however, the dressing does not need to be reapplied after the first 24 hours. The exception to this is in areas of friction or if drainage will get on the patient's clothing.

■ No return appointment is necessary.

Acne Surgery

BACKGROUND AND HISTORY

Acne surgery is performed on comedones and, occasionally, pustules. Open comedones or "blackheads" are removed purely for cosmetic purposes. Removal does not shorten the resolution of the acne lesions. Removal of closed comedones or "whiteheads" does shorten the resolution time, as acne surgery prevents them from rupturing and becoming larger papules or pustules (Strauss, 1999).

INDICATIONS

Acne surgery may be performed on most patients with comedonal or pustular acne. Pretreatment with a topical retinoid by the patient for approximately 1 month greatly improves the removal of comedones (Baran, 1998; Strauss, 1999).

CONTRAINDICATIONS

Care should be taken with patients who may develop postinflammatory hyperpigmentation or those who may bruise easily. They should be informed of the possible risks of bruising and hyperpigmentation.

POTENTIAL COMPLICATIONS

- Discomfort from the procedure

- Immediate swelling and pinpoint bleeding

- Small amounts of bruising

- Postinflammatory hyperpigmentation

- Rupture of the comedo if improper technique is used (Baran, 1998; Strauss, 1999).

Standard Precautions   Every practitioner should use standard precautions at all times when interacting with patients, especially when performing procedures. Determining the level of precaution necessary requires the practitioner to exercise clinical judgment based on the patient's history and the potential for exposure to body fluids or aerosol-borne pathogens (for further discussion, see Chapter 2).

PATIENT PREPARATION

- Explain the procedure to the patient or the patient's guardian, or both, and be prepared to answer any questions.

- The patient or guardian must give informed consent before start of the procedure.

 Materials Utilized to Perform Acne Surgery _____

- Alcohol pads

- No. 11 blade or a 25-gauge needle

- Unna-type comedo extractor

- 4 × 4-inch gauze

Procedure for Performing Acne Surgery

1. Clean the area with an alcohol pad.

2. Use a No. 11 blade or 25-gauge needle to open the pore of the comedo or pustule gently.

3. Place the Unna-type comedo extractor flat against the skin.

4. Apply pressure downward while gently sliding toward the comedo or pustule (Fig. 24-6).

Note: The extractor may need to be moved in all four quadrants to ensure all the comedonal contents are removed.

5. Stop any bleeding with direct pressure with 4 × 4-inch gauze.

FIGURE 24-6. Acne surgery. (Redrawn from Pfenninger JL, Fowler GC: Procedures for Primary Care Physicians. St. Louis, Mosby–Year Book, 1994, p 55.)

Note: The patient may want to wash his or her face before leaving the office.

FOLLOW-UP CARE AND INSTRUCTIONS

- Instruct the patient to wash the area with soap and water as usual.

- Advise the patient that topical retinoids and alpha-hydroxy acids may need to be avoided for 24 hours to prevent irritation of the open areas.

- No return appointment is necessary.

REFERENCES

Baran R, Chivot M, Shalita AR: Acne. In Baran R, Maibach HI (eds): Textbook of Cosmetic Dermatology, 2nd ed. London, Martin Dunitz, 1998, pp 433-444.

Bennett RG: Curettage. In Fundamentals of Cutaneous Surgery. St. Louis, CV Mosby, 1988a, pp 532-552.

Bennett RG: Electrosurgery. In Fundamentals of Cutaneous Surgery. St. Louis, CV Mosby, 1988b, pp 553-590.

Bennett RG: The skin biopsy. In Fundamentals of Cutaneous Surgery. St. Louis, CV Mosby, 1988c, pp 517-531.

Fitzpatrick TB, Bernhard JD, Cropley TG: The structure of skin lesions and fundamentals of diagnosis. In Fitzpatrick TB, Eisen AZ, Wolff K, et al (eds): Dermatology in General Medicine, 5th ed. New York, McGraw-Hill, 1999, pp 13-41.

Graham GF: Cryosurgery. In Fitzpatrick TB, Eisen AZ, Wolff K, et al (eds): Dermatology in General Medicine, 5th ed. New York, McGraw-Hill, 1999, pp 2980-2987.

Ho VCY: Benign epithelial tumors. In Fitzpatrick TB, Eisen AZ, Wolff K, et al (eds): Dermatology in General Medicine, 5th ed. New York, McGraw-Hill, 1999, pp 873-890.

Hruza GJ: Dermatologic surgery: Introduction and approach. In Fitzpatrick TB, Eisen AZ, Wolff K, et al (eds): Dermatology in General Medicine, 5th ed. New York, McGraw-Hill, 1999, pp 2923-2937.

Lowry DR, Androphy EJ: Warts. In Fitzpatrick TB, Eisen AZ, Wolff K, et al (eds): Dermatology in General Medicine, 5th ed. New York, McGraw-Hill, 1999, pp 2484-2497.

Moy RL: Suturing techniques. In Usatine RP, Moy RL, Tobinick EL, et al (eds): Skin Surgery: A Practical Guide. St. Louis, CV Mosby, 1998, pp 88-100.

Moy RL, Usatine RP: Complications and their prevention. In Usatine RP, Moy RL, Tobinick EL, et al (eds): Skin Surgery: A Practical Guide. St. Louis, CV Mosby, 1998a, pp 287-299.

Moy RL, Usatine RP: Elliptical excision. In Usatine RP, Moy RL, Tobinick EL, et al (eds): Skin Surgery: A Practical Guide. St. Louis, CV Mosby, 1998b, pp 120-136.

Pollack SV, Kobayashi T: Cosmetic electrosurgery. In Coleman WP III, Hanke CW, Alt TH, et al (eds): Cosmetic Surgery of the Skin: Principles and Techniques, 2nd ed. St. Louis, CV Mosby, 1997, pp 272-286.

Randle HW, Roenigk RK: Indications for Mohs micrographic surgery. In Roenigk RK, Roenigk HH (eds): Dermatologic Surgery: Principles and Practice, 2nd ed. New York, Marcel Dekker, 1996, pp 703-730.

Russell BA, Amonette RA, Swanson NA: Mohs micrographic surgery. In Fitzpatrick TB, Eisen AZ, Wolff K, et al (eds): Dermatology in General Medicine, 5th ed. New York, McGraw-Hill, 1999, pp. 2988-2991.

Schultz BC: Skin biopsy. In Roenigk RK, Roenigk HH (eds): Dermatologic Surgery: Principles and Practice, 2nd ed. New York, Marcel Dekker, 1996, pp 177-190.

Schwartz RA, Stoll HL Jr: Epithelial precancerous lesions. In Fitzpatrick TB, Eisen AZ, Wolff K, et al (eds): Dermatology in General Medicine, 5th ed. New York, McGraw-Hill, 1999, pp 823-839.

Seabury-Stone M, Lynch PJ: Viral warts. In Sams WM, Lynch PJ (eds): Principles and Practice of Dermatology, 2nd ed. New York, Churchill Livingstone, 1996, pp 127-133.

Siegel DM, Moy RL, Usatine RP: Wound care. In Usatine RP, Moy RL, Tobinick EL, et al (eds): Skin Surgery: A Practical Guide. St Louis, CV Mosby, 1998, pp 278-286.

Siegel DM, Usatine RP: The punch biopsy. In Usatine RP, Moy RL, Tobinick EL, et al (eds): Skin Surgery: A Practical Guide. St Louis, CV Mosby, 1998a, pp 101-119.

Siegel DM, Usatine RP. The shave biopsy. In Usatine RP, Moy RL, Tobinick EL, et al (eds): Skin Surgery: A Practical Guide. St Louis, CV Mosby, 1998b, pp 55-76.

Stasko T: Complications of cutaneous procedures. In Roenigk RK, Roenigk HH (eds): Dermatologic Surgery: Principles and Practice, 2nd ed. New York, Marcel Dekker, 1996, pp 149-175.

Strauss JS, Thiboutot DM: Diseases of the sebaceous glands. In
Fitzpatrick TB, Eisen AZ, Wolff K, et al (eds): Dermatology in General
Medicine, 5th ed. New York, McGraw-Hill, 1999, pp 769-784.
Tobinick EL, Usatine RP: Choosing the type of biopsy. In Usatine RP,
Moy RL, Tobinick EL, et al (eds): Skin Surgery: A Practical Guide.
St Louis, CV Mosby, 1998, pp 40-54.
Usatine RP: Electrosurgery. In Usatine RP, Moy RL, Tobinick EL, et al
(eds): Skin Surgery: A Practical Guide. St Louis, CV Mosby, 1998a,
pp 165-199.
Usatine RP: Hemostasis. In Usatine RP, Moy RL, Tobinick EL, et al (eds):
Skin Surgery: A Practical Guide. St Louis, CV Mosby, 1998b, pp 31-39.
Zalla MJ, Roenigk RK: Excision. In Roenigk RK, Roenigk HH (eds):
Dermatologic Surgery: Principles and Practice, 2nd ed. New York,
Marcel Dekker, 1996, pp 191-207.

BIBLIOGRAPHY

Pollack SV, Grekin RC: Electrosurgery and electroepilation. In
Roenigk RK, Roenigk HH (eds): Dermatologic Surgery: Principles and
Practice, 2nd ed. New York, Marcel Dekker, 1996, pp 219-231.
Sinclair RD, Tzermias C, Dawber R: Cosmetic cryosurgery. In Baran R,
Maibach HI (eds): Textbook of Cosmetic Dermatology, 2nd ed.
London, Martin Dunitz, 1998, pp 691-700.
Usatine RP, Moy RL: Anesthesia. In Usatine RP, Moy RL, Tobinick EL,
et al (eds): Skin Surgery: A Practical Guide. St. Louis, CV Mosby, 1998,
pp 20-30.
Usatine RP, Tobinick EL: Cryosurgical techniques. In Usatine RP,
Moy RL, Tobinick EL, et al (eds): Skin Surgery: A Practical Guide.
St. Louis, CV Mosby, 1998, pp 137-164.
Zacarian SA: Complications, indications and contraindications in
cryosurgery. In Roenigk RK, Roenigk HH (eds): Dermatologic Surgery:
Principles and Practice, 2nd ed. New York, Marcel Dekker, 1996,
pp 259-272.

Chapter 25

Incision and Drainage of an Abscess

Patrick C. Auth and George S. Bottomley

PROCEDURE GOALS AND OBJECTIVES

Goal: To incise and drain an abscess successfully while observing standard precautions and with the minimal degree of risk to the patient.

Objectives: The student will be able to ...

- Describe the indications, contraindications, and rationale for performing incision and drainage of an abscess.

- Identify and describe common complications associated with incision and drainage of an abscess.

- Describe the essential anatomy and physiology associated with the performance of incision and drainage of an abscess.

- Identify the materials necessary for performing incision and drainage of an abscess and their proper use.

- Identify the important aspects of post-procedure care after incision and drainage of an abscess.

BACKGROUND AND HISTORY

The world's oldest medical manuscript is a small clay tablet written in Sumerian around 2100 BC. A portion of it translates as, "If a man, his skull contains some fluid, with your thumb press several times at the place where the fluid is found. If the swelling gives way (under your finger) and (pus) is squeezed out of the skull, you shall incise, scrape the bone and (remove) its fluid ..." (Manjo, 1977). Advances made over the last 4100 years in the use of minor surgical procedures to treat abscesses are discussed in this chapter.

INDICATIONS

■ A localized collection of infection that is tender and is not resolving spontaneously. The cardinal signs of infection (pain, fever, redness, swelling, and loss of function) are usually present.

CONTRAINDICATIONS

■ Facial furuncles should not be incised or drained if they are located within the triangle formed by the bridge of the nose and the corners of the mouth. These infections should be treated with antibiotics and warm compresses, as the risk of septic phlebitis with intracranial extension can follow incision and drainage of a furuncle in this area.

■ Abscesses that occur very near the rectum or genitalia must be carefully evaluated, and consideration should be given to referring these patients to a general surgeon for treatment.

■ Patients with diabetes, debilitating disease, or compromised immunity should be observed after incision and drainage of an abscess.

POTENTIAL COMPLICATIONS

■ Cellulitis or re-collection of pus: Bacteremia and septicemia are complications of an inadequately treated abscess. In patients with diabetes or disease that interferes with immune function, an abscess on an extremity can be complicated by severe cellulitis or gangrene, with subsequent loss of the affected extremity.

■ Perianal abscess incision and drainage frequently results in a chronic anal fistula up to 50% of the time in adults.

■ An abscess in the palmar aspect of the hand can extend from superficial to deep tissue via the palmar fascia.

■ Deep infection is suspected when the simple incision and drainage fails to reduce the erythema, pain, pus, or swelling. More extensive surgical debridement, hospitalization, and intravenous antibiotics may be necessary in a patient with deep palmar abscess.

REVIEW OF ESSENTIAL ANATOMY AND PHYSIOLOGY

An abscess is a focal circumscribed accumulation of purulent materials (pus and other inflammatory tissue). An acute or "hot" abscess has all the characteristics of a classic inflammatory episode, producing redness, heat, pain, and swelling. It is a suppurative reaction caused by the invasion of pyogenic (pus-forming) bacteria into a tissue or organ. Grossly (on the skin or surface of an organ), abscesses appear as focal, round, or ovoid areas of swelling covered by skin or other tissue. On palpation, there is usually an area where the covering is thin and comes to a head (point), and when palpated that area is more easily compressible or fluctuant due to its liquid or gel-like contents.

A dry abscess is one that resolves without rupture. A sterile abscess is one from which bacteria cannot be cultured. A chronic or cold abscess lacks the redness, heat, pain, and swelling of an acute abscess and usually is associated with liquefactive necrosis of tuberculous lesions.

CLINICAL EVALUATION

The patient usually complains of pain and swelling. Abscesses commonly occur in the perianal region. A subcutaneous abscess is often seen. Evaluation includes a search for the underlying cause of the abscess—that is, infection secondary to puncture wound or foreign body, exposure to unusually pathogenic organisms, a faulty or overwhelmed immune system, the presence of hyperglycemia, bacteremic spread from another focus, and development of a deep abscess in badly contused muscle tissue in which there was no preceding penetration of skin. When a sweat gland or hair follicle forms an abscess, it is called a furuncle or boil. When the furuncle extends into the subcutaneous tissue, it is referred to as a carbuncle. Paronychia is an abscess that involves the nail. Perifollicular abscesses are commonly found on the extremities, buttocks, breasts, or in hair follicles. A subcutaneous abscess is often seen. When signs and symptoms of localized infection or an abscess are present, incision and drainage should be considered.

THERAPY

A small abscess may respond to warm compresses or antibiotics and may drain spontaneously. If done properly, such treatment renders antibiotics unnecessary.

If the abscess enlarges, the inflammation, collection of pus, and walling off of the abscess cavity render such conservative treatments ineffectual.

In nonlactating women, a breast abscess that is not subareolar is rare and should prompt a biopsy in addition to incision and drainage of the abscess. Indications include a localized collection of pus that is tender and is not resolving spontaneously.

A culture should be obtained by aspiration or swabbing of the abscess cavity, because unusual organisms may have caused the abscess. The infection may also warrant the administration of antibiotics.

ETIOLOGY

Healthy skin and its protective mechanisms are usually successful at fending off potentially pathogenic microorganisms. If, however, this barrier is interrupted through trauma (mechanical, chemical, or thermal) to the stratum corneum, inflammation, or through the often more ingenious mechanisms of infectious agents themselves, skin infections and abscesses develop. Most often, *Staphylococcus aureus* is the causative agent in abscesses, but some abscesses are due to *Streptococcus* species or a combination of microorganisms, including gram-negative and anaerobic bacteria. The flora found in the affected area usually causes the abscess. Puncture wounds or the presence of foreign bodies are common underlying causes of abscess formation. The skin of the debilitated, elderly, diabetic (hyperglycemic state), or otherwise immunocompromised patient may also offer a damaging agent easier access.

Histologically, an abscess is a central area of pus composed of dead white blood cells, bacteria, degenerating tissue debris, and proteins from the immune response to the bacteria. Surrounding this is a zone of healthy neutrophils. Depending on the age of the abscess, peripheral to this is a circumferential area of vascular dilation, macrophages, fibroblasts, and fibrocytes in varying stages of development and collagen. Ultimately, a connective tissue capsule surrounds the area, which inhibits the penetration of anti-infective agents. A diffuse abscess is a localized accumulation of pus that is not well encapsulated.

Abscesses can interfere with normal function of nearby tissue, either by expansion and subsequent pressure on adjacent structures (such as an abscess adjacent to the trachea) or through expulsion of its contents and seeding of bacteria into surrounding areas or the vascular system, with resultant septicemia.

In the treatment of abscesses, the important anatomic structures underlying the abscess must be appreciated and anticipated before an incision is performed. The location of the abscess is critical to the direction of the incision. The abscess locations listed here are in close proximity to major vessels and should be aspirated with an 18-gauge needle attached to a 10-mL syringe before drainage to avoid inadvertent incision into an artery:

■ Peritonsillar and retropharyngeal regions

■ Anterior triangle of the neck

■ Supraclavicular fossa

- Deep in the axilla

- Antecubital space

- Groin

- Popliteal space

Standard Precautions   Every practitioner should use standard precautions at all times when interacting with patients, especially when performing procedures. Determining the level of precaution necessary requires the practitioner to exercise clinical judgment based on the patient's history and the potential for exposure to body fluids or aerosol-borne pathogens (for further discussion, see Chapter 2).

PATIENT PREPARATION

- Advise the patient regarding the potential benefits and risks associated with the procedure.

- Be sure to describe the care required to pack the wound after the procedure.

- Provide an opportunity for the patient to ask questions and receive answers.

- Assist the patient into a comfortable supine position that affords complete access to the abscess site.

 ## Materials Utilized for Performing Incision and Drainage of an Abscess

- Alcohol or povidone-iodine (Betadine) wipe

- 1% to 2% lidocaine (Xylocaine) without epinephrine

- 19- to 22-gauge needle

- Three or four towels for drapes

- No. 11 or No. 15 scalpel blade

- Scalpel handle

- Kelly clamps

- Adson forceps

- Curved hemostats

- 4 × 4-inch gauze pads

- Sterile gloves

- 500 mL of normal saline solution
- ¼- to ½-inch Nu-Gauze strip for packing the wound
- Bandage scissors
- Dressing of choice to cover wound

Procedure for Performing Incision and Drainage of an Abscess

 ### Skin Preparation

1. Apply a single layer of povidone-iodine to the abscess and allow to air-dry before performing the incision.

 ### Drapes

1. Place drapes to ensure isolation of the abscess and the prepared surrounding skin.

 ### Anesthesia

1. Use a regional field block anesthetic technique to anesthetize the abscess by injecting a ring of anesthetic agent approximately 1 cm away from the erythematous border of the abscess around its perimeter.

Note: This will allow the lesion to be anesthetized circumferentially. The onset of action of the anesthetic is approximately 5 to 10 minutes. Complete anesthesia is difficult to provide, especially when breaking the septum within the cavity of the abscess with a hemostat.

2. After alcohol preparation of the skin, superficially infiltrate the skin in a linear course across the abscess and then traverse the second linear course directly perpendicular to the first. Be careful to remain superficial to the abscess cavity.

 ### Incising and Drainage

1. Make the incision along the relaxed skin tension lines (Langer's lines) to reduce scarring (Fig. 25-1).

2. Open the abscess widely by extending the incision across its full dimension (Fig. 25-2). If more drainage is desired, make a second incision perpendicular to the first, forming a cruciate pattern.

Note: This technique typically results in a less aesthetically pleasing scar when fully healed.

3. Obtain a specimen for culture as soon as the purulent material is expressed from the abscess cavity.

Note: If a culture is obtained, it should be from the abscess cavity and not from the superficial skin over the abscess. Alternatively, the abscess cavity can be aspirated with a large-bore (18-gauge) needle before the incision is made. The aspirated contents can then be sent for the

FIGURE 25-1. Skin tension lines of the body surface. (Adapted from Trott AT: Wounds and Lacerations. Emergency Care and Closure, 2nd ed. St. Louis, Mosby–Year Book, 1998, p 17.)

FIGURE 25-2. (Redrawn from Rosen P, Barkin R, Sternback G: Essentials of Emergency Medicine. St. Louis, Mosby–Year Book, 1991, p 645.)

continued

FIGURE 25-3.

Hemostat

Syringe with irrigation needle

FIGURE 25-4.

FIGURE 25-5. (Redrawn from Rosen P, Barkin R, Sternback G: Essentials of Emergency Medicine. St. Louis, Mosby–Year Book, 1991, p 645.)

appropriate cultures in more complicated cases. It is rarely helpful in routine cases.

4. Explore the abscess cavity thoroughly. This can be accomplished with a sterile cotton-tipped applicator or with hemostats. Insert the blunt end of the hemostat into the abscess cavity and spread the hemostat to break up the septum and loculations within the abscess, thus releasing any further pockets of purulent material (Fig. 25-3).

5. Thoroughly irrigate the cavity with normal saline before any gauze is inserted to pack the cavity (Fig. 25-4).

6. After complete drainage of the cavity, insert iodoform gauze into the abscess cavity, with 1 cm of gauze exiting from the cavity (Fig. 25-5), and then pack the cavity with packing material, such as iodoform gauze. The length and width of the gauze depend on the abscess size.

Note: The iodoform gauze serves two purposes: it prevents the incision from sealing over and provides for adequate drainage of the abscess cavity. The iodoform gauze is removed and reinserted every 12 to 24 hours by either the patient or a caregiver.

Note: Healing should progress from the inside out, that is, epithelialization of the abscess cavity should occur before healing of the incision site to minimize the chance of recurrence.

7. Apply a sterile dressing over the abscess site to absorb drainage and prevent foreign materials from entering the wound.

8. Instruct the patient or caregiver on the procedure for packing the wound and twice daily changes at home until healthy closure of the wound occurs.

SPECIAL CONSIDERATIONS

Primary management of abscesses should be incision and drainage and routine culture. Usually incision and drainage is sufficient treatment to cure an abscess. Antibiotic therapy is not indicated for the typical abscess in patients with normal defenses. However, additional treatment may be necessary for patients in the following situations:

- Abscesses to be treated with oral antibiotic therapy are those that are surrounded with lymphangitis or a large area of cellulitis. The cellulitis is determined by tenderness peripheral to the area of the abscess as well as increased warmth and redness, as opposed to the nontender induration palpated around an abscess that is well localized and that would not benefit from the addition of oral antibiotics. When surrounding cellulitis is present or when the patient has risk factors mentioned previously, dicloxacillin (250 to 500 mg every 6 hours) may be used. Alternative antibiotics can be used, but they must cover *Staphylococcus* organisms until the culture results have been returned and a more specific antibiotic treatment is determined.

- Purulent material from immunosuppressed patients (including diabetic patients) should be cultured, with the patient placed on oral antibiotics pending the culture results. Antibiotics may be used in conjunction with surgical incision and drainage in patients who are immunocompromised (i.e., those who have diabetes, leukemia, or acquired immune deficiency syndrome or those who are undergoing chemotherapy). This purulent material should be examined by Gram stain, and the specimen should be sent for culturing (both aerobic and anaerobic) and sensitivity testing before any antibiotic treatment is started.

- Aspiration is used for diagnostic confirmation. The rationale to drain the abscess is to avoid incision of a mycotic aneurysm and imminent exsanguination. The aspiration confirms that the material within the cavity is purulent and not serosanguineous or pure blood.

- In nonlactating women, a breast abscess that is not subareolar is rare and should prompt the consideration of a biopsy in addition to incision and drainage of the abscess. A culture should be obtained by aspiration or swab of the abscess cavity, because unusual organisms may have caused the abscess. The infection may also warrant the administration of antibiotics.

PAIN RELIEF

If the packing is tight in the abscess cavity, the pain can be sufficient to warrant the use of acetaminophen or nonsteroidal anti-inflammatory drugs. Narcotics are rarely needed beyond the initial incision and drainage procedure. The procedure alone may provide sufficient pain relief from a tense abscess so that no pain medication is needed.

FOLLOW-UP CARE AND INSTRUCTIONS

- Advise the patient that following removal of the iodoform pack, the patient is to apply warm wet soaks to the area four to six times a day for 5 to 7 days.
- A nonadherent dressing (Adaptic, Telfa) should be applied over the wound and covered with sterile gauze.

IMMOBILIZATION

- Advise the patient that in some areas of the body (particularly hand and foot injuries involving joints), motion may interfere with healing.
- Instruct the patient to elevate an injured extremity to help improve venous and lymphatic drainage and control swelling and pain and focal edema control.

ANALGESICS

- Usually a nonsteroidal analgesic provides sufficient pain relief.

GENERAL FOLLOW-UP CARE

- Advise the patient to keep the wound clean and dry.
- Instruct the patient about how to remove the dressing 2 days after the procedure, replace with a dry, sterile dressing, and change the dressing daily.
- Some patients can be taught to change their own packing, replace the dressings, and advance the drain.
- Instruct the patient to watch for signs of recurrence of the abscess or for evidence of further infection such as cellulitis.
- Instruct the patient to notify the clinician immediately if any of the following occurs: re-collection of pus in the abscess, fever and chills,

increased pain or redness, red streaks near the abscess, increased swelling in the area.

REFERENCE

Manjo G: The Healing Hand: Men and Women in the Ancient World. Cambridge, Mass, Harvard University Press, 1977, pp 58-59.

BIBLIOGRAPHY

Goroll HA, Mulley AG: Primary Care Medicine, 5th ed. Philadelphia, Lippincott Williams & Wilkins, 2006, pp 1242-1243.

Kelly WN: Essentials of Internal Medicine. Philadelphia, Lippincott Williams & Wilkins, 2001, pp 570-574.

Lawrence PF: Essentials of General Surgery, 4th ed. Philadelphia, Lippincott Williams & Wilkins, 2006, pp 167-168, 330-301.

Simon RR, Brenner BE: Emergency Procedures and Techniques, 4th ed. Baltimore, Lippincott Williams & Wilkins, 2002, pp 416-419.

Chapter 26

Wound Dressing Techniques

Paul F. Jacques

PROCEDURE GOALS AND OBJECTIVES

Goal: To apply wound dressings correctly, which will optimize conditions for healing.

Objectives: The student will be able to …

- Describe the indications and contraindications for applying a dressing over a wound.
- Identify the common complications associated with wound dressings.
- Describe the types of wounds.
- Describe the three biologic phases of wound healing.
- Identify the appropriate types of dressings and the rationale for their use.
- List the complications of dressing application and recognize the associated signs and symptoms.
- Describe the patient wound follow-up care instructions.

BACKGROUND AND HISTORY

There are several types of skin lesions that benefit from the application of dressings: wounds from trauma or surgical intervention; ulcers from an arterial, venous, diabetic or pressure-type cause; or burn injury. This chapter presents some of the basic principles of dressing techniques for wounds. The sources in the bibliography are provided for more in-depth information for the clinician who works in a setting where wound management is an ongoing responsibility.

Research and technology have significantly enhanced the medical community's ability to optimize healing and thus better treat wounds. Many new dressing materials are available, and much more is known and understood about the body's mechanisms of wound healing. When trauma occurs, either by accident or surgical intervention, the goal of managing the wound is to optimize the healing potential while preventing possible complications such as infection or deformity.

During the Middle Ages, Henri de Mondeville (1260-1320) made a major stand on the principle of cleanliness to avoid suppuration, a popular belief that remained in effect for centuries. In 1460, Heinrich von Pfolspeund wrote a book regarding trauma titled *Bundth-Ertznel,* which means "bandage treatment." Von Pfolspeund had considerable war experience, where he developed a breadth of knowledge about war-related traumatic wounds. He subscribed to the belief that only certain types of wounds should be closed and that for most war wounds, oil of turpentine should be poured into the wound, with the resulting suppuration being a sign of healing. Von Pfolspeund wrote that wounds should be bound with clean white cloths, for if not clean, harm would result. He also advocated that physicians wash their hands before tending to individual patients.

In 1545, Ambroise Paré, a military surgeon, was accustomed to treating wounds with boiling oil. The custom was to pour boiling oil into the wound to stop suppuration. When Paré's supply of boiling oil ran out he simply dressed the wounds with clean cloths and minimal medication. He was dumbfounded to find on the following morning that the soldiers treated without the boiling oil were relatively free of pain, afebrile, and resting comfortably. Paré spent the rest of his life advocating keeping medications out of wounds and letting nature work. His expression, "I dressed him, and God healed him," made medical history.

It was during the 19th century that a better understanding of wound healing emerged, and antiseptic surgery was introduced in 1867. With the development of general anesthesia in 1847, surgeons were better able to carry out more deliberate surgical procedures. However, at that time, pus was still believed to be necessary to the healing of wounds. The brilliant work of Louis Pasteur in France and the discovery of bacteria as the source of infection changed the management of surgical cases. A British surgeon, Joseph Lister, concluded that microorganisms were the cause of the high mortality rate and implemented the use of carbolic acid (a powerful antiseptic). With the advent of spraying carbolic acid into the wound and around the

Figure 26-1. The ideal dressing.

surgical operative site, Lister's patient mortality rate dropped precipitously. The theory of asepsis was developed and is the standard of care today.

Today, there are more than 2000 brands of wound dressings. The clinician should be aware of the major types and categories of dressings and the indications for each.

INDICATIONS

A wound dressing decreases the risk of infection, and the correct material covering the wound optimizes the healing process. The ideal dressing accomplishes the following:

■ Maintains a high degree of humidity between the wound and the dressing

■ Provides a thermal insulation for the wound, which provides a better environment for cellular growth (Fig. 26-1)

■ Removes excess exudate and toxic substances from the wound

■ Allows gas exchange

■ Is impermeable to bacteria to prevent infection

■ Does not leave particulate material or contaminants within the wound

Dressings are also indicated for the following:

■ To apply the aesthetic principle of hiding the injury

■ To protect the wound from accidental trauma, abrasions, self-inflicted "picking," or other irritations

■ To provide support, immobilization, and compression

There is no single ideal product available that provides all these functions at once, but the clinician should consider carefully which characteristics of the dressing are the most important for the patient's wound. The wound treatment plan should consider factors such as the cause, severity, environment, size and depth, anatomic location, volume of exudate, and the risk or presence of infection. Patient considerations such as medical status, preferences, level of comfort, and cost-benefit analysis must also be taken under advisement. The final factors to consider are the availability, durability, adaptability, cost, and uses of the wound care products.

CONTRAINDICATIONS

Ultimately, the dressing should not cause pain or traumatize the wound with removal. It is essential to avoid applying a dressing that may compromise the blood supply to the tissue within and surrounding the wound. There are no other significant contraindications to dressing a wound. Relative contraindications include the following:

- Skin sensitivity to the dressing and related products (i.e., allergies to tape, adhesives, latex, iodoform gauze, povidone, neomycin or bacitracin) should be discussed with the patient before application of the dressing of choice.

- Persistent povidone application to a wound causes damage to the normal tissue and inhibits healing, and thus should be avoided.

- Decreased circulation in the affected area: Dressings can interfere with circulation in a digit or extremity if applied too tightly. Therefore, only material that stretches should be applied when the dressing will encircle the extremity.

- Application of gauze dressings, such as gauze squares (2 × 2-inch or 4 × 4-inch squares), directly on a wound: The gauze can adhere to the wound as the epithelial cells intertwine within the gauze. Removal of the dressing can cause removal of the eschar (scab) and new epithelial cells from the wound as well as cause the patient some significant discomfort. If a dressing has become adherent to a wound, it should be soaked in normal saline for approximately 10 minutes before removal is attempted. Some dressing materials have been designed to adhere less to wounds than does traditional gauze, and these should be considered when the potential for wound adherence is high.

- When dealing with elderly patients, carefully consider the texture and integrity of the skin before applying an adhesive tape directly to the skin. With the aging process, there is a loss of collagen within the dermis and an increased friability of the skin. Therefore, adhesives can readily tear the "normal" aged skin when removal of the adhesive tape is warranted to change the dressing. The way to keep a dressing in place is to use a gauze roll or elastic roll over the dressing and around the body part affected and apply tape only to the gauze or elastic roll ends or edges.

- When treating infants and children, be sure to reinforce the wound dressing with additional gauze covering the wound, thereby making it more difficult for the child to remove the dressing.

REVIEW OF ESSENTIAL ANATOMY AND PHYSIOLOGY

WOUND TYPES

The material used for a dressing depends on the type, size, and location of the wound. The wound types include closed, open (full- or partial-thickness), necrotic, infected, granulating, and epithelializing.

Closed and Open Wounds

For a closed wound, in which the skin integrity is intact, there is no evidence that a dressing decreases the risk of infection. Nonadherent gauze dressing absorbs exudate and prevents irritation. For an open wound, the objective is to encourage clean granulation by creating a moist environment without slough.

Necrotic Wounds

Necrotic wounds must be surgically debrided, if possible, to remove non-viable tissue, because necrotic tissue impedes the healing process. If the patient is not a surgical candidate, the use of hydrocolloids or hydrogels can facilitate debridement. Contact with the exudate causes the hydrophilic particles of the hydrocolloids to swell and form an impermeable gel. Rehydrating necrotic tissue separates from the normal tissues and sloughs off. Separation may take a few weeks depending on the size of the lesion. Hydrocolloids (DuoDerm) absorb exudate and produce a moist environment without maceration of the surrounding tissues.

Infected Wounds

Infected wounds should be treated with normal saline irrigation. Minor infections are adequately treated with saline bathing. Alginates are used for more extensive infected wounds. These products contain calcium and sodium alginic acid prepared in a fiber form. Moisture causes the calcium alginate to convert to a soluble sodium salt and produces a hydrophilic gel. The gel is easily removed with saline irrigation or by bathing. Dressing removal is easy and comfortable for the patient.

Granulating Wounds

Granulating wounds require a moist environment, and removal of the dressing should not damage the tissue. Impregnated gauze [Xeroform] works well as long as the dressing is not allowed to dry out, in which case it then debrides the wound of new granulation tissue when the dressing is pulled off. Hydrocolloids or hydrogels with a transparent film covering are good alternatives to impregnated gauze.

Epithelializing Wounds

Epithelializing wounds (abrasions) should be treated in the same manner as granulating wounds, being careful not to remove the new epithelial layer when changing the dressing. Therefore, they should be covered with a nonadherent dressing (Telfa), a biosynthetic sheet, or a transparent film.

WOUND HEALING

There are three stages in the healing process of a wound, regardless of whether the wound is surgical or traumatic in nature.

Inflammatory (0 to 6 Days)

Edema, erythema, heat, and pain characterize the inflammatory phase, which begins at the time of injury and lasts 4 to 6 days. Hemostasis controls bleeding, and polymorphonuclear leukocytes control bacterial growth. After about 4 days, macrophages migrate into the wound area and produce chemo-attractants and growth factors, which facilitate wound healing.

Proliferative (4 to 24 Days)

In an open wound, granulation tissue is generated, which produces red, beefy, shiny tissue with a granular appearance. This tissue consists of macro-phages, fibroblasts, immature collagen, blood vessels, and ground substance. As the granulation tissue proliferates, fibroblasts stimulate the production of collagen, which gives tissue its tensile strength and structure.

As the wound fills with granulation tissue, its margins contract, decreasing the wound's surface area. During epithelialization, cells migrate from the wound margins, ultimately sealing it. Epithelialization can occur only in the presence of viable, vascular tissue. When this phase is complete, a scar forms.

Maturation (21 Days to 24 Months)

During the maturation phase, the collagen fibers reorganize, remodel, and mature, gaining tensile strength. The maximal tensile strength that is regained is approximately 80%.

POOR WOUND HEALING

Advanced age, diabetes mellitus, immunosuppression, radiation therapy, vitamin deficiency, malnutrition, cancer, vascular insufficiencies, or wound infection are some of the more common causes of poor wound healing. If a wound is not healing readily, the clinician should undertake a comprehensive evaluation of the patient, looking for systemic inhibitors of wound healing.

Environmental factors can impede the healing of a wound, such as recurrent trauma or pressure on the site of the wound (which may occur with bending the affected area), edema that impedes oxygen flow to and from the wound, necrotic tissue within the wound, and patient incontinence, which can expose the wound to urine or feces. Poorly healing wounds are at increased risk for infection, hemorrhage, dehiscence, evisceration, and fistula formation.

PREVENTION OF INFECTION IN WOUNDS

Clinicians must wash their hands before and after dressing a wound. A study conducted in April 2000 demonstrated a 16% compliance with hand washing before patient interaction and a 25% hand-washing rate after patient contact. Nosocomial infections can be prevented only by increased compliance with effective hand washing (Bishoff, 2001).

The skin is the barrier against infection. When the skin is compromised, through trauma or surgical intervention, the patient is at risk for bacterial growth within the wound. The longer the wound is exposed to air particles, dirt, water, and so forth, the risk of infection increases exponentially. The appropriate surgical management, such as debridement, irrigation, or suturing, should be undertaken before wound dressings are applied. Debridement refers to the removal of tissue that is likely to impede the healing process, such as necrotic and unnecessary fibrinous tissue or damaged tissue that is unlikely to survive. This is typically performed as a surgical procedure and its description is beyond the scope of this chapter. Irrigation involves cleaning the wound to minimize contamination by infectious and foreign materials. Typically, large quantities of normal saline solutions are used, and large-capacity syringes can be used to spray the solution with sufficient pressure to irrigate structures that may be difficult to reach. Wound closure and wound contamination classification are covered in depth in Chapter 23.

There are four steps in the prevention of wound infection in the trauma patient. First and foremost is adequate and timely resuscitation of the patient. Hypoxia or hypovolemia, or both, increase the risk of infection. Second is early wound care, which includes debridement, hemostasis, irrigation, and primary wound closure. Third is the application of antibiotics. Although most wounds do not require antibiotic therapy, if antibiotics are indicated, they should be administered early, using an agent that provides appropriate coverage of the most likely infecting microbes. In addition, achieving adequate concentrations of the antibiotic for bactericidal effects is essential. The fourth stage is tetanus immune prophylaxis when indicated (see Chapter 23). These basic infection prevention principles are also applicable for non-traumatic wounds.

Standard Precautions   Every practitioner should use standard precautions at all times when interacting with patients, especially when performing procedures. Determining the level of precaution necessary requires the practitioner to exercise clinical judgment based on the patient's history and the potential for exposure to body fluids or aerosol-borne pathogens (for further discussion, see Chapter 2).

PATIENT PREPARATION

■ Inform the patient about the procedure of wound dressing.

■ Explain to the patient exactly what is being done and why, and answer any questions that he or she might have.

Materials Utilized for Performing Wound Dressing

Note: Dressings should have the following characteristics: softness, permeability, sterility, and elasticity.

Primary Dressings
■ Alginates

Note: These products are derived from brown seaweed. Alginates (AlgiDerm, AlgiSite, Dermastat) are absorbent and conform to the shape of a wound because they are provided in the shape of a rope (twisted fibers) or pads. An alginate interacts with wound exudate to form a soft gel that maintains a moist healing environment. Alginates can absorb up to 20 times their weight. These products absorb heavy exudate from a deep, draining wound, regardless of whether the wound is infected (Fig. 26-2).

Use alginate in presence of heavy exudate with or without the presence of infection.

Use collagen with or without the presence of infection.

Collagen particles or gel

FIGURE 26-2. Alginate is used in the presence or absence of infection.

FIGURE 26-3. The biosynthetic dressing.

■ Biosynthetic dressings

Note: Biosynthetic dressings (E-Z Derm, Glucan II) were developed as temporary coverings for burns. A biosynthetic dressing may be a gel or a semiocclusive sheet that can be left in place for 1 to 10 days, depending on the clinical situation. Biosynthetic dressings facilitate wound healing by re-epithelialization. These dressings may be used to treat partial-thickness wounds, such as tears, burns, abrasions, and some pressure ulcers (Fig. 26-3).

■ Collagens

Note: Collagen dressings may be used as primary dressing for partial- and full-thickness wounds, regardless of whether they are infected (see Fig. 26-2). During wound healing, collagen encourages the deposition and organization of newly formed collagen fibers and granulation tissue in the wound bed. It stimulates new tissue development and wound debridement. With the use of collagen, a secondary dressing needs to be applied to absorb exudate. Collagen dressing products are available as sheets, pads, particles, and gels (Fibracol Plus, Kollagen Medifil, hyCURE).

■ Foams

Note: Foam dressings (Curafoam Plus, Sof-Foam Dressing, 3M Reston Self-Adhering Foam, Tielle hydropolymer dressing) are absorbent, nonadhering, and lint free. Foams may be either hydrophilic or hydrophobic and are nonocclusive unless they have a film coating. They are used as either a primary dressing, directly on the wound to provide absorption and insulation, or as a secondary dressing overlying a wound packing. Foams may require a secondary dressing to hold them in place if they do not have an adhesive border or film coating as an additional bacterial barrier. (Fig. 26-4).

■ Hydrocolloids

Note: Hydrocolloids (DuoDerm, ExuDerm, OriDerm hydrocolloid, 3M Tegasorb hydrocolloid dressings) are occlusive or semiocclusive dressings that can be composed of gelatin, pectin, or carboxymethylcellulose (see Fig. 26-4). These types of dressings provide a moist healing environment that allows clean wounds to granulate or necrotic lesions to debride autolytically. These types of products are manufactured in various shapes, sizes, and forms, such as wafers, pastes, and powders. Hydrocolloid

Epidermis

Full-thickness wound is
through the epidermis,
dermis, subcutaneous
tissue, and possibly
muscle/bone.

Dermis

Subcutaneous tissue

Secondary dressing

Hydrocolloid paste or gel
(no infection)

Hydrogel (with or without
infection)

With or without necrosis

Secondary dressing

Foam

FIGURE 26-4. The foam
dressing.

dressings are self-adhesive, provide light to moderate absorption capacity,
minimize skin trauma, and may be used underneath a compression product
such as Unna boots. However, they are not recommended for infected
wounds or wounds with heavy exudate or exposed tendons or bones.
Another benefit of this type of dressing is that it protects the lesion from
contamination and can be left in place 1 to 10 days, depending on the type
of lesion and placement.

■ Hydrogels

Note: Hydrogels are water or glycerin-based amorphous gels (Curasol, SK
Integrity amorphous hydrogel, 3M Tegagel hydrogel wound filler products).
The gels can be applied to wounds directly, or gauze or sheets impregnated
with the hydrogel are available. They do not absorb exudate because of
their high water content. These dressings maintain a moist wound
environment, thereby promoting granulation and epithelialization or
autolytic debridement of necrotic lesions. They are indicated for the
management of partial- and full-thickness wounds, deep wounds, wounds

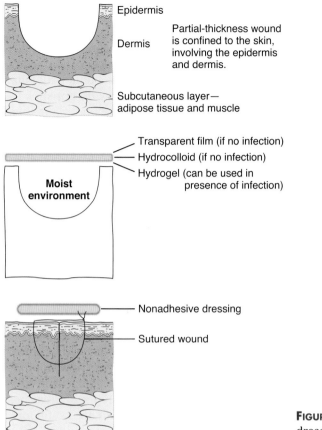

Epidermis

Partial-thickness wound is confined to the skin, involving the epidermis and dermis.

Dermis

Subcutaneous layer— adipose tissue and muscle

Transparent film (if no infection)

Hydrocolloid (if no infection)

Hydrogel (can be used in presence of infection)

Moist environment

Nonadhesive dressing

Sutured wound

FIGURE 26-5.   The hydrogel dressing.

with necrosis, slough, minor burns, and tissue damaged by radiation (Fig. 26-5). These dressings are applied and removed easily and can be used when infection is present.

Secondary Dressings

■ Transparent films

Note: Transparent films (OpSite, Bioclusive transparent dressing, Polyskin II, 3M Tegaderm transparent dressing) are adhesive, semipermeable, polyurethane membrane dressings that vary in thickness and size. These films are waterproof and impermeable to bacteria, yet they permit water vapor to cross the barrier. Transparent films allow direct observation of the wound and do not require a secondary dressing. The limitations are that they should not be used on fragile skin or with infected wounds.

■ Dressing gauze

Note: Gauze dressings are manufactured in many forms. They can be used as primary, secondary, or securing dressings. Gauze for cleaning, debriding, packing, and covering usually is available in the form of packets containing sterile 4 × 4-inch or 2 × 2-inch squares. Nonadherent gauze [Telfa pads] are an important improvement in gauze dressings because they do not stick to wounds and facilitate exudate transmittal away from the wound. Gauze also comes impregnated with many different substances, such as oil emulsions, petrolatum, saline, scarlet red, sodium chloride, water, Xeroform, or zinc-saline solution. Some impregnated gauze dressings serve as occlusive dressings and prevent drainage from the wound.

■ Flexible collodion

Note: Flexible collodion is a preparation of nitrocellulose dissolved in alcohol and ether. It is a plastic-like substance that is applied aseptically to a wound and forms a thin, clear sealant layer of plastic over the wound. This product is a good choice for scalp lacerations, where gauze dressing is difficult to apply.

■ Dressing stabilizer (wrapping or rolling gauze)

Note: Rolls of dressing material are used to hold other materials against a wound. The ideal roll gauze has some elastic properties; it is used to add bulk and cushion to the dressing (Kling, Kerlix). Another type of wrapping gauze that is categorized as a dressing stabilizer is tubular gauze used to stabilize a dressing circumferentially (Tube-gauze). These types of dressings are applied using a stainless steel metal-cage applicator and are useful for dressing digits.

■ Tape

■ ACE bandage

■ Tube gauze

■ Cleansing materials

■ Irrigation set

■ Normal saline

■ Hydrogen peroxide

■ Povidone-iodine

Note: Antiseptic agents such as povidone-iodine can injure skin, delaying healing; therefore, they should be used only when necessary and used sparingly on damaged skin.

Procedure for Performing Wound Dressing

1. Wash hands and put on clean sterile gloves.

2. Clean the wound.

Note: Clean wounds with dirt or grease contamination with mild soap and irrigate with water to remove the detergent. Irrigate deep wounds to remove excessive exudate, slough, or loose necrotic tissue (see Chapter 23). Closed wounds should be cleansed gently with normal saline or hydrogen peroxide to remove clotted blood from the wound edge, which can contribute to scarring or infection, or both. Excessive exposure to hydrogen peroxide can injure damaged skin, so an effort should be made to limit exposure to intact, dry skin surfaces only.

3. Determine the appropriate primary dressing based on the factors described previously. Maintain aseptic technique when applying dressings (see Chapter 3).

4. Apply the secondary dressing to absorb excessive exudate as well as to provide a cushion (Figs. 26-6 and 26-7).

5. Secure the dressing in a fashion that will provide flexibility and not restrict the movement of the patient, unless such restriction is warranted by the nature of the wound (Fig. 26-8).

6. Make sure that the tape is wide enough and long enough to adhere the gauze to the skin.

FIGURE 26-6. Application of tubular gauze.

7. Wounds overlying flexor surfaces on the extremities or digits will be unduly stressed with flexion of the joint; therefore, range of motion should be

continued

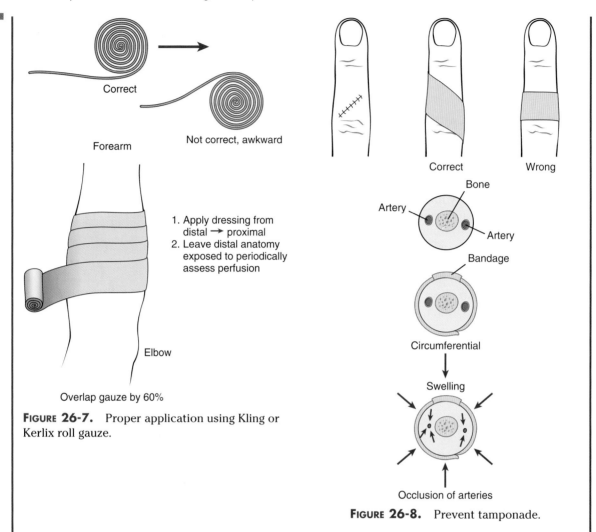

Figure 26-7. Proper application using Kling or Kerlix roll gauze.

Figure 26-8. Prevent tamponade.

somewhat restricted to prevent dehiscence (Fig. 26-9). Splints or bulky dressings should be considered to reduce the range of motion of the affected joint.

8. Apply dressings to cover sutured wounds.

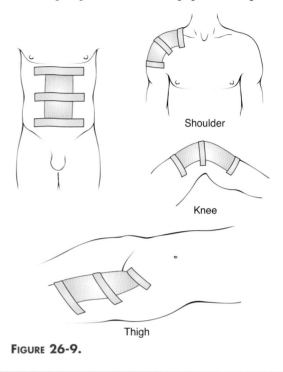

Tape applied to a dressing must be wide/long enough to keep the dressing in place. Dressings should allow for movement of the body without hindering range of motion or dislodging the dressing.

Shoulder

Knee

Thigh

FIGURE 26-9.

FOLLOW-UP CARE AND INSTRUCTIONS

■ When indicated, the patient or caregiver should undertake dressing changes. Carefully explaining the procedure helps to facilitate timely, appropriate, and effective wound management. Noncompliance or the inadequate communication of information can result in poor healing, infection, pain, and disfiguring scars.

■ Instruct the patient to change the dressing after cleansing the wound, if the dressing becomes wet or dirty, or after a certain amount of time has passed, typically 2 to 3 days.

■ Instruct the patient to clean the wound gently approximately three times a day using some hydrogen peroxide on cotton swabs or gauze and then gently blot the wound dry. Dried blood or superficial coagulum should be removed from the wound edges to prevent widening of the final scar.

■ Reassure the patient that body hygiene can be maintained by showering but that the shower spray should not spray directly on the wound.

Advise against bathing in a tub because of the possibility of an infection developing in the wound.

- Instruct the patient to observe the wound edges for increased redness or increased tenderness and to contact the office for assessment.

- Make the patient aware of what to expect concerning the progress of the wound over time. Normal wound healing often exhibits characteristics that can be confused with wound infections; therefore, describe in detail what the wound should look like and feel like in the course of the normal healing process. The normal healing process often involves a limited inflammatory response that produces erythema and tenderness for a few days.

- Additionally, make the patient aware of the signs and symptoms of a wound infection, which include erythema, pain, warmth, edema, discharge, throbbing, fever, regional adenopathy, and spreading erythema.

- Patients not able to perform dressing changes or evaluate the progress of their wounds may be candidates for visiting nursing services.

- Wound infections may require interventions that vary by factors such as severity and the proximity to other organ systems. Infections in closed wounds may require that sutures be removed or incision and drainage be performed. Some infections may require aggressive systemic antibiotic therapy, especially those that are spreading by vascular or lymphatic systems or are following tissue lines such as fascia or muscle.

- Infected wounds should be cleaned with normal saline solution at least four times a day and the dressing changed.

- Instruct the patient to wash his or her hands with soap and water before and after tending to the wound.

- Instruct the patient to use the same primary and secondary dressing materials as used by the health care provider.

- When a wound is free of infection, sutures have been removed, all skin surfaces are dry, and the wound is no longer draining, the use of dressings can be discontinued. At this point, dressings may be still be used when indicated as padding to protect the fragile, newly healed tissues from damage due to physical trauma. However, in most cases, dressings can be discontinued when the indications for them, primarily protection of the wound, are no longer present.

CONCLUSION AND RESOURCES

Wound management of the chronic wound is a complex topic with extensive ongoing research to identify etiologic factors and to develop better materials and methods of dealing with the chronic wound. The June 2005 issue of The

Nursing Clinics of North America provides thirteen excellent articles on wound care.

Surgical Materials Testing Laboratory (SMTL) sponsors a website (www.dressings.org) that contains an exhaustive list of wound care products. SMTL provides dressings datacards as well as technical papers and test reports. The datacards contain information on many wound care products and detail the indications, contraindications, methods of use, frequency of change, warnings, presentation of the product, and sizes of the dressing products. The datacards also include a bibliography for each product.

SMTL is sponsored by the government of Wales to provide information to the National Healthcare Service. SMTL is a not-for-profit organization that sponsors the Wound Management Practice Resource Centre, which is yet another great resource that can be found online (www.smtl.co.uk/WMPRC/index.html).

REFERENCE

Bischoff WE, Reynolds TM, Sessler CN, et al: Handwashing compliance by health care workers: The impact of introducing an accessible, alcohol-based hand antiseptic. Arch Intern Med 60:1017-1021, 2001.

BIBLIOGRAPHY

Felciano DV, Moore EE, Mattox KL: Trauma. Norwalk, Conn, Appleton & Lange, 1996.

Grossman JA: Minor Injuries and Disorders: Surgical and Medical Care. Philadelphia, JB Lippincott, 1984.

Hess CT, Salcido R: Wound Care, 3rd ed. Springhouse, Pa, Springhouse, 2000.

Pieper B (ed): Wound Care. The Nursing Clinics of North America, vol 40, no. 2. Philadelphia, Saunders, June 2005.

Trott AT: Wounds and Lacerations: Emergency Care and Closure, 2nd ed. St. Louis, Mosby–Year Book, 1997.

Wardrope J, Edhouse J: The Management of Wounds and Burns, 2nd ed. Oxford, England, Oxford University Press, 1999.

Westaby S: Wound Care. St. Louis, CV Mosby, 1998.

Schwartz SI: Principles of Surgery, 7th ed. New York, McGraw-Hill, 1999.

Chapter 27

Cryosurgery

P. Eugene Jones and Theresa E. Hegmann

PROCEDURE GOALS AND OBJECTIVES

Goal: To perform cryosurgery on a lesion successfully, using techniques that will facilitate wound healing and minimize the likelihood of complications.

Objectives: The student will be able to …

- Describe the indications, contraindications, and rationale for performing cryosurgery.

- Identify and describe common complications associated with the use of cryosurgery on skin lesions.

- Describe the essential anatomy and physiology of the skin as it pertains to the performance of cryosurgery.

- Identify the materials and tools necessary for performing cryosurgery on skin lesions.

- Identify the important aspects of post-procedure care after cryosurgery on small skin lesions.

BACKGROUND AND HISTORY

The therapeutic use of cold for treatment of injuries and inflammation dates back as early as 2500 BC, when Egyptians appreciated its adjunctive value. Over the centuries, famous physicians such as Hippocrates and Napoleon's chief army surgeon Dominique Jean Larrey used cold for analgesia and hemorrhage control (Graham, 1999). The modern era of cryosurgery began when James Arnott developed the application of cold for a variety of conditions. He achieved a temperature of $-24°$ C with a salt and crushed ice brine to treat neuralgia and for palliative care in terminally ill cancer patients. The first dermatologic application of cryosurgery was in New York in 1899 when the dermatologist A. C. White applied liquefied air via cotton-tipped applicators to warts, nevi, and premalignant and malignant skin lesions (Graham, 1999). Liquid nitrogen was introduced as a cryogen about 1948. By 1962, Irving Cooper developed a more modern apparatus that facilitated cryosurgical spray application techniques (Grekin, 1990).

Biologic effects on the skin and subcutaneous tissue are achieved by selective destruction of tissue as heat is transferred from the skin to a heat sink (typically liquid nitrogen). The subzero temperatures achieved result in intra- and extracellular ice crystal formation, disruption of cell membrane integrity, pH changes, and thermal shock (Kuplik, 1997). The degree of tissue damage depends on the rate of cooling and the minimum temperature achieved, so to achieve maximal tissue destruction effect, longer freeze times, slow thaw times, or a series of freeze-thaw cycles can be used (Gage, 1978; Andrews, 2004). Generally, these more aggressive approaches to cryosurgery are unnecessary for benign skin lesions. Milder freezing techniques destroy the more sensitive cells of the epidermis, while leaving the dermis and underlying structures intact. This leads to dermo-epidermal separation and is usually sufficient for treating many common benign lesions. Post-treatment inflammation may trigger an immune reaction that contributes to destruction of the target lesion.

INDICATIONS

Cryosurgery is indicated for many common benign skin conditions, and for certain malignant conditions in carefully selected patients for whom the diagnosis has been definitively established. Specific lesions that may be treated with cryosurgery are listed in Table 27-1. Lesions with more sharply demarcated borders tend to be more responsive to cryosurgery. Common skin conditions that respond well to the technique include seborrheic keratoses, skin tags, sun-damaged skin (e.g., actinic keratoses and solar lentigines), and skin lesions caused by viral infection (e.g., common warts, condyloma acuminatum, and molluscum contagiosum).

The technique has several advantages over other surgical modalities in selected patients with appropriate lesions. These include its technical ease, portability, and the brief period of time required for treatments, all of which

Table 27.1	**Lesions Treatable with Cryosurgery**	
BENIGN LESIONS	PRECANCEROUS LESIONS OR TUMORS OF UNCERTAIN BEHAVIOR	MALIGNANT LESIONS
Acne vulgaris	Actinic cheilitis	**Basal cell carcinoma**
Angiolymphoid hyperplasia	Actinic keratosis	**Bowen's disease**
Angiokeratoma	Keratoacanthoma	**Kaposi's sarcoma**
Angioma, cherry and spider	Lentigo maligna	**Squamous cell**
Chondrodermatitis nodularis chronica helicis	Bowenoid papulosis	**carcinoma**
Condyloma acuminata (venereal warts)	Leukoplakia	**Actinic keratosis with squamous cell carcinoma**
Dermatofibroma		
Disseminated superficial actinic porokeratosis		
Granuloma faciale		
Granuloma fissuratum		
Hemangioma		
Hidradenitis suppurativa		
Keloid		
Leishmaniasis		
Lentigines, lentigo simplex, solar lentigo		
Lichen planus		
Lichen sclerosis et atrophicus		
Lichen simplex chronicus		
Lymphocytoma cutis		
Molluscum contagiosum		
Mucocele		
Myxoid cyst		
Nevi		
Porokeratosis of Mibelli		
Prurigo nodularis		
Psoriatic plaques		
Pyogenic granuloma		
Rosacea		
Sebaceous hyperplasia		
Seborrheic keratosis		
Skin tags (acrochordons)		
Syringoma		
Venous lake		
Verrucae, including common warts, plantar warts, and flat warts		
Other		

From Drake LA, Ceilley RI, Cornelison RL, et al: Guidelines of care for cryosurgery. J Am Acad Dermatol 31:648-653, 1994.

make it ideal for clinic settings. Additionally, minimal patient preparation is required, there is low risk of infection or other major complications, and there is no need for expensive supplies or injectable anesthesia.

Because of the ease of application and relatively minimal associated risks, cryosurgery is especially useful in the following subsets of patients:

■ Elderly, high-risk surgical patients

- Patients allergic to local anesthetics

- Patients with coagulopathies and pacemakers (Drake, 1994)

CONTRAINDICATIONS

Cryosurgery is absolutely contraindicated in patients with the following:
- Lesions requiring tissue pathology for diagnostic reasons

- Lesions located in a body area with compromised circulation

- Lesions known or suspected to be melanoma, sclerosing basal cell carcinoma, or recurrent basal cell or squamous cell carcinomas

- Previous adverse reaction to cryosurgery

Relative contraindications to cryosurgery include:
- Lesions overlying nerves (Arndt, 1997)

- Lesions located in pretibial areas, eyelid margins, nasolabial fold, ala nasi, or on hair-bearing areas

- Lesions of dark-skinned individuals; treatment in these individuals may leave hypopigmented scars

- Patient history of cold intolerance, cold urticaria, cryoglobulinemia, or Raynaud's disease

- Autoimmune disease or concurrent treatment with immunosuppressive drugs

POTENTIAL COMPLICATIONS

- Immediate complications can include dizziness or vasovagal syncope, blister formation, edema, bleeding, and pain. Treating lesions of the scalp, forehead, or temple may produce a transient headache (Arndt, 1997). Occasionally, large, bloody post-procedural bullae may be seen, though facial lesions typically crust over without vesicle or bulla formation.

- Delayed complications can include infection, hemorrhage, and excessive formation of granulation tissue (Young, 1997). It is not uncommon for verruca vulgaris lesions to recur as a larger circumferential lesion after cryosurgery. Patients should be cautioned about the possible appearance of these "ring warts" at previously treated sites.

- Prolonged and possibly permanent complications include post-procedure hypopigmentation, alopecia in hair-bearing areas, and atrophy. Patients may also note altered sensation, hyperpigmentation or, rarely, hypertrophic scarring; these changes, though sometimes protracted, are usually temporary.

Table 27.2	**Cryogens and Their Effective Celsius Temperature**
CRYOGEN	TEMPERATURE (°C)
Ice	0
Salt ice	−20
CO_2 slush	−20
CO_2 snow	−70
CO_2 solid	−78.5
Liquid nitrous oxide	−89.5
Liquid nitrogen	−20 (swab)
Liquid nitrogen	−195.8 (spray/probe)

■ Damage to underlying structures can be prevented by avoidance of overfreezing, and by continually moving the skin back and forth while performing cryosurgery in order to avoid freezing the skin to underlying bone, cartilage, or tendon tissue.

REVIEW OF ESSENTIAL ANATOMY AND PHYSIOLOGY

Knowledge of local neurovascular anatomy is imperative before performing cryosurgery. When in doubt, the clinician should consult an anatomy reference before proceeding. Areas of concern include the skin near the medial epicondyle of the elbow and the lateral aspects of the digits and the angle of the mandible, as nerves are more superficial in these areas and are prone to freeze injury (Habif, 1996). The pretibial area is also problematic, as patients—especially the elderly—may experience slow wound healing in this area after cryosurgery. Cryotherapy is contraindicated in areas of the body with compromised circulation, such as a lower extremity lesion in a patient with peripheral vascular disease. Patient selection criteria include lesion location, skin color and type, size and number of lesions, response to previous therapy, condition of the skin and subcutaneous tissue, and coexisting medical conditions. Because melanocytes are more sensitive to cold injury, post-inflammatory hypopigmentation is more common in darker skin. Cryogens and their effective Celsius temperatures are noted in Table 27-2.

Standard Precautions   Every practitioner should use standard precautions at all times when interacting with patients, especially when performing procedures. Determining the level of precaution necessary requires the practitioner to exercise clinical judgment based on the patient's history and the potential for exposure to body fluids or aerosol-borne pathogens (for further discussion, see Chapter 2).

PATIENT PREPARATION

■ Thoroughly explain the procedure and its attendant risks, as well as alternative treatment options available to the patient. Document informed consent by having the patient sign a consent form, or by dictation into the procedure note, depending on local policies and procedures.

- Ensure patient comfort in a seated or supine position, if possible. Choosing a supine position may help prevent syncopal episodes.

- The application of liquid nitrogen can be painful, particularly for children; therefore, additional efforts may be necessary to prepare children psychologically before the procedure is performed.

- Use of precryosurgery anesthesia with topical agents such as lidocaine-prilocaine (EMLA) or lidocaine (ELA-Max) cream is worth considering, especially in pediatric patients, unless contraindicated.

- Outlining the lesion with a surgical marking pen may be helpful, as freezing may temporarily obliterate visual lesion margins.

Materials Utilized for Performing Cryosurgery

Sterile Cotton-Tipped Applicator/Swab Method
- Liquid nitrogen

- Styrofoam cup

- Cotton-tipped applicator (with a solid, not hollow, handle)

- Gloves

Spray Method
- Liquid nitrogen spray gun

- Gloves

- Spray extension (necessary to treat difficult-to-reach lesions) (Fig. 27-1)

Cryoprobe Method
- Liquid nitrogen spray gun

- Probes (see Fig. 27-1)

- Gloves

- Probe extension (necessary to treat difficult-to-reach lesions; see Fig. 27-1)

FIGURE 27-1. Materials used to perform cryosurgery.

Procedure for Performing Cryosurgery

Note: Because longer time and depth of freeze destroys more tissue, care must be exercised to not overtreat. It is better to treat conservatively and re-treat a lesion at a later date than to overtreat once and risk permanent hypopigmentation or damage to underlying structures.

    Note: Lesion thickness typically dictates length and depth of freeze. For example, a large, flat, thin seborrheic keratosis should be frozen in sections and not from the center out, as this results in too deep a freeze. Thicker lesions, such as a hyperkeratotic verruca, require more prolonged freezing that typically results in hemorrhagic bulla formation beneath the lesion (Habif, 1996). The depth of freeze achieved typically approximates 1.5 times the lateral spread of the visible cutaneous ice ball (Torre, 1979). See "Special Considerations" for more information on recommended freeze duration.

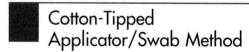

Cotton-Tipped Applicator/Swab Method

Note: The cotton-tipped applicator/swab method is useful on smaller lesions and around the eye or ear canal where unconcentrated spray may be deleterious.

1. Pour enough liquid nitrogen from holding tank into a disposable polystyrene (Styrofoam) cup to cover cotton tip of applicator when dipping applicator into cup.

2. With gloved fingertips, loosen tight weave of the cotton tip on the swab to allow absorption of more liquid nitrogen. If desired, the cotton tip may be twisted to a point to allow more focal application of the liquid nitrogen to small lesions.

3. Dip swab in liquid nitrogen and apply swab tip to lesion (Fig. 27-2).

continued

FIGURE 27-3. Spray method.

FIGURE 27-2. Swab method.

4. Repeat dipping and application procedure until an ice ball extends 1 to 2 mm beyond the clinical lesion, lasting from 5 to 30 seconds (see "Special Considerations").

FIGURE 27-4. Cryoprobe method.

 ## Spray Method

Note: This method is more useful for larger or multiple lesions.

1. Hold the spray tip 1 to 2 cm from the lesion surface and gently squeeze the trigger mechanism (Fig. 27-3).

2. Apply spray in a pulsatile, rotary, spiral, or paintbrush fashion.

3. For better control, maintain an intermittent, pulsatile spray rather than a continuous spray. Cones or a disposable ear speculum can be used to confine spray to a specific focal point.

 ## Cryoprobe Method

Note: More commonly used for malignant lesions such as superficial or nodular basal cell carcinoma, the cryoprobe technique requires additional training and experience before it can be used clinically.

1. Select the appropriate probe based on the size and shape of the lesion (see Fig. 27-1).

2. Precool the tip to prevent skin adhesion.

3. Apply the tip to the lesion with direct pressure for the specified period (Fig. 27-4) (Arndt, 1997).

Table 27.3 Comparison of Freeze Times for Benign and Malignant Lesions and Range of Expected Cosmetic Results Using Intermittent Spray

LESION	FREEZE TIME (sec)	RANGE OF EXPECTED COSMETIC RESULTS
Acne scarring	10	Good to fair
Actinic keratoses	5-10	Excellent to good
Chondrodermatitis	30	Good to fair
Granuloma faciale	30	Good to fair
Hemangioma	60+	Good to fair
Hypertrophic scarring	20	Good to fair
Keratoacanthoma	30	Excellent to good
Lentigines	10	Excellent to good
Lentigo maligna	60-120	Excellent to good
Morphea-type BCC	90-120	Good to fair
Nevi	10	Good to fair
Nodular BCC	60-90	Excellent to good
Sebaceous hyperplasia	5-10	Excellent to good
Seborrheic keratoses	10	Good to fair
Superficial BCC	60	Excellent to good

BCC, basal cell carcinoma.

From Freedberg IM, Eisen AZ, Wolff K, et al (eds): Fitzpatrick's Dermatology in General Medicine, vol II, 5th ed. New York, McGraw-Hill, 1999, p 2982.

SPECIAL CONSIDERATIONS

Tissue damage increases with longer freeze-thaw cycles. Thinner lesion depth (e.g., actinic keratoses, lentigines) requires less freezing, whereas thicker lesion depth (e.g., dermatofibromas, keloids) requires more. Freeze times refer to the interval after the initial ice ball margin, or halo, forms, and range from 5 to 10 seconds for skin tags, actinic keratoses, and solar lentigos, to 20 to 30 seconds for dermatofibromas or hypertrophic scars and keloids. Some examples of typical freeze times for different types of lesions are presented in Table 27-3.

Treating twice with a slow thaw between cycles is more destructive to cells than a single treatment with a rapid thaw. Continuous freezing for longer than 30 seconds after an adequate ice ball is achieved around the target area should be avoided when treating benign lesions, as it may cause scarring (Andrews, 2004). Cryosurgery of malignant lesions requires additional expertise and training acquired under the tutelage of an experienced cryosurgeon. Ice ball margins of 5 mm are needed for treatment of malignant lesions in order to ensure adequate tissue destruction. A thermocoupled temperature probe needle device positioned under the base of the lesion facilitates appropriate length and depth of tissue freeze until sufficient experience is acquired.

FOLLOW-UP CARE AND INSTRUCTIONS

Lesion care after cryosurgery should include the following:

■ Instruct the patient to gently wash the area with soap and water twice daily.

■ Severe residual pain is not uncommon after cryosurgery to thicker tissue areas such as the palms, soles, and anatomically confined areas such as periungual tissue (Habif, 1996). Post-procedure pain may be treated with over-the-counter acetaminophen or ibuprofen, if not contraindicated.

■ Advise the patient not to use gauze or an occlusive dressing because of the possibility of prematurely removing the eschar.

■ Recommend polymyxin B sulfate-bacitracin zinc (Polysporin) or other similar topical ointment to soften hardened eschar.

■ Inform the patient that, after cryosurgery, it is common for a blister to form. This blister may be hemorrhagic at the treated site and dries, crusts, and peels along with the lesion.

■ Reassure the patient that erythema and edema are common immediately after cryosurgery.

■ Tell the patient to expect crusting to separate in approximately 10 days.

References

Andrews MD: Cryosurgery for common skin conditions. Am Fam Physician 69:2365-2372, 2004.

Arndt KA, Wintroub BU, Robinson JK, LeBoit PE (eds): Primary Care Dermatology. Philadelphia, WB Saunders, 1997.

Drake LA, Ceilley RI, Cornelison RL, et al: Guidelines of care for cryosurgery. J Am Acad Dermatol 31:648-653, 1994.

Gage AA: Experimental cryogenic injury of the palate: Observations pertinent to cryosurgical destruction of tumors. Cryobiology 21:157-169, 1978.

Graham GF: Cryosurgery. In Freedberg IM, Eisen AZ, Wolff K, et al (eds): Fitzpatrick's Dermatology in General Medicine, 5th ed. New York, McGraw-Hill, 1999, pp 2980-2987.

Grekin RC: Physical modalities of dermatologic therapy. In Arnold HL, Odom RB, James WD (eds): Andrews' Diseases of the Skin: Clinical Dermatology, 8th ed. Philadelphia, WB Saunders, 1990 pp 1008-1015.

Habif TP: Clinical Dermatology: A Color Guide to Diagnosis and Therapy, 3rd ed. St. Louis, Mosby–Year Book, 1996.

Jones SK, Darville JM: Transmission of virus by cryotherapy and multi-use caustic pencils: A problem to dermatologists? Br Dermatol 121:481, 1989.

Kuplik EG: Cryosurgery for cutaneous malignancy. Dermatol Surg 3:1081-1087, 1997.

Torre D: Understanding the relationship between lateral spread of freeze and depth of freeze. J Dermatol Surg Oncol 5:51-53, 1979.

Young R, Sinclair S: Practical cryosurgery. Aust Fam Physician 26:1045-1047, 1997.

Chapter 28

Treating Ingrown Toenails

Sue M. Nyberg

PROCEDURE GOALS AND OBJECTIVES

Goal: To treat problems associated with an ingrown toenail by removing all or part of the affected nail.

Objectives: The student will be able to ...

- Describe the indications, contraindications, and rationale for removing an ingrown toenail.

- Identify and describe common complications associated with removing an ingrown toenail.

- Describe the decision process used to determine when to remove an ingrown toenail.

- Describe the essential anatomy and physiology associated with removal of an ingrown toenail.

- Identify the materials necessary for performing removal of an ingrown toenail and their proper use.

- Identify the important aspects of post-procedure care after removal of an ingrown toenail.

BACKGROUND AND HISTORY

The management of an ingrown toenail is one of the most common procedures that the primary care practitioner is asked to perform. The ingrown toenail can be painful, causing limitation in function and mobility in many patients. Typically, only the great toe is affected, and either the medial or lateral border may be involved. In their protective role, nails bear the brunt of daily activities. Walking, running, wearing shoes, or participating in sports are just a few of the stresses that feet must endure. The most frequent underlying cause of an ingrown toenail is improper trimming of the nail, resulting in impingement, inflammation, and even infection in the surrounding and over-lying skin of the nail fold. Improperly fitted (e.g., high-heeled, narrow-toe) shoes that compress the toes together are also a significant contributing factor to the development of ingrown toenails. Other injuries to the nail bed that change the shape of the nail or a congenitally increased curvature of the lateral edges of the nail plate may also result in an ingrown nail.

Patients present with pain along the margin of the toenail that is aggravated by any type of pressure, especially when wearing shoes. Erythema and swelling are usually present and, if infection has occurred, pustular drainage may be noted. Conservative measures such as elevation of the nail plate with a small cotton wick, frequent soaking, wearing loose-fitting shoes, and selective trimming of the nail may be attempted; however, either partial or total removal of the nail remains the definitive treatment (Peggs, 1994).

INDICATIONS

The most common indication for the removal of a nail is onychocryptosis (ingrown nail).

Other indications include the following:

- Onychomycosis (fungal infection of the nail)

- Chronic, recurrent paronychia (inflammation of the nail fold)

- Onychogryposis (deformed, curved nail) (Peggs, 1994)

CONTRAINDICATIONS

Relatively few contraindications to the procedure exist but include a bleeding diathesis or an allergy to local anesthesia (Peggs, 1994). In these rare situations, conservative measures should be attempted first, with consideration of referral to a specialist if operative treatment is still indicated.

POTENTIAL COMPLICATIONS

Infection is a possible complication; however, it should be easily treatable with appropriate antibiotics and frequent soaks. If the nail bed is not

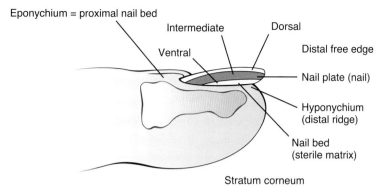

FIGURE 28-1. Anatomy of the nail and nail bed. (Redrawn from Pfenninger JF, Fowler GC: Procedures for Primary Care Physicians. St. Louis, Mosby–Year Book, 1994, p 40.)

cauterized (ablated), the nail will regrow and symptoms may return. If the nail bed is cauterized, there is still a potential for regrowth and return of symptoms (approximately 10% with phenol ablation).

REVIEW OF ESSENTIAL ANATOMY AND PHYSIOLOGY

Nails are derived by keratinization of cells from the nail matrix, which is located at the proximal end of the nail plate (Fig. 28-1). The nail plate consists of the nail root embedded in the posterior nail fold, a fixed middle portion, and a distal free edge. The whitish nail matrix of proliferating epithelial cells grows in a semilunar pattern. It extends outward past the posterior nail fold and is called the *lunula* (Swartz, 1998). Sensory supply to the great toe is through the digital nerves that have an extensor and plantar branch on both the medial and lateral aspects of the toe.

Standard Precautions Every practitioner should use standard precautions at all times when interacting with patients, especially when performing procedures. Determining the level of precaution necessary requires the practitioner to exercise clinical judgment based on the patient's history and the potential for exposure to body fluids or aerosol-borne pathogens (for further discussion, see Chapter 2).

PATIENT PREPARATION

- Explain the procedure to the patient to help alleviate as much anxiety as possible.

- Reassure the patient that the procedure is not painful except for the initial injection.

- Indicate the need for the patient's cooperation in keeping the foot still.

Materials Utilized to Remove an Ingrown Toenail

- Local anesthetic without epinephrine (vasoconstricting agents should never be used in anesthetizing a digit)

- 5-mL syringe with a 1- to 1½-inch, 25- to 27-gauge needle

- Povidone-iodine (Betadine) swabs

- Sterile drape

- Rubber band or small Penrose drain

- Straight hemostats

- Sterile straight scissors

- Sterile periosteal elevator

- Sterile gauze pads

- Sterile cotton-tipped applicators

- Phenol solution (88%) if permanent ablation of nail bed is desired

- Isopropyl alcohol

- Antibiotic ointment

- Rolled or tubular gauze dressing

Procedure for Removing an Ingrown Toenail

1. Place the patient in a supine position.

2. Scrub the digit with povidone-iodine and drape the toe in a sterile fashion.

Anesthesia (see Chapter 22)

3. Withdraw approximately 5 mL of local anesthetic (without epinephrine) into syringe.

4. Inject the anesthetic in a ring fashion around the toe. The initial injection should be proximal to the edges of the medial nail fold on the dorsal surface of the toe. There are four digital nerves that should be anesthetized: both extensor and plantar branches of the medial and lateral nerves.

5. Inject approximately 1 mL of anesthetic around each nerve site, starting dorsally and directing the needle gently in a plantar direction, injecting around the plantar digital nerve.

6. Repeat the procedure on the lateral side of the toe.

7. After the toe is anesthetized (approximately 5 to 10 minutes), apply a tourniquet to the base of the toe (either a rubber band or small Penrose drain clamped with a hemostat).

Cut nail in
this fashion to
begin removal

FIGURE 28-2. Toenail removal.

Toenail Removal

8. For partial nail removal, first cut the nail lengthwise with sterile scissors or nail cutters, 4 to 5 mm from the affected nail fold (Fig. 28-2).

Note: If the entire nail is to be removed, cutting the nail in half in a lengthwise manner facilitates easier removal.

9. Loosen and lift the nail with a narrow periosteal elevator, flat edge of the scissors, or any similar instrument. If the entire nail is to be removed, the nail can first be cut in half with sterile scissors or nail cutters.

10. Gradually separate the nail from the underlying nail bed by applying gentle, upward pressure, taking care to minimize trauma to the underlying nail bed. It is important to ensure that the proximal nail underneath the cuticle is fully loosened.

Ablation of the Nail Matrix

11. If permanent removal of the nail is desired to prevent recurrent problems, the matrix of the nail bed must be ablated.

12. Dry the nail bed with sterile gauze and apply an 88% phenol solution to the nail matrix with a sterile cotton-tipped applicator for approximately 3 minutes.

Caution: Care must be taken not to expose surrounding tissue to the phenol solution.

13. Neutralize the area with isopropyl alcohol.

14. Remove the tourniquet.

Post-Procedure Care

15. Apply antibiotic ointment to the nail bed and apply a sterile gauze pad to the site.

16. Wrap the toe with rolled or tubular gauze

FOLLOW-UP CARE AND INSTRUCTIONS

■ Instruct the patient to keep the foot elevated for 24 to 36 hours, with gradual return to ambulation.

■ Over-the-counter analgesics are generally sufficient for pain relief.

■ Advise the patient to change the dressing in approximately 24 hours and to soak the toe in warm water twice a day for several days.

■ Instruct the patient to report back to the office with any signs of infection (fever, increasing swelling or erythema, pustular drainage).

■ To prevent recurrence of the ingrown nail, advise the patient to wear low-heeled shoes with adequate room for the forefoot and toes.

■ Instruct the patient not to trim the nails too short and to trim in a flat, straight-across fashion.

REFERENCES

Peggs JF: Treatment of ingrown toenails. In Pfenninger JL, Fowler GC (eds): Procedures for Primary Care Physicians. St. Louis, Mosby–Year Book, 1994, p 38-43.
Swartz MH: Textbook of Physical Diagnosis: History and Examination, 3rd ed. Philadelphia, WB Saunders, 1998, p 94.

Chapter 29

Draining Subungual Hematomas

Darwin Brown

PROCEDURE GOALS AND OBJECTIVES

Goal: To drain a subungual hematoma successfully with a minimal degree of risk and discomfort to the patient.

Objectives: The student will be able to ...

- Describe the indications, contraindications, and rationale for draining a subungual hematoma.

- Identify and describe common complications associated with draining a subungual hematoma.

- Describe the essential anatomy and physiology associated with draining a subungual hematoma.

- Identify the materials necessary for draining a subungual hematoma and their proper use.

- Identify the important aspects of post-procedure care after draining a subungual hematoma.

BACKGROUND AND HISTORY

Subungual hematoma is an injury that is common to the nail bed of fingers and toes. The vast majority are caused by simple trauma, which can result in bleeding into the space between the nail bed and fingernail. The subungual hematoma may also occur as a result of repetitive, indirect trauma to the distal end of the nail plate, typically from a tight-fitting shoe.

The patient often presents with intense pain secondary to the pressure produced by the hematoma. The primary goal of treatment is to relieve the pressure created by the hematoma. Drainage of the hematoma provides dramatic pain relief for the patient and decreases the secondary pressure effects to the digit. If the pressure is not relieved, damage to the nail matrix and the germinal layer may occur, causing delayed regrowth or dystrophy of the nail plate (Donnelly, 1992). The procedure itself is simple and can be performed safely in the practitioner's office.

Clinicians who perform this procedure should familiarize themselves with the anatomy of the nail bed and surrounding structures. The procedure is easy to perform with basic training and can be one of the more rewarding clinical treatments encountered in primary care or urgent care settings.

INDICATIONS

This procedure is indicated for relief from the acute pain associated with visible, painful subungual hematomas.

CONTRAINDICATIONS

All patients presenting with nail trauma must be carefully assessed by history, physical examination, and, when indicated, radiography. Based on the clinical impression from these data, a decision can be made about the appropriateness of proceeding with the draining of the hematoma. Potential contraindications include the following:

■ Crushed or fractured nails

■ Fracture of the distal phalanx, which can inadvertently be converted to an open fracture by draining the hematoma

■ Suspected subungual melanoma

■ Artificial acrylic nails are flammable and cautery should be avoided (Buttaravoli, 2005)

■ Hematomas involving 50% or more of the nail may indicate laceration of the underlying nail bed (Zook, 1999; Van Beek, 1990). It has been generally recommended that these patients be referred for nail removal and repair of the laceration (Simon, 1987; Melone, 1985; Wang, 2001). Others, however, recommend leaving the nail in place because insufficient data exist supporting improved cosmetic outcomes with removal of the nail (Buttaravoli, 2005; Fieg, 2002; Meek, 1998).

POTENTIAL COMPLICATIONS

Significant complications associated with this procedure are rare. Patients should be informed that there is potential for nail bed deformities to persist even after healing of the injury has occurred.

- The most likely complication resulting from a subungual hematoma is permanent nail deformity, especially if a nail bed injury is missed. Meek and White (1998) noted that from the perspective of many patients, nail deformity resulting from a subungual hematoma is considered minimally important.

- Infection of any remaining hematoma is uncommon but can occur. Using sterile technique and covering the site with a dressing after the procedure is completed can minimize the risk of this complication.

- Use of a cautery may result in an inadvertent burn to the nail bed after penetrating the nail, causing permanent damage.

- Functional deficits (numbness) are also a rare complication.

The procedure itself has no significant complications.

REVIEW OF ESSENTIAL ANATOMY AND PHYSIOLOGY

The nail anatomy is shown in Figure 29-1. The nail plate is produced by the underlying matrix or nail bed. The nail plate and the underlying nail bed are supported by the distal phalanx. The nail plate is not directly innervated;

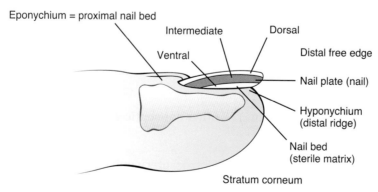

FIGURE 29-1. Anatomy of the nail and nail bed. (Redrawn from Pfenninger JF, Fowler GC: Procedures for Primary Care Physicians. St. Louis, Mosby–Year Book, 1994, p 40.)

however, the nail bed is richly innervated. The nail bed consists of all the tissue directly beneath the nail that functions in nail generation and migration. The arterial blood supply to the nail bed comes from two terminal branches of the volar digital artery (Zook, 1999).

Standard Precautions   Every practitioner should use standard precautions at all times when interacting with patients, especially when performing procedures. Determining the level of precaution necessary requires the practitioner to exercise clinical judgment based on the patient's history and the potential for exposure to body fluids or aerosol-borne pathogens (for further discussion, see Chapter 2).

PATIENT PREPARATION

- Describe the procedure to the patient and reassure him or her that there is rarely any more pain than what is already being experienced.

- Ask the patient if they have artificial acrylic nails, because the answer will determine the technique to be used.

- Anesthesia usually is not needed and is often more painful than the procedure.

- If the hematoma is to be evacuated using a large-bore needle or scalpel blade, a digital block may be useful (see Chapter 22), as this method is more painful than cautery because of the pressure applied to the nail (Concannon, 1999). However, this is rarely required.

- Inform the patient that, depending on the selected technique, an irritating odor may occur.

- The patient should be instructed to hold the digit very still during the procedure.

 ## Materials Utilized for Draining a Subungual Hematoma

- Gloves

- Face shield

- Povidone-iodine (Betadine) or other antiseptic-germicidal solution

- Alcohol wipes

- Cautery (battery-operated or electrocautery unit), No. 11 scalpel, 18-gauge needle, or a paper clip and hemostat

- Lighter to heat paper clip

- Sterile gauze

■ Antibiotic ointment

■ Bandage

Procedure for Draining a Subungual Hematoma

1. Place the patient in a sitting or supine position in which he or she can rest comfortably during the procedure without risk of further injury should lightheadedness occur. Examine the injured digit to determine the extent of injury.

2. Note the size of the hematoma.

3. Assess for fractures of the digit, especially the distal phalanx.

4. If a nondisplaced fracture is suspected, splint in an anatomic position until swelling improves.

Note: Radiographs should be obtained whenever you suspect a fracture.

5. Allow the affected digit to soak in an antiseptic solution such as povidone-iodine.

Note: Care must be taken to use aseptic technique in preparation for evacuation.

6. Clean the nail with alcohol.

Caution: **Alcohol is a highly flammable material. Wash off alcohol with sterile water or allow the alcohol to dry before placing hot cautery or flame near the nail.**

7. Burn a small hole in the nail using a conventional hand-held cautery or the straightened end of a paper clip (Fig. 29-2).

8. If using a paper clip, hold it with a hemostat.

9. Heat the straightened portion of the paper clip with a lighter until the tip is red hot.

Figure 29-2.   (Redrawn from Pfenninger JF, Fowler GC: Procedures for Primary Care Physicians. St. Louis, Mosby–Year Book, 1994, p 48.)

Figure 29-3.   (Redrawn from Pfenninger JF, Fowler GC: Procedures for Primary Care Physicians. St. Louis, Mosby–Year Book, 1994, p 48.)

10. Apply the hot tip with gentle pressure to the nail over the site of the hematoma (Fig. 29-3).

Note: It may take two or three attempts to burn through the nail with the heated paper clip.

continued

11. Make a 1- to 2-mm hole, which is large enough to allow for long-term drainage.

Note: A sudden burst of blood may occur if the pressure beneath the nail is great enough.

12. Alternatively, with an 18-gauge needle or a No. 11 scalpel blade, use a rotary motion to bore a hole through the nail to the hematoma. Consider using a digital block for this method if the patient is unable to tolerate pressure on the nail (see Chapter 22).

Note: After the blood has drained, the associated pain should improve significantly. If pain does not subside significantly, underlying fractures should be reconsidered.

13. Clean the area with alcohol wipes.

14. Apply antibiotic ointment and a light dressing to the nail.

SPECIAL CONSIDERATIONS

For young children, providing parents or guardians more information on the procedure can be helpful. Also, secure immobilization may be needed when performing this procedure in this population.

FOLLOW-UP CARE AND INSTRUCTIONS

Advise the patient of the proper follow-up care after this procedure.

- The affected digit should be soaked in warm, soapy water two or three times a day.

- A light dressing should be kept over the area until the evacuation site closes completely.

- The patient should notify the practitioner if pain persists. The practitioner should also be notified if there is a change in sensation, purulent or foul-smelling drainage, fever, or erythema of the skin surrounding the area.

- The patient should understand that the nail and discomfort should improve progressively over the following few days.

- If any change occurs or the injury is not improving as expected, the patient should call or return to the office.

REFERENCES

Buttaravoli PM, Stair TO: Common Simple Emergencies. Published online by Longwood Information (accessed July 1, 2005). Available at: www.ncemi.org/cse/cse1007.htm

Concannon MJ: Common Hand Problems in Primary Care. Philadelphia, Hanley & Belfus, 1999, p 119.

Donnelly RE: Step-by-step procedures for treating common nail problems. Part I: Paronychia and subungual hematoma. J Am Acad Phys Assist 5:145-150, 1992.

Fieg EL: Management of nail bed lacerations. Am Fam Physician 65:1997-1998, 2002.

Meek S, White M: Subungual haematomas: Is simple trephining enough? J Accid Emerg Med 15:269-271, 1998.

Melone CP, Grad JB: Primary care of fingernail injuries. Emerg Med Clin North Am 3:255-261, 1985.

Simon R, Wolgin M: Subungual haematoma: Association with occult laceration requiring repair. Am J Emerg Med 5:302-304, 1987.

Van Beek AL, Kassan MA, Adson MH, et al: Management of acute fingernail injuries. Hand Clin 6:23-35, 1990.

Wang QC, Johnson BA: Fingertip injuries. Am Fam Physician 63:1691-1696, 2001.

Zook EG, Brown RE: The perionychium. In Green DP, Hotchkiss RN, Pederson WC (eds): Green's Operative Hand Surgery, 4th ed, vol II. Philadelphia, Churchill Livingstone, 1999, pp 1354, 1356.

BIBLIOGRAPHY

Chang P: Nail bed repair. In Blair WF (ed): Techniques in Hand Surgery. Baltimore, Williams & Wilkins, 1996.

Kaya TI, Tursen U, Baz K, Ikizoglu G: Extra-fine insulin syringe needle: An excellent instrument for the evacuation of subungual hematoma. Dermatol Surg 29:1141-1143, 2003. (Describes a different technique for removal of subungual hematoma.)

Skinner PB Jr: Management of traumatic subungual hematoma. Am Fam Physician 71:856, 2005. (Describes a slight variation in technique.)

Chapter 30

Anoscopy

Sue M. Nyberg

Procedure Goals and Objectives

Goal: To examine the anus and rectum thoroughly, with minimal discomfort to the patient, and obtain accurate information while maintaining patient modesty.

Objectives: The student will be able to …

- Describe the indications, contraindications, and rationale for performing anoscopy.

- Identify and describe potential complications associated with performing anoscopy.

- Describe the essential anatomy and physiology associated with the performance of anoscopy.

- Describe how to perform a digital rectal examination.

- Identify the materials necessary for performing anoscopy and their proper use.

- Properly perform an anoscopy.

BACKGROUND AND HISTORY

Anorectal disorders are a common source of discomfort for many patients, and adequate visualization of the anorectal canal is important for appropriate diagnosis and treatment of these conditions. Anoscopy is a relatively simple procedure to perform, but adequate patient education and clinical skill are required to reduce the patient's anxiety and embarrassment about the procedure. This procedure is performed in ambulatory, emergency, and inpatient settings and is commonly carried out before colonoscopy.

INDICATIONS

Indications for performing anoscopy include, but are not limited to, the evaluation of the following:

■ Rectal bleeding

■ Anorectal pain

■ Pruritus

■ Anal discharge

■ Prolapse of the rectum

■ Mass detected in the rectal vault on digital examination

Therapeutic procedures may be performed along with routine anoscopy and include biopsy of suspicious lesions, removal of foreign bodies, and collection of a specimen for culture.

CONTRAINDICATIONS

Relatively few contraindications to the procedure exist; however, in the following situations, further patient education or referral to a specialist may be necessary if the examination is indicated:

■ Presence of severe rectal pain

■ Anoscopic examination in patients with perirectal abscess, acutely thrombosed hemorrhoid, or acute anal fissure, as severe discomfort may result as well as, in the case of anal fissure, possible bleeding

■ Patient unwilling to have the procedure performed

■ Patient not able to cooperate appropriately so that an adequate examination can be performed

■ Presence of severe anal stricture

POTENTIAL COMPLICATIONS

- Anal or perianal tears may occur but are usually mild and respond to conservative measures (Fry, 1985).

- Bleeding is rare but may occur with an anal tear or in the presence of internal hemorrhoids and usually responds to conservative measures unless a coagulation defect is present.

REVIEW OF ESSENTIAL ANATOMY AND PHYSIOLOGY

Understanding the anatomy of the anus and surrounding tissues facilitates accurate diagnosis and treatment of anorectal disorders. Careful visual inspection of the perianal region may reveal evidence of hemorrhoids, skin tags, fissures, dermatitis, abscesses, fistulous openings, or lesions. A thorough digital examination before anoscopy should evaluate the competency of the external anal sphincter and assess for palpable lesions.

The rectum is the distal 10- to 12-cm portion of the alimentary tract continuous proximally with the sigmoid colon and distally with the anal canal (Fig. 30-1). The rectum ends anteroinferior to the tip of the coccyx by turning sharply posteroinferiorly (the anorectal flexure) as it perforates the pelvic diaphragm (levator ani) to become the anal canal. The most distal point of the anal canal is the anal verge. The anal verge, the dentate line, and the anorectal ring are the three main anatomic points of reference.

- The anal verge, the external boundary of the anal canal, is the junction between the anal and perianal skin.

- The dentate line, the cephalad border of the anatomic anal canal, is a true mucocutaneous junction. Squamous epithelium is located distal to the dentate line, and columnar epithelium is located proximal to the dentate line in the rectum. At this junction is a circular ring of glands

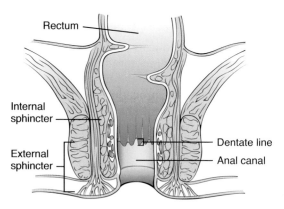

FIGURE 30-1. Anatomy of the rectum.

that secrete mucus to lubricate the anal canal. The dentate line lies approximately 1 to 2 cm above the anal verge.

■ The anorectal ring, 1 to 2 cm above the dentate line, is the upper border of the anal sphincteric complex and is easily palpable during digital examination.

The superior rectal artery, the continuation of the inferior mesenteric artery, supplies the proximal portion of the rectum. The two middle rectal arteries, usually arising from the inferior iliac arteries, supply the middle and inferior portions of the rectum, and the inferior rectal arteries, arising from the internal pudendal arteries, supply the anorectal sphincter muscles and anal canal. It is important to remember that the internal hemorrhoidal plexus arises above the dentate line and that the external hemorrhoidal plexus arises below the dentate line.

Both sympathetic and parasympathetic nerves innervate the rectum. The external sphincter (a voluntary skeletal muscle) and the levator ani muscles are innervated by the inferior rectal branch of the internal pudendal nerve (S2, S3, S4) as well as by fibers from the fourth sacral nerve. The internal sphincter (an involuntary muscle approximately 2.5 cm in length) is innervated by both sympathetic and parasympathetic nerves. It is generally accepted that either an intact functional external sphincter or anorectal ring (pubo-rectalis muscle that encircles the very distal rectum) can provide nearly perfect anal continence. The internal sphincter plays little part in maintaining voluntary anal continence. This is important when counseling patients who are considering surgical treatment of anal fissures (Surrell, 1994).

Standard Precautions   Every practitioner should use standard precautions at all times when interacting with patients, especially when performing procedures. Determining the level of precaution necessary requires the practitioner to exercise clinical judgment based on the patient's history and the potential for exposure to body fluids or aerosol-borne pathogens (for further discussion, see Chapter 2).

PATIENT PREPARATION

The only patient preparation needed is adequate education about the purpose of the examination and the technique used. Many patients have a degree of embarrassment about undergoing the examination and should be reassured that they will be appropriately draped. Although the procedure may be slightly uncomfortable and may cause an urge to defecate, it should not be painful (unless predisposing conditions are present). No bowel preparation is usually necessary.

Materials Utilized for Anoscopy

- Anoscope: The anoscope is a cylindrical instrument with a removable obturator, made of clear polyethylene or reusable metal (Fig. 30-2). Some anoscopes have their own attached light source; if not, another external light source must be used.

- Water-soluble lubricant

- Disposable gloves

- Light source (directed or worn on the head)

- Appropriate culture swabs (when indicated)

- Monsel's solution

- Large-tipped cotton swabs

FIGURE 30-2.   An anoscope.

Procedure for Anoscopy

 ## Position

1. Place the patient in a lateral decubitus or dorsal lithotomy position with appropriate draping.

 ## Inspection

1. Know the anatomy of the anus and surrounding tissues to facilitate accurate diagnosis and treatment of anorectal disorders.

2. Make a careful visual inspection of the perianal region to reveal any evidence of fissures, dermatitis, abscesses, fistulous openings, or lesions.

3. Ask the patient to bear down during inspection; this may reveal prolapsing hemorrhoids.

 ## Digital Rectal Examination

A thorough digital examination should be performed before anoscopy.

1. With a gloved, lubricated finger, gently press on the anal verge and ask the patient to relax. This should allow the finger to enter the anal canal.

2. The examiner should then evaluate the competency of the external anal sphincter by asking the patient to simulate interrupting a bowel movement.

3. After the patient relaxes, the examiner should also assess the rectal canal for any palpable lesions or masses. Finally, the prostate gland should be assessed in the male patient. The examiner should rotate the finger a full 360 degrees to ensure that all rectal structures are fully evaluated.

4. Generally, internal hemorrhoids and the dentate line are not palpable.

5. Any stool present on the examining finger should be examined for occult blood (Fry, 1985).

 ## Anoscopy

1. After lubricating the anoscope, gently spread the patient's buttocks and gently insert the anoscope into the anal canal. Slowly advance the anoscope until the flange at the base rests on the perianal skin.

2. Remove the obturator and inspect the mucosa of the perianal canal thoroughly for suspected pathology (Fig. 30-3).

FIGURE 30-3. (From Wigton RS: Gastrointestinal procedures. In Mosby's Primary Care Procedures, CD-ROM series. St. Louis, CV Mosby, 1999.)

3. Repeat the procedure, if needed, to ensure adequate inspection of the entire canal (Fry, 1985).

4. If a biopsy is necessary, one of a variety of long-handled biopsy instruments may be used.

5. Control any bleeding with Monsel's solution and pressure (Moesinger, 2000).

FOLLOW-UP CARE AND INSTRUCTIONS

Examination findings should be discussed thoroughly with the patient. Complications are rare with this procedure, and follow-up care should be based on the treatment of any condition found during the examination. The patient should be instructed to notify the provider if significant, unexpected bleeding or pain occurs after the procedure.

REFERENCES

Fry RD, Kodner IJ: Anorectal disorders. Clin Symp 37:2-5, 1985.
Moesinger RC: Gastrointestinal procedures. In Chen H, Sonnenday CJ (eds): Manual of Common Bedside Surgical Procedures. Philadelphia, Lippincott Williams & Wilkins, 2000, pp 159-160.
Surrell JA: Clinical anorectal anatomy and examination. In Pfenninger JL, Fowler GC (eds): Procedures for Primary Care Physicians. St. Louis, Mosby–Year Book, 1994, pp 898-901.

BIBLIOGRAPHY

Moore KL, Dalley AF: Clinically Oriented Anatomy, 4th ed. Philadelphia, Lippincott Williams & Wilkins, 1999.
Varma JR: Clinical anorectal anatomy and examination. In Pfenninger JL, Fowler GC (eds): Procedures for Primary Care Physicians. Philadelphia, Mosby–Year Book, 1994, pp 902-905.

Chapter 31

Flexible Sigmoidoscopy

Dawn Morton-Rias

PROCEDURE GOALS AND OBJECTIVES

Goal: To perform flexible sigmoidoscopy on a patient safely and accurately.

Objectives: The student will be able to …

- Describe the indications, contraindications, and rationale for performing flexible sigmoidoscopy.

- Identify and describe common complications associated with performing flexible sigmoidoscopy.

- Describe the essential anatomy and physiology associated with the performance of flexible sigmoidoscopy.

- Identify the materials necessary for performing flexible sigmoidoscopy and their proper use.

- Describe the steps associated with the safe performance of a flexible sigmoidoscopy examination.

BACKGROUND AND HISTORY

The need to examine and evaluate the rectum and colon has existed for centuries. Hippocrates mentioned the use of a rectal speculum for the diagnosis and treatment of anal disorders. Early instrumentation of the lower bowel was hampered by the lack of light. Several inventors experimented with endoscopic illumination, but Max Nitze of Germany (1879) and Howard Kelly of the United States (1895) are credited with the development of modern rigid proctosigmoidoscopy. Early proctosigmoidoscopy involved visual inspection of the lower bowel through a rigid scope inserted into the patient's anus and advanced to the rectum and sigmoid colon. Later, distal illumination, proximal illumination, and air insufflation expanded the visualization capabilities. Overholt of the United States reported the first experiences with fiberoptic flexible sigmoidoscopy by successfully examining the colon beyond the 25-cm limit of rigid sigmoidoscopy.

Modern flexible sigmoidoscopy involves the visual inspection and evaluation of the anal canal, rectum, and variable portions of the sigmoid colon. The procedure facilitates evaluation of lower bowel pathology, such as rectal bleeding, pain, constipation or diarrhea, and pathologic findings identified on digital or radiologic examination of the colon. Rigid sigmoidoscopy, considered optimal for visualization, biopsy, or culture of large surfaces, was not a welcome clinical intervention. Patient comfort was secondary to the evaluative and diagnostic benefits obtained from the procedure. Screening and diagnostic benefits of rigid sigmoidoscopy were minimal because of a lack of public awareness of the value of the test, limited clinical training of physicians to perform sigmoidoscopy properly, a high cost-benefit ratio in asymptomatic patients, and, perhaps most important, poor patient perception and dissatisfaction with rigid sigmoidoscopy. Consequently, rigid sigmoidoscopy has not been well utilized. This remains so even today.

According to the American Society for Gastrointestinal Endoscopy, Standards for Training and Practice Committee, flexible sigmoidoscopy, which also involves direct visualization and evaluation of the lower colon, enables detection of three to four times as many precancerous polyps and is more widely accepted by patients. Both flexible and rigid sigmoidoscopy are appropriate for evaluation of colonic symptoms, and yet neither substitute for full colonoscopy when the latter is indicated. Modern biotechnology has facilitated the integration of instrument flexibility, illumination, and therapeutic as well as photographic capabilities into the modern flexible sigmoidoscopy.

Colorectal cancer is the third most common cancer and the third leading cause of cancer death in both sexes, accounting for approximately 10 percent of cancer deaths overall (Jemal, 2005). Screening and surveillance guidelines endorsed by federal agencies and professional medical societies call for enhanced use of flexible sigmoidoscopy in conjunction with a complete history and physical examination, digital examination, and fecal occult blood assessment in the early detection and treatment of colon cancer. Evidence exists that a reduction in mortality from colorectal carcinoma is feasible through early detection and removal of polyps. Flexible sigmoidoscopy is a valuable screening tool in the early detection of changes in colonic mucosa, even before symptoms become evident. The 60-cm sigmoidoscope can reach to the splenic flexure and therefore directly identify about one half of colonic lesions (either cancers or polyps). An additional 20% of neoplasms are found if abnormal sigmoidoscopies are followed by colonoscopic examination of the entire colon. It allows direct visualization of changes, polyps, and other lesions and direct sampling. Flexible sigmoidoscopy is a reliable and cost-effective procedure that yields accurate findings when proper techniques are used.

Flexible sigmoidoscopy is safely and effectively performed by primary care physicians, physician assistants, nurse practitioners, and clinical nurse specialists. All health care providers are strongly encouraged to acquire proper training and supervision in performing this procedure. It is recommended that providers perform at least 20 flexible sigmoidoscopies under direct supervision by a physician trained in the technique before attempting to perform the procedure independently. Flexible sigmoidoscopy is a therapeutic and diagnostic procedure that is best used in conjunction with other screening and diagnostic practices. The screening protocol includes assessment of risk, a digital examination, assessment of occult blood, and sigmoidoscopy. Full colonoscopy and barium radiography of the colon may be indicated. Flexible sigmoidoscopy is not simply a one-time test. The optimal screening interval after a negative sigmoidoscopy has not been determined; the American Gastroenterological Association guidelines recommend repeat screening after 5 years (Winawer, 2003). Continuity of care and follow-up are key to realization of the benefit of this diagnostic procedure.

INDICATIONS

Specific indications for flexible sigmoidoscopy include evaluation and diagnosis of the following:
- Frank rectal bleeding

- Occult blood

- Hemorrhoidal inflammation

- Anal fissures

- Polyps

- Inflammatory conditions of the colon

In addition, flexible sigmoidoscopy is indicated for the following:
- To monitor inflammatory bowel disease.

- For follow-up and further evaluation of findings identified through barium enema radiography.

- Current cancer screening guidelines outlined by the American Cancer Society recommend baseline flexible sigmoidoscopy for all adults by age 50 (Smith, 2001).

- The American Society for Gastrointestinal Endoscopy recommends baseline and annual flexible sigmoidoscopy for individuals with a positive family history of familial polyposis, for individuals who have a first-degree relative with a history of colonic neoplasia, and for those with a positive family history of hereditary nonpolyposis or colon cancer.

- Some surgeons recommend flexible sigmoidoscopy before hernia repair to rule out a colonic tumor.

CONTRAINDICATIONS

Flexible sigmoidoscopy is a relatively safe procedure with few contraindications. Some sources suggest that polypectomy is not recommended using flexible sigmoidoscopy because of possible hemorrhage and risk of electrocautery-induced explosion. Others suggest that removal of polyps that are smaller than 0.5 cm during flexible sigmoidoscopy is safe and acceptable.

Contraindications to flexible sigmoidoscopy include:
- Fulminant colitis

- Severe or acute diverticulitis

- Toxic megacolon

- Acute peritonitis

- Poor bowel preparation

- Poor patient cooperation

- Severe cardiopulmonary disease

As with any diagnostic or therapeutic procedure, one must always weigh the importance of the information to be obtained against the risks associated with the procedure.

POTENTIAL COMPLICATIONS

Complications are rare but they can occur.
- Minor complications from flexible sigmoidoscopy include spotting and minor bleeding from the site.

- The most serious complication of flexible sigmoidoscopy is perforation of the bowel. This may occur if the instrument is pushed directly through the mucosa, usually in an area of sharp flexion or through a diverticulum, which has been mistaken for bowel lumen.

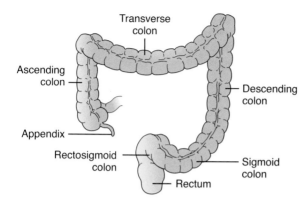

FIGURE 31-1. Anatomy of the large intestine and rectum.

■ Tears at the site of an anastomosis in patients who have undergone rectal surgery is also a possible complication.

■ A perforation or tear of the lumen requires surgical repair.

These complications may be avoided by taking a complete history, using proper technique, obtaining supervision and training, and using a reduced pace and rate of examination.

REVIEW OF ESSENTIAL ANATOMY AND PHYSIOLOGY

The anal canal is the terminal end of the gastrointestinal tract (Fig. 31-1). It is a tubular structure of approximately 3 to 4 cm in length. The anorectal junction is an important landmark, characterized by a change in the pinkish mucosa to pale squamous epithelium. This landmark will not be observed if the instrument is advanced too rapidly. The rectum is the fixed terminal portion of the large intestines. The rectum is generally 15 cm long, and its inferior portion is continuous with the anal canal. The rectal mucosa is generally pink, moist, and glistening. The lumen of the rectum has three shelflike projections called the superior, middle, and inferior valves of Houston. These values are composed of mucous membranes, circular muscle, and fibrous tissue. The entrance to the sigmoid colon is marked by the presence of haustrations that are seen as small mucosal projections into the lumen. These haustrations appear to divide the sigmoid lumen into compartments. Branches of the inferior mesenteric artery and sigmoid arteries provide the arterial blood supply of the sigmoid colon. Venous drainage is achieved via the inferior mesenteric vein. Lymphatic drainage is achieved via the intermediate colic lymph nodes on the branches of the left colic arteries and left inferior mesenteric lymph nodes around the inferior mesenteric artery.

Standard Precautions   Every practitioner should use standard precautions at all times when interacting with patients, especially when performing procedures. Determining the level of precaution necessary requires the practitioner to exercise clinical judgment based on the patient's history and the potential for exposure to body fluids or aerosol-borne pathogens (for further discussion, see Chapter 2).

PATIENT PREPARATION

■ Explain the procedure to the patient, allowing an opportunity for the patient to ask questions and for them to be answered satisfactorily.

■ Obtain informed consent for the procedure.

Preparation before the procedure may include:
■ A liquid diet for 24 hours before the procedure

■ One or two bowel-cleansing enemas before the procedure. Patients are encouraged to use a commercially prepared enema product. Harsh laxatives may irritate the mucosa and cause retention of soft or watery stool, which may interfere with the quality of the examination. Complete and meticulous bowel preparation must be achieved to avoid explosion of combustible gases.

■ Patients are to continue taking their prescribed medications.

■ Patients are generally advised to discontinue use of aspirin, non-steroidal anti-inflammatory agents, and blood thinners before the procedure because these agents generally interfere with coagulation.

■ Prophylactic antibiotic therapy may be prescribed for patients with cardiac valvular disease.

■ The patient must be aware of the indications and expected outcomes as well as the logistics of the examination before positioning and draping.

Materials Utilized to Perform a Flexible Sigmoidoscopy

■ A standard, small-caliber, flexible fiberoptic sigmoidoscope, either 35 or 60 cm in length (Fig. 31-2), and an appropriate light source

Note: The basic unit consists of a control head, flexible insertion tube, and maneuverable tip. The most important features of the scope are flexibility, optics, and a small outside diameter with the largest internal biopsy channel possible. Durability as well as ease of cleaning and maintenance are essential. The coated glass fibers allow transmission of images longitudinally and transmit light to the distal end of the scope as well as to the proximal end. Smaller channels within the scope allow for the insufflation of air that is

FIGURE 31-2. Schematic diagram of a fiberoptic sigmoidoscope. (Redrawn from Pfenninger JL, Fowler GC: Procedures for Primary Care Physicians. St. Louis, Mosby–Year Book, 1994, p 916.)

necessary for distention of the lumen, water infiltration, and fulguration apparatus. These are useful for aspiration of retained liquid stool, mucus, or enema water. The water, suction, and air controls are located on the control head and the scope. The exterior of the scope is housed in a plastic sleeve.

- Large, cotton-tipped swabs, to push aside stool or to assess mucosal integrity

- Culture and biopsy materials, so that lesions and suspicious mucosa may be adequately sampled

- Appropriate draping materials to protect patient modesty

- Unsterile gloves

- Water-soluble lubricant

- Suction machine

- Containers with and without water

- Forceps

Procedure for Performing a Flexible Sigmoidoscopy

Note: Flexible sigmoidoscopy is an outpatient procedure. The success of the examination relies on provider technique and rapport with the patient, as well as patient comfort, preparation, and cooperation.

Note: Sedation is rarely necessary. Low-dose intravenous diazepam may be indicated for patients with significant apprehension or anal disease or for children.

continued

1. Place the patient in any one of three positions: knee-chest position, an inverted position, or left Sims' position. Some prefer the left Sims' position in that it is perceived to be a less embarrassing position. The knee-chest position as well as the inverted position allows for greater access, as the bowel tends to move away from the pelvis. Encourage the patient in the knee-chest position or inverted position to remain still and to keep the hips straight.

2. Dim the room lighting; an assistant should be available in the examination room.

3. Begin the procedure with a well-lubricated digital examination of the anus.

Note: This examination also serves to ensure proper rectal clearance as well as to relax the rectal sphincter and lubricate the anal canal.

4. Palpate the anal region for abnormalities, fissures, and inflammation of internal or external hemorrhoid tissue. Palpate the ischioanal fossae and perineum between the thumb and forefinger.

5. Insert the examining finger farther to palpate the anterior wall and then sweep down to the posterior wall.

Note: This step in effect becomes a bidigital examination because while the index finger is within the anus, the thumb is palpating the tissue of the perineum, ischioanal fossae, and coccygeal areas. In addition, this step allows the provider to assess the anal diameter to determine if the selected caliber scope is appropriate.

6. The distal 10 to 15 cm of the scope may be lubricated, but care should be used to avoid lubrication of the tip, as this will cloud the lens.

7. To minimize the patient's discomfort, a common approach for insertion of the scope involves gradual replacement of

FIGURE 31-3. (Redrawn from Wigton RS: Gastrointestinal procedures. In: Mosby's Primary Care Procedures, CD-ROM series. St. Louis, CV Mosby, 1999.)

the examining digit during withdrawal with the insertion of the scope (Fig. 31-3).

8. While advancing the scope, you will feel a slight "give" as the scope passes the anal canal and enters the rectum.

9. Advancement, as well as deflection, of the scope via the hand-held control knobs must be slow and gradual.

10. Small turns of the control knobs result in significant movement of the scope. You may observe a "red out" during advancement of the scope. This finding suggests that the lens of the scope is pressed against the lumen, and the instrument must be retracted slightly.

11. Avoid excessive suctioning during the procedure, as the mucosal wall may be suctioned directly to the scope and may become dry and erythematous as well.

12. Use the least amount of air insufflation as possible for visualization to minimize distention and avoid patient discomfort.

Note: Overinsufflation may cause the mucosa to become less flexible and may cause perforation or serosal lacerations.

Note: The normal healthy mucosa is pink and glistening. Plaques, lesions, masses, and polyps must be noted.

Note: Transition to the rectum is generally evident by recognition of three prominent haustral folds, the valves of Houston. These angulations must be successfully negotiated, and this component of the examination is considered most technically challenging.

Note: Dutta and Kowalewski (1987) suggest the following general rules for insertion of the flexible fiberoptic sigmoidoscope.

- Clockwise torque decreases bowel angulation; counterclockwise torque does the reverse.

- Slight suction may aid in negotiation of sharp angulation in the bowel.

- If spasm occurs, pause and then resume.

- If you reach sharp curves, withdraw a bit before advancing the scope.

13. Throughout the procedure, sampling, culture, and biopsy specimens may be obtained. Use the largest forceps available that will fit through the scope. Survey samples should be obtained from fold edges because they yield the greatest results.

14. Under rare circumstances and with specialized and specific training and certification, small polyps may be removed via electrosurgery under endoscopic conditions.

15. Small sessile polyps (5 mm or less) may be removed with hot biopsy forceps.

Note: Some providers attempt polypectomy of larger lesions through mechanical debulking.

Note: Dutta and Kowalewski's 10 overall golden rules for flexible sigmoidoscopy are as follows:

- Never attempt the procedure on an uncooperative or unwilling patient.

- Always obtain written consent.

- Talk with your patient before, during, and after the procedure.

- Allow yourself enough time.

- Do not spend 20 minutes inserting the scope. The best visualization of colonic mucosa may be on the way out.

- Proper bowel preparation is essential. Postpone the test if necessary.

- Do not insist on inserting the instrument the full 60 cm; 30 to 40 cm may be all that is possible.

- Never advance the scope blindly.

- The 90- to 180-degree deflection available on most scopes is very helpful. Use it.

- Use less air; suction as necessary.

16. Withdraw the scope gradually, and carefully inspect the colon during this process.

Note: Withdrawal of the scope is a crucial part of the examination. The examiner must ensure that the steering knob is not locked, and he or she must use torque combined with in-and-out movements to deflect and observe while exiting.

17. When the tip of the sigmoidoscope is withdrawn from the anus, be careful that it does not strike anything, as the anus can be easily damaged.

18. Reinsert the scope 5 to 6 cm to remove the remaining air. Take care not to suck the mucosa into the scope. The patient can be instructed to tell the examiner when all the air has been removed.

19. Inspect the anal canal thoroughly using either an anoscope or the sigmoidoscope. This can also be performed at the beginning of the procedure.

SPECIAL CONSIDERATIONS

Flexible sigmoidoscopy of infants, children, teenagers, and elders requires attention to positioning, preparation, and communication. Infants and children may be understandably apprehensive and may require mild sedation. Special attention to concerns and an explanation of details may be necessary in preparing teenagers and young adults. Teenagers and young adults may be particularly sensitive to traffic within the examination suite. Hence, attention should be paid to limiting exposure. Elders, patients with limited mobility, and those with circulatory compromise may prefer or require left lateral (Sims') positioning for enhanced patient comfort. Full disclosure, communication, and rapport remain key in attending the needs of special populations.

FOLLOW-UP CARE AND INSTRUCTIONS

Flexible sigmoidoscopy is a relatively safe and benign procedure. Post-procedure complications are rare but may include the following:

- Patients may complain of mild cramping and bloating from distention of the colon. Patients may also notice spotting after biopsy. These reactions are normal.

- Instruct the patient to seek immediate medical attention if he or she experiences severe abdominal pain, significant abdominal distention, nausea, vomiting, fever, chills, or a rectal bleed of greater than $\frac{1}{2}$ cup after the procedure.

REFERENCES

Dutta S, Kowalewski E: Flexible Sigmoidoscopy for Primary Care Physicians. New York, Alan R. Liss, 1987.

Jemal A, Murray T, Ward W, et al: Cancer statistics, 2005. CA Cancer J Clin 55:10, 2005.

Smith RA, von Eschenbach AC, Wender R, et al: American Cancer Society guidelines for the early detection of cancer: Update of early detection guidelines for prostate, colorectal, and endometrial cancers. Also: Update 2001—Testing for early lung cancer detection. CA Cancer J Clin 51:38, 2001.

Winawer S, Fletcher R, Rex D, et al: Colorectal cancer screening and surveillance: Clinical guidelines and rationale—Update based on new evidence. Gastroenterology 124:544, 2003.

BIBLIOGRAPHY

ASGE guideline: colorectal cancer screening and surveillance, American Society for Gastrointestinal Endoscopy. Gastrointestinal Endoscopy Vol. 63, No. 4, 2006. Available at: www.gieoumal.org.

Charette A: Patient information: Flexible sigmoidoscopy: USDA Nutrition Center on Aging at Tufts University. Available at: www.uptodate.com

Clinical Abstracts—Guidelines for Colorectal Cancer Screening. Available at: http://www.medscape.com

Fincher RK, Osgard EM, Jackson JL, et al: A comparison of bowel preparations for flexible sigmoidoscopy: Oral magnesium citrate combined with oral bisacodyl, one hypertonic phosphate enema, or two hypertonic phosphate enemas. Am J Gastroenterol 94:2122-2127, 1999.

Gitnick G: Gastroenterology: Medical Outline Series. New York, Medical Examination, 1985.

Hellinger M: Screening and detection of colorectal cancer. Cancer Control 5:17-18, 1998.

Jednak MA, Nostrant TT: Screening for colorectal cancer. Prim Care 25:293-308, 1998.

Johnson BA: Flexible sigmoidoscopy: Screening for colorectal cancer. Am Fam Phys 59:313-324, 327-328, 1999.

Katon K, Keeffe E, Melnyk C: Flexible Sigmoidoscopy. New York, Grune & Stratton, 1985.

Lewis JD, Asch DA, Ginsberg GG, et al: Primary care physicians' decisions to perform flexible sigmoidoscopy. J Gen Intern Med 14:297-302, 1999.

Levin TR, Conell C, Shapiro JA, et al: Complications of screening flexible sigmoidoscopy. Gastroenterology 123:1786, 2002.

Lichtenstein P, Holm NV, Verkasalo PK, et al: Environmental and heritable factors in the causation of cancer. N Engl J Med 343:78-85, 2000.

Manoucheri M, Nakamura DY, Lukman RL: Bowel preparation for flexible sigmoidoscopy: Which method yields the best results? J Fam Pract 49:273, 2000.

Moore K: Clinically Oriented Anatomy. Baltimore, Williams & Wilkins, 1985.

National Institute of Diabetes and Digestive and Kidney Diseases: NIH Publication No. 95-1133. December, Bethesda, Md, 1992.

Painter J, Saunders DB, Bell GD, et al: Depth of insertion at flexible sigmoidoscopy: Implications for colorectal cancer screening and instrument design. Endoscopy 31:227-231, 1999.

Rex D: Colonic disease: Advances in screening, management and perspectives on health care utilization. Paper presented at the annual meeting of the American College of Gastroenterology, October 15, 1999. Available at: http://www.medscape.com/viewarticle/423637

Ruffin M, Gorenflo D, Woodman B: Predictors of screening for breast, cervical, colorectal and prostatic cancer among community-based primary care practices. J Am Board Fam Pract 13:1-10, 2000.

Schoen RE, Weissfeld JL, Bowen NJ, et al: Patient satisfaction with screening flexible sigmoidoscopy. Arch Intern Med 160:1790-1796, 2000.

Schoenfeld P, Piorkowski M, Allaire J, et al: Flexible sigmoidoscopy by nurses: State of the art 1999. Gastroenterol Nurs 22:254-261, 1999.

Shaukat MS, Ramirez FC: The utilization of flexible sigmoidoscopy by family practitioners after residency training. Gastrointest Endosc 52:45-47, 2000.

Society of American Gastrointestinal Endoscopic Surgeons (SAGES) Patient Information—Flexible Sigmoidoscopy. Available at: http://www.medscape.com

Stewart BT, Keck JO, Duncan AV, et al: Difficult or incomplete flexible sigmoidoscopy: Implications for a screening programme. Aust N Z J Surg 69:2-3, 1999.

Taylor T, Williamson S, Wardle J, et al: Acceptability of flexible sigmoidoscopy screening in older adults in the United Kingdom. J Med Screen 7:38-45, 2000.

Tuggy M: Virtual reality flexible sigmoidoscopy simulator training: Impact on resident performance. J Am Board Fam Pract 11:426-433, 1998.

Wallace MB, Kemp JA, Meyer F, et al: Screening for colorectal cancer with flexible sigmoidoscopy by nonphysician endoscopists. Am J Med 107:286-287, 1999.

Zubarik R, Eisen G, Zubarik J, et al: Education improves colorectal cancer screening by flexible sigmoidoscopy in an inner city population. Am J Gastroenterol 95:509-512, 2000.

Chapter 32

Removal of Cerumen and Foreign Bodies from the Ear

Tammy Dowdell Ream

PROCEDURE GOALS AND OBJECTIVES

Goal: To remove cerumen impaction or foreign bodies from the auditory canal while observing standard precautions and with the minimal degree of risk to the patient.

Objectives: The student will be able to …

- Describe the indications, contraindications, and rationale for performing cerumen or foreign body removal.

- Identify and describe common complications associated with cerumen or foreign body removal.

- Describe the essential anatomy and physiology associated with performance of cerumen or foreign body removal.

- Identify the necessary materials for performing cerumen or foreign body removal and their proper use.

- Identify the important aspects of post-procedure care following cerumen or foreign body removal.

BACKGROUND AND HISTORY

Cerumen is a normal substance produced and found in the external auditory canal. Cerumen serves as protective coating, trapping fine dust and repelling water away from the tympanic membrane. The acidic nature of cerumen is not suitable for bacterial growth, thus aiding in prevention of otitis externa development. Fine hair located in the auditory canal moves the cerumen out of the external meatus, preventing obstruction. Many factors can interfere with this physiologic process, leading to cerumen impaction and obstruction, including a narrowed auditory canal or external meatus, overproduction of cerumen, or use of cotton-tipped applicators in the canal. Although commonly asymptomatic, cerumen impaction can lead to tinnitus, vertigo, and the perception of fullness or pain (Tintinalli, 2004). The most common cause of conductive hearing impairment is cerumen impaction.

It is not unusual to see patients with complaints of a foreign body in the ear in the primary care setting. Foreign bodies found in the auditory canal may include insects, beans, beads, cotton, and other things. Children frequently place small items in the ear. Insects may crawl or fly into the canal. If an insect remains alive in the canal, patients may complain that they can feel it moving or hear it. Patients may be asymptomatic but more commonly report some discomfort due to the presence of the foreign body. This discomfort may be quite severe if there is an infection present or if there is a live insect. Occasionally, the presenting complaint is a change in hearing or sense of fullness.

INDICATIONS

Cerumen removal is indicated when the patient is symptomatic or a cerumen impaction is noted on physical examination, preventing needed visualization. Any foreign body present in the auditory canal is an indication for removal.

CONTRAINDICATIONS

Removal of cerumen impaction or a foreign body from the auditory canal is generally a simple procedure, but there are times when patients should be referred to an otolaryngologist for evaluation. The use of a microscope or removal of the cerumen or foreign body under general anesthesia may be necessary in the following cases:

- Uncooperative patient

- Suspected tympanic membrane rupture

- Inability to visualize the tympanic membrane when rupture is suspected

- Contact of the foreign body with the tympanic membrane

POTENTIAL COMPLICATIONS

- Tympanic membrane perforation
- Ossicle damage
- Abrasion of the canal
- Movement of the foreign body further into the canal
- Temporary vertigo
- Tinnitus

REVIEW OF ESSENTIAL ANATOMY AND PHYSIOLOGY

The ear is made up of the external, middle and inner divisions (Fig. 32-1). The inner ear includes the cochlea and semicircular canals. The middle ear is protected by the tympanic membrane and includes the bony structures (incus, stapes, and malleus) utilized in normal hearing. The external ear is made up of the pinna and external auditory canal.

Prior to removal of a cerumen impaction or foreign body, an examination is required to evaluate the tympanic membrane and external auditory canal. Minor movement of the pinna is painful in the patient with otitis externa and otoscopic evaluation will reveal erythema and swelling of the canal. The

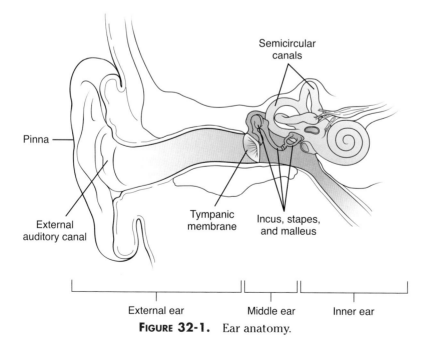

Semicircular canals

Pinna

External auditory canal

Tympanic membrane

Incus, stapes, and malleus

External ear   Middle ear   Inner ear

FIGURE 32-1.   Ear anatomy.

tympanic membrane will not be visualized if a cerumen impaction is present. Evidence of tympanic membrane rupture is an indication for otolaryngology referral.

Standard Precautions   Practitioners should use standard precautions at all times when interacting with patients. Determining the level of precaution necessary requires the practitioner to exercise clinical judgment based on the patient's history and the potential for exposure to bodily fluids or aerosol-borne pathogens (for further discussion, see Chapter 2).

PATIENT PREPARATION

- Discuss the proposed procedure with the patient, including the associated risks.
- Advise the patient to remain still during the procedure.
- Warn the patient that the procedure may be uncomfortable but if it becomes painful the removal attempt will be stopped.
- The patient should be placed in an upright and comfortable position.
- Discuss any concerns the patient expresses regarding the procedure.

Materials Utilized to Perform Cerumen or Foreign Body Extraction

- Syringe (metal ear syringes are available [Fig. 32-2], but any 30- to 60-mL syringe will work)
- Otoscope
- Body temperature water

FIGURE 32-2. Metal ear syringe.

FIGURE 32-3.   Cerumen spoon **(A)**, cerumen loop **(B)**, and right-angle hook **(C)**.

- Cerumen spoon (Fig. 32-3A)
- Cerumen loop (see Fig. 32-3B) or right-angle hook (see Fig. 32-3C)
- Alligator forceps
- Lidocaine or mineral oil for live insects
- Cup-shaped forceps for round foreign bodies
- Small-diameter suction tip if suction is available
- Magnet if the foreign body is metal
- Cyanoacrylate glue (super glue) and a wooden cotton swab

Procedure for Cerumen and Foreign Body Extraction

 ### Cerumen Removal

1. After confirming the presence of cerumen impaction with an otoscopic examination, place the patient in an upright, comfortable position.

2. Place a waterproof barrier–backed absorbent pad across the patient's neck and shoulder, on the side of the affected ear.

3. Fill the large syringe with body temperature water.

4. Have the patient or an assistant hold a basin under the affected ear to collect the fluid during irrigation unless using an ear wash system with suction built in.

5. Place the syringe tip (you also may attach an 18-gauge intravenous catheter or butterfly catheter tubing to the syringe) into the lateral canal (Fig. 32-4).

6. Irrigate, targeting the superior canal surface, allowing the fluid to flow behind the impaction and pushing it toward the canal orifice.

7. The canal and tympanic membrane should be inspected frequently during the procedure for injury or rupture.

8. Repeat as needed until the impaction is removed or the patient voices pain.

continued

FIGURE 32-4. Irrigation.

9. If irrigation is not successful, manual removal with a cerumen spoon may be attempted. This is generally more uncomfortable for the patient.

10. Using the otoscope to visualize the cerumen, place the cerumen spoon into the canal. Your aim is to put the spoon at one edge of the impaction and pull it distally. It is vital the patient remain still during this maneuver to prevent tympanic membrane rupture or abrasion of the canal.

11. If the cerumen does not dislodge easily, reattempt irrigation after inspection. Frequently the manual attempt loosens the impaction, allowing irrigation to be successful.

12. After the cerumen is removed, a final inspection of the canal and tympanic membrane is mandated.

Foreign Body Removal

1. After confirming the presence of a foreign body with an otoscopic exam, place the patient in a comfortable position.

2. The foreign body type drives the approach for removal. Irrigation is not an option for absorbent material (e.g., beans).

3. If a live insect is present, warm oil or lidocaine may be dropped into the canal to immobilize or kill the insect (Hall, 2003). Lidocaine may also provide an anesthetic effect (Tintinalli, 2005).

4. Insert the cerumen loop or right-angle hook into the canal through the otoscope.

Caution: **Do not make a blind insertion.**

5. Aim the instrument at the superior edge of the foreign body, sliding it behind and then pulling the material toward the external orifice.

6. Alligator forceps are useful for items that are soft and easily grasped (e.g., cotton).

7. Round material (e.g., beads) are removed more easily with cup-shaped forceps to prevent movement of the body toward the tympanic membrane.

8. If suction is available, a small-diameter suction tip may be placed against the object for removal.

9. Metal objects may be removed with a magnet (Hall, 2003).

10. Skilled clinicians have used cyanoacrylate glue (super glue) applied to the wooden end of a cotton swab. Insert the wooden tip into the canal, placing it against the foreign body until the glue dries, and then withdraw the swab and foreign body together.

Caution: **It is important that the glue not come in contact with the patient's skin.**

11. After the foreign body is removed, a final inspection of the canal and tympanic membrane is mandated to evaluate for canal or tympanic membrane damage.

SPECIAL CONSIDERATIONS

- Any infection should be treated promptly, but the tympanic membrane may appear slightly erythematous immediately following irrigation.

- There are commercial ear irrigation systems available that provide irrigation with simultaneous suction.

- Home dental irrigation units have been used but are not recommended. The narrow irrigation stream may cause a tympanic membrane rupture. Backsplash is also increased with these units.

FOLLOW-UP CARE AND INSTRUCTIONS

- If tympanic membrane rupture occurs, otolaryngologist evaluation should be scheduled within 1 to 2 weeks; treat for pain and provide reassurance (Tintinalli, 2004).

- To decrease the risk of development of resultant otitis externa, dry the auditory canal after the irrigation by placing 2 or 3 drops of isopropyl alcohol into the canal (in the absence of tympanic membrane perforation) or using a warm blow dryer on a low setting (Jacker, 2005).

- If the patient had decreased hearing due to cerumen impaction, improved hearing is usually noted immediately following removal of the cerumen.

- The patient should be instructed to report any signs or symptoms of infection to the clinician as soon as they are noted. These include, but are not limited to, localized pain, erythema, and swelling.

REFERENCES

Hall KL, Curry RW Jr: Selected disorders of the ear, nose, and throat. In Taylor RB (ed): Family Medicine: Principles and Practice, 6th ed. New York, Springer-Verlag, 2003, pp 612-621.

Jacker RK, Kaplin MK: Ear, nose, and throat. In Tierny LM Jr, McPhee JJ, Papadakis MA (eds): Current Medical Diagnosis and Treatment, 44th ed. New York, Lange Medical Books/McGraw-Hill, 2005, pp 177-214.

Tintinalli A, Lucchesi M: Common disorders of the external, middle, and inner ear. In Tintinalli JE, Kelen GD, Stapczynski JS (eds): Emergency Medicine: A Comprehensive Study Guide, 6th ed. New York, McGraw-Hill, 2004, pp 1464-1471.

BIBLIOGRAPHY

Gates GA, Rees TS: Otologic changes and disorders. In Cassel CK, Leipzig RM, Cohen HJ, et al (eds): Geriatric Medicine: An Evidence Based Approach, 4th ed. New York, Springer-Verlag, 2003.

LeBlond RF, DeGowin RL, Brown DD: The head and neck. In DeGowin's Diagnostic Examination, 8th ed. New York, McGraw-Hill, 2004 pp 191-338.

Mantooth R: Foreign Bodies, Ear. Accessed 7/6/05. Available at: http://www.emedicine.com/emerg/topic185.htm

MDchoice, Inc: Wax Blockage. Accessed 7/6/05. Available at: http://www.drkoop.com/ency/93/000979.html

Pray WS, Pray JJ: Earwax: Should it be removed? US Pharm 5:21-27, 2005.

Chapter 33

Trauma-Oriented Ocular Examination, Corneal Abrasion, and Ocular Foreign Body Removal

Jonathon W. Gietzen

PROCEDURE GOALS AND OBJECTIVES

Goal: To perform a trauma-oriented ocular examination, treat corneal abrasion or ulceration, and perform ocular foreign body removal safely and with minimal degree of risk to the patient.

Objectives: The student will be able to ...

- Describe the indications, contraindications and rationale for performing a trauma-oriented ocular examination.

- Identify the common precautions and potential complications associated with the performance of a trauma-oriented ocular examination.

- Describe the essential anatomy and physiology associated with the performance of a trauma-oriented ocular examination.

- Identify the materials necessary for performing a trauma-oriented ocular examination.

- Demonstrate the essential steps necessary to perform a trauma-oriented ocular examination, identification of corneal injury, and safe and complete ocular foreign body removal.

- Identify the important aspects of post-procedure patient care, including recommended treatment strategies.

BACKGROUND AND HISTORY

Ocular trauma is a commonly encountered condition in the primary care setting. Ocular trauma can occur as part of work, hobby, recreation, or leisure activities, usually of an accidental nature. It is estimated that each year in emergency departments in the United States almost 900,000 patients are treated for eye injuries. The rate of eye injuries is approximately 3.15 per 1000 population (95% confidence interval [CI], 2.66-3.63), with the injury rate among males being 4.52 per 1000 (95% CI, 3.77-5.20) (McGwin, 2005; Harwood-Nuss, 2005; Moeller, 2003).

The most common injuries to the eye are contusion or abrasion (44.4%), foreign body (30.8%), burns (10.2%), and conjunctivitis (9.9%). Lacerations and punctures account for 1.8% and 0.5% of ocular traumas, respectively. The settings for these injuries include home (44.6%), public places (23.6%), and industrial locations (20.3%). The most prevalent causes of injury are foreign body (44.6%), struck against or by an object (33%), and burns (12%). The most common patient is a male in his 20s to 30s (McGwin, 2005; Harwood-Nuss, 2005; Moeller, 2003).

In the primary care setting a rapid and systematic approach to examination of the patient with ocular trauma enables the clinician to accurately delineate the type, location, and degree of ocular impairment. This examination is frequently performed in primary care settings (Harwood-Nuss, 2005; Janda, 1991)

Once the clinician has accurately assessed the eye injury, an appropriate treatment plan can be developed. Many uncomplicated or simple corneal abrasions and/or superficial corneal foreign bodies are easily removed in the primary care setting. Primary care clinicians should be able to perform basic care for the most common eye injuries. They should also know when the patient's condition is beyond their scope of practice and when to refer the patient to either an optometrist or an ophthalmologist (Harwood-Nuss, 2005; Janda, 1991; Bunuel-Jordana, 2004).

INDICATIONS

A trauma-oriented eye examination is indicated for any potential eye injury, including blunt force, suspected scratch or abrasion, suspected foreign body, or any acute visual disturbance (Harwood-Nuss, 2005; Janda, 1991). Properly performed, the examination adds little additional risk to the patient's vision (Harwood-Nuss, 2005). Symptoms of a corneal abrasion include foreign body sensation, tearing, pain, and photophobia. Symptoms range from mild foreign body sensation to severe pain. The degree of pain appears to be strongly associated with the degree of damage to the cornea. Symptoms typically begin instantly after the injury and can last from minutes to days. Conjunctival injection and eyelid swelling may be present (Harwood-Nuss, 2005; Janda, 1991; Ophthalmology, Cornea [www.emedicine.com]).

FIGURE 33-1. Fox shield.

CONTRAINDICATIONS (or, when to refer to an ophthalmologist for emergent treatment)

RUPTURED GLOBE

Patients with a high level of suspicion for a ruptured globe, globe laceration, or intraocular foreign body should not be examined further and the clinician should immediately refer the patient to an ophthalmologist. Suspect a penetrated globe if the patient was in a situation in which the particle may have had a high velocity (e.g., grinding metal) when it struck the eye (McGwin, 2005; Harwood-Nuss, 2005; Janda, 1991).

If the globe is ruptured, do not use topical agents on the eye. Make the patient comfortable as soon as possible. Cover *both* eyes with a Fox shield (Fig. 33-1) or other dressing (e.g., flattened paper cup) to reduce the movement of the injured eye (Harwood-Nuss, 2005).

An actively draining globe laceration often demonstrates ocular hypotony (intraocular pressure [IOP] < 5 mm Hg). Although a trained ophthalmologist or optometrist may roughly estimate hypotony due to a draining globe by having the patient close his or her eyes and gently applying light pressure with the thumbs to feel the eyes, this is not recommended. The injured eye may feel "softer" than the non-injured eye. Some authors question the benefit of checking IOP in the setting of an obvious globe injury as it may increase risk for infection or extension of the injury (Fig. 33-2) (Harwood-Nuss, 2005; Janda, 1991; Lima-Gomez, 2004).

If the penetrated globe is leaking aqueous humor, application of fluorescein may demonstrate a dark blue stream of fluid leaking from the site

A   Schiøtz manometer   B   Tonopen

FIGURE 33-2. Measuring intraocular pressure with a Schiøtz manometer **(A)** and Tonopen **(B)**.

FIGURE 33-3. Eyelid laceration.

of the injury, through the pool of fluorescein (Seidel sign) (Harwood-Nuss, 2005; Janda, 1991). An eye with a laceration to the globe without active aqueous humor leak may have a positive Seidel sign if the eye is gently pressed after the fluorescein has been applied.

EYELID LACERATION

Almost every patient with eyelid lacerations should be evaluated immediately and treated by an ophthalmologist (Fig. 33-3). Vertically oriented lacerations in the medial portion of the lower eyelid are of particular concern as

Figure 33-4. Use of the Morgan lens to flush the eye.

they may involve the tear ducts. These repairs are best left to either an ophthalmologist or plastic surgeon (Janda, 1991). The only exception to this is superficial, horizontally oriented (parallel to the eyelid) lacerations. These may be safely repaired in the primary care setting.

Caustic Splash Exposure

Caustic or other serious splash injuries require rapid dilution of the offending chemical. The clinician should treat the condition first and then assess the patient after the eye has been adequately flushed. Flushing should begin as soon as possible, including flushing of the eye at home in the sink or shower or outside with a garden hose. The lids should be held open during the flushing either manually or with a Morgan lens, which is a special contact lens that can be attached to a fluid source to flush the eye thoroughly (Fig. 33-4) (Harwood-Nuss, 2005; Janda, 1991).

CAUTIONS AND CONSIDERATIONS

The clinician must follow standard infection control precautions. Patients who have received a direct blow to the eye may present with pupillary abnormalities, which may be misinterpreted as a sign of intracranial pathology (Harwood-Nuss, 2005). Patients with severe eye injuries often present with a significant degree of nausea and vomiting. Rectal, intravenous, or intramuscular anti-emetics may reduce the nausea and indirectly calm the patient to reduce the likelihood of further eye damage (Harwood-Nuss, 2005).

Patients with prior corneal flap surgical procedures may have dislodgement of this flap with trauma (e.g., finger in eye) (Fig. 33-5). This should be carefully examined and cleaned judiciously and the flap made to lie back in its normal position. Refer the patient to the on-call ophthalmologist prior to discharge.

Contact lens wearers presenting with a corneal ulceration are at risk for *Pseudomonas* infection. A *Pseudomonas* infection of the cornea can cause

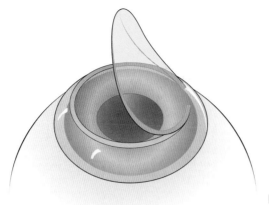

Figure 33-5. Dislodgement of corneal flap following surgical procedure.

permanent vision disability or loss in as short a time period as 24 hours (Harwood-Nuss, 2005; Moeller, 2003; Alberti, 2001). Patients with exposure to organic debris in the eye are at increased risk for infection. A broad-spectrum topical antibiotic should be prescribed (Moeller, 2003; Alberti, 2001).

When considering imaging the eye, do not perform a magnetic resonance image (MRI). MRI is not recommended because it may inadvertently move a metallic foreign body into or around in the eye, causing further damage. Plain radiography and/or computed tomography (CT) are recommended, as neither causes further injury to the eye.

Cooperation with this procedure is essential. The inebriated patient, confused elderly, children, and others who may be cognitively impaired or unable to control their responses to a recommended procedure may need sedation. These patients may necessitate a consultation with an ophthalmologist before any further examination or treatment is attempted.

COMMON COMPLICATIONS

The patient may experience increased eye pain, photophobia, nausea, and/or vomiting due to the eye examination. This is primarily due to how the body responds to the intraocular injury. Judicious use of topical anesthetics; darkening the room; and use of either oral, intravenous, intramuscular, or rectal anti-emetics can be useful to reduce overall patient discomfort (e.g., eye pain, nausea and vomiting, and/or the anxiety accompanying eye injury) (Harwood-Nuss, 2005). Anti-emetics can reduce further eye injury because uncontrolled vomiting increases intraocular pressure and increased intraocular pressure may cause additional bleeding to occur in patients who have bled into their eye.

REVIEW OF ESSENTIAL ANATOMY AND PHYSIOLOGY

The eye is a complex organ, with six extraocular muscles and four cranial nerves that work in tandem. It can allow for blinking to prevent desiccation (with muscles other than the six extraocular), to adjust near and far vision and pupillary response to light stimulus. Together the eyes produce images at the occipital lobe of the brain. Bilateral visual input is essential for proper visual cortex data interpretation. The overlapping of both left and right visual fields compensates for visual loss on one side, thus enabling adequate visual function in a person who has experienced significant visual field loss, to retain a reasonable visual field. The eye possesses several features that serve to protect it from innocuous conditions, such as dry eyes, to a "blow out" injury:

- The ability to produce tears, to heal the surface of the eye rapidly

- The ability to adjust intraocular pressure

- Accommodating for direct injury with the ability for the orbit to give in or "blow out" and the eye to change shape to absorb impact forces

It is important to know and understand terms related to the anatomy of the eye (Fig. 33-6). This knowledge is useful when examining the patient, documenting the findings, and discussing the case with other clinicians. The anterior chamber is the area bounded in front by the cornea and in back by

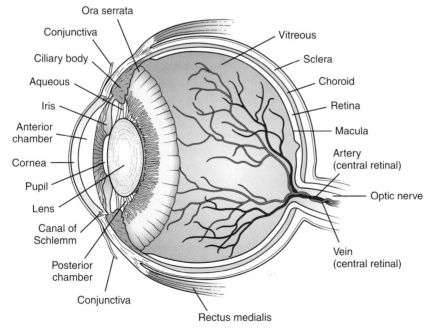

FIGURE 33-6. Anatomy of the eye.

the iris, and is filled with aqueous fluid. The aqueous fluid is a clear, watery solution in the anterior and posterior chambers. The canal of Schlemm is the passageway for the aqueous fluid to exit the eye to maintain normal intra-ocular pressures. The choroid, which carries blood vessels, is the inner coat between the sclera and the retina. Its main function is to deliver nutrients and remove waste products. The conjunctiva is a clear membrane covering the white of the eye (sclera). It functions as protection from external injury.

The cornea is a clear, transparent portion of the outer coat of the eyeball through which light passes to the lens, modulating light refraction and providing further protection. The corneal epithelium of the eye heals from most injuries in 1 or 2 days without any further consequences. The clinician must realize that the cornea is an avascular structure; oral medication will be delivered to it indirectly, primarily through the tears. Thus, topical medications are the drug of choice for most eye injuries, providing the direct application of the medication to the site where it is needed. The iris gives our eyes color and it functions like the aperture on a camera, enlarging in dim light and contracting in bright light. The aperture itself is known as the pupil. The lens helps to focus light on the retina.

The macula is a small area in the retina that provides our most central, acute vision. The optic nerve conducts visual impulses to the brain from the retina. The posterior chamber is the area behind the iris, but in front of the lens, that is filled with aqueous. The pupil is the opening, or aperture, of the iris. The retina is the innermost coat of the back of the eye, formed of light-sensitive nerve endings that carry the visual impulse to the optic nerve. The retina may be compared to the film of a camera. The sclera is the white of the eye; it serves to provide support and strength to the eye. The vitreous is a transparent, colorless mass of soft, gelatinous material filling the eyeball behind the lens, providing greater structural support to the eyes.

PATIENT PREPARATION

- The patient is often seated at the edge of an examination table. The patient could also be placed in a recumbent position in an eye or ENT chair, if available, to facilitate the examination.

- Darkening the room as much as possible reduces any photophobia.

- A calm and assured demeanor helps the patient to relax.

- The patient should be made aware that the anesthetic drops may initially burn.

- The fluorescein may cause the patient's vision to turn yellow/orange.

- Some topical antibiotics burn slightly when applied. The patient should be educated that slight burning is normal and that he or she likely is not experiencing an allergy or problem from the drop or ointment prescribed.

Materials Utilized for Trauma-Oriented Ocular Examination, Corneal Abrasion, and Ocular Foreign Body Removal (Janda, 1991)

- Vision chart (near point, distance)
- Anesthetic drops (e.g., Alcaine)
- Fluorescein strips
- Black light or cobalt blue light
- Magnifier (slit lamp, ophthalmoscope, or other magnification source)
- Cotton-tipped swabs
- Corneal spud, or small-gauge needle on 1- to 3-mL syringe
- Corneal burr
- Normal saline or equivalent for eye rinse
- Tissue or wash cloth
- Fox shield
- Universal precautions: gloves, hand washing soap or similar solution, sharps container
- Emesis basin

Procedure for Examination of an Injured Eye (Harwood-Nuss, 2005; Bunuel-Jordana, 2004)

1. Obtain a history of the injury, detailing how and when the injury occurred, what agents were involved (i.e., chemical, blunt or sharp instrument, and so on), and what, if anything, has been applied to the injured eye. This will help you decide what type of injury or foreign body may be present.

2. Identify medication allergies, especially to anesthetics, fluorescein, and topical antibiotics.

3. A distance and/or near point vision examination is useful to demonstrate visual acuity. Record whether the examination was performed with or without corrective lens(es). Perform this examination prior to any additional procedures in order to demonstrate existing vision deficits. Record findings of right eye (OD), left eye (OS), and both eyes (OU).

Note: Patients with significant visual disturbance (e.g., native refractive disorder, blood in anterior chamber, or other changes in the vitreous) may find their visual acuity improved when looking through a pinhole occluder. Patients in whom visual acuity fails to improve with a pinhole occluder may have more significant defects in the retina, macula, or optic nerve.

continued

4. Position the patient for examination in sitting or semi-recumbent position. Ultimately the best position is the position in which the patient is most comfortable and the clinician has the best access to perform the visual examination.

5. Explain the procedure to the patient using non-medical terms at the patient's level of understanding.

6. Examine the eye for deformity, pupil reaction, extra-ocular movements, fundus, and obvious foreign body. This examination can be performed with a slit lamp, ophthalmoscope, or magnifying lens.

Note: Many foreign bodies will be found on the surface of the cornea, others might be stuck on the inner portion of the eyelid, and still others might be found penetrated into the cornea. The minority will have penetrated the globe. If a superficial foreign body is identified, decide which method you will use to remove the foreign body (see "Procedure for Foreign Body Removal from the Eye").

7. Apply 1 or 2 anesthetic drops into the affected eye.

8. Moisten fluorescein strip with anesthetic drop or normal saline (Fig. 33-7)

9. Instruct the patient to hold his or her head straight and to gaze upward nasally. Apply strip to lower part of conjunctiva just above the lower lid.

10. Ask the patient to blink the affected eye.

11. Visualize the cornea with black light or cobalt blue light. As the patient's tears break up or dilute the fluorescein, you may need the patient to blink to redistribute the fluorescein over the cornea.

12. Instruct the patient to hold his or her head straight and gaze upward, nasally and temporally, while you simultaneously evert the lower lid to increase the visual field.

Figure 33-7. Application of fluorescein to the eye using fluorescein strip.

13. To evert the upper eyelid, have the patient look downward but not close the eyes (Fig. 33-8). Apply a cotton-tipped applicator against the mid-portion of the lid, parallel to the surface. Gently grasp the eyelashes, lift upward and flip the lid back over the cotton applicator. This should enable an increased visual field for the cornea as well as expose the undersurface of the upper lid. Instruct the patient to hold his or her head straight and to gaze downward nasally and temporally to allow you to view the upper portion of the cornea.

14. Occasionally, it may be beneficial to expose more of the eye to increase your view of the corneal surface. If it is necessary to do so, with the cotton applicator still in place, rotate the tip of the applicator toward the superior portion of the upper lid. This will effectively raise the lid a few more degrees. This technique is called double lid eversion.

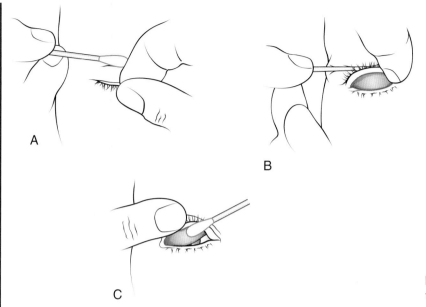

A

B

C

FIGURE 33-8. Everting the eyelid (see text).

Findings

If several scratches (oftentimes linear) are found on the cornea, be careful to inspect the inner surface of the eyelids (usually superior lid) for a foreign body (Fig. 33-9). If a corneal abrasion is identified without an offending foreign body, the foreign body or mechanism that caused the injury may no longer be present in the eye or may have floated into the fornices (corners) of the orbit. If foreign body is suspected, but not visualized, carefully swab the fornices using a saline-moistened, cotton-tipped swab (Fig. 33-10). Estimate the depth and length of the abrasion. Report the abrasion location relative to normal eye landmarks, such as nasal, temporal, pupil, or as points on a watch face (e.g., 3-mm superficial corneal abrasion located at 3 o'clock on the right eye medial to the border of the iris).

FIGURE 33-9. Corneal scratches.

continued

FIGURE 33-10. Swabbing the fornices using a saline-moistened, cotton-tipped applicator.

FIGURE 33-11. Dendritic keratitis.

Some patients with prior corneal damage develop recurrent corneal ulcerations. A typical presentation involves the reporting of eye symptoms upon arising in the morning with no recent history of trauma. The erosion will be in the same location as the initial eye injury and has an appearance similar to a typical corneal abrasion. The cause of post–eye trauma ulcer formation is failure of the ocular basement membrane to adhere properly. The patient should be treated with standard treatment for corneal abrasion. Some authors suggest nighttime use of ointments to help moisten the eye. One controlled study revealed long-term, treatment actually increased the likelihood of recurrent corneal ulceration (Eke, 1999). If a clinician suspects a pattern of recurrent ulceration, referral to an optometrist or ophthalmologist is in order to identify the cause. Causes of recurrent corneal ulceration include granulation tissue abnormalities, subclinical infection, or residual tissue overgrowth requiring debridement (Roberts, 1996).

If the appearance of the lesion on the surface of the cornea resembles a stellate or an irregular branching pattern, the patient may have a viral infection. A fluorescein examination might reveal dendritic keratitis, which is characteristic of ocular viral infections (Fig. 33-11). The treatment includes (topical, systemic) preparations with good antiviral activity. Lack of good response to topical antibiotics should cause the clinician to reflect on the accuracy of the previous diagnosis and to consider whether this finding was missed initially.

Procedure for Foreign Body Removal from the Eye

1. Foreign body removal may be as simple as flushing the eye; however, if more than a simple flushing is required, the eye should be anesthetized prior to using any device to remove the foreign body.

2. Surface foreign bodies may be easily removed with a moistened cotton swab.

3. Superficial metallic foreign bodies may be removed using either a small-gauge needle (e.g., 25-gauge needle on a 1-mL syringe) (Fig. 33-12) or a corneal spud, which is specially designed to remove corneal foreign objects (Fig. 33-13).

4. The patient's gaze should be directed so that the foreign body is clearly visible. Approaching the patient's eye from the side and inferiorly distracts the patient from the procedure and minimizes anxiety and blinking reflexes.

5. The needle should be held with bevel up, and approach the cornea at a flat angle. The needle tip should scoop the foreign body while removing little or none of the surrounding corneal tissue.

6. Metallic foreign bodies often leave a rust ring in the cornea that should be removed either immediately or within a few days using a device called a corneal burr (see Fig. 33-13). Not removing the rust ring may cause a disturbance in the patient's vision and may delay healing of the corneal tissue (Fig. 33-14). Sometimes the rust ring can be left for a day or two and removed during re-examination. The rust actually causes the cornea to soften a bit in that area, so the burr procedure may be somewhat easier to perform at that time.

FIGURE 33-12. Removal of superficial metallic foreign body using a small-gauge needle.

A   Corneal spud   B   Corneal burr

FIGURE 33-13. Corneal spud **(A)** and corneal burr **(B)**.

continued

FIGURE 33-14. Rust ring in the cornea created by metallic foreign body.

Concluding the Examination

Rinse the eye generously with normal saline or equivalent to remove the fluorescein dye and also flush out any offending debris. Instruct the patient that the fluorescein dye will drain through the tear ducts into the nose and may be present in the nasal discharge for the next few hours and that it may stain white clothing.

SPECIAL CONSIDERATIONS

Update tetanus immunization if the patient's last tetanus was given more than 10 years ago or no record of the last immunization exists. Use precaution not to leave anesthetic drops unattended. Patients might ask to take extra anesthetics with them for pain control. It is important to educate your patients that even short-term repeated use of the drops can cause the cornea to soften and slough off (Harwood-Nuss, 2005; Moeller, 2003). If the rust ring from the metallic foreign body cannot be removed completely, refer the patient to an eye care practitioner for definitive care.

It is important to emphasize the need to practice eye injury prevention strategies. Patients who may be at greater risk for potential eye injuries need to know the possible long-term consequences, such as recurrent, nonhealing ulcer. Children are at high risk for ocular re-injury; therefore, it is essential that parents understand and implement eye-protecting sports gear. Clinicians should have information available to share with their patients regarding the distribution of protective eyewear. (McGwin, 2005; Michael, 2002).

Cycloplegic drops are sometimes prescribed in an effort to help reduce pain by limiting the constriction and dilation movement of the ciliary muscle in the pupil; however, continued use of some of these medications may contribute to the development of hallucinations. If this occurs, ask the patient to call for advice. Typically advise the patient to stop the cycloplegic drops, and follow up in the next few days. The hallucinations usually stop after several hours but may take up to a day.

FOLLOW-UP CARE AND INSTRUCTIONS

There are four main goals in the treatment of corneal abrasions: controlling pain, reducing risk for secondary infections, promoting corneal re-epithelization, and risk avoidance to reduce reoccurrence (Moeller, 2003).

PAIN CONTROL

The anesthetic will wear off after a short period of time, so eye pain will return. Topical non-steroidal anti-inflammatory drugs are often prescribed for pain reduction and appear to be effective (Moeller, 2003; Alberti, 2001; Kaiser, 1997; Harris, 2005; Solomon, 2000). Patching the eye is no longer largely recommended due to studies showing no benefit to pain control and possibly increased rates of infection. Advising the patient to wear sunglasses may improve overall vision comfort during healing (Moeller, 2003; Michael, 2002; Kaiser, 1997; Flynn, 1998; Patterson, 1996; Cullum, 1994; Hulbert, 1991; Kirkpatrick, 1993; Kaiser, 1995). Bandage contact lenses are usually prescribed by the optometrist or ophthalmologist if the condition is severe enough to have considered patching to prevent lid/epithelium interaction.

REDUCE SECONDARY INFECTION

Often a topical antibiotic drop or ointment is prescribed (Moeller, 2003; Alberti, 2001). Patients who develop a corneal ulcer from contact lens use often grow *Pseudomonas*; therefore, patching is contraindicated. Patching a patient with a pseudomonal ulcer will create the ideal *Pseudomonas* breeding environment. In a short time (24 to 48 hours), a patient may develop permanent visual impairment or blindness due to the *Pseudomonas* bacteria burrowing into the deeper portion of the eye. Ideally, these patients should be treated with a broad-spectrum antibiotic that is effective against a wide variety of bacteria, including *Pseudomonas*. A follow-up examination the next day with the ophthalmologist or optometrist is essential (Alberti, 2001; Roberts, 1996; Gorbach, 2001; Tierney, 2005; Dambro, 2005). Patients with deep corneal abrasions, abrasion from contaminated organic material, or corneal abrasion from contact lens use need to follow up with an optometrist or ophthalmologist to ensure proper healing. Deep corneal abrasions may require a prescription of narcotic analgesics for pain control.

RE-EPITHELIZATION

A follow-up visit for a patient with a superficial corneal abrasion or uncompli-cated foreign body is usually not necessary. Educate the patient that the symptoms will resolve in 1 or 2 days. Larger abrasions may take up to a week to heal fully. If in doubt, the patient should return to the primary care clinic daily and if more seriously injured, the patient should be followed daily by optometry or ophthalmology (Harwood-Nuss, 2005; Moeller, 2003; Bunuel-Jordana, 2004). Contact lens wearers should refrain from using their contact lens(es) until the eye has healed, plus another 5 to 7 days to let the eye "rest." This will avoid the risk of reaction in the eye, which would cause the patient to not be able to wear contact lenses in the future. This is another reason why contact lens wearers should have a current prescription for their glasses. Before prescribing topical steroids, consult with an eye care practitioner about the use of this medicine in any situation (Moeller, 2003).

REDUCE REOCCURRENCE

Avoidance of reoccurrence via the use of appropriate eye protection, such as safety guards on equipment and safety glasses or goggles (e.g., American National Standards Institute [ANSI] certified lens for paintball, carpentry work, and racquetball) should be reinforced (McGwin, 2005; Harwood-Nuss, 2005; Moeller, 2003; Michael, 2002).

PATIENT DISCHARGE INSTRUCTIONS FOR CORNEAL ABRASION

Inform the patient that most eye injuries heal fully over a few days. The patient should also be given the following instructions:

- Use ice compresses and oral painkillers to relieve pain.

- Use ointment or eye drops exactly as prescribed.

- Return in 1 day for re-examination of the eye (if the patient is unable to return, make arrangements to communicate with the patient).

- Avoid touching or rubbing the eye, especially when waking up.

- Don't wear contact lenses until the eye has healed and the patient has finished all ointments or drops for at least 1 day, preferably as long as a week, to allow the eye to "rest."

- The patient should visit his or her eye care practitioner prior to resuming contact lens wear.

- Avoid exposure to bright light. Sunglasses or a hat with a brim may be helpful to avoid glare.

- To avoid future injury, advise the patient to wear appropriate eye protection, such as safety goggles, when working near materials that could become airborne and cause eye damage, or sports glasses, when playing sports (FIRST Consult [www.firstconsult.com]).

■ Advise the patient to call for advice or return for a recheck if he or she experiences increasing pain that doesn't respond to medications prescribed, a change in vision or change in vision tolerance (e.g., bright lights, increased eye watering or tearing), new discharge from the eye, or failure of the eye to improve or completely heal in 1 or 2 days.

REFERENCES

Alberti MM, Bouat CG, Allaire CM, Trinquand CJ: Combined indomethacin/gentamycin eyedrops to reduce pain after traumatic corneal abrasion. Eur J Ophthalmol 11:233-239, 2001.

Bunuel-Jordana L, Fiore DC: Is ophthalmologic follow-up for corneal abrasions needed? Am Fam Physician 70:32, 2004.

Cullum RD, Benjamin C: The Wills Eye Manual, 2nd ed. Philadelphia, JB Lippincott, 1994.

Dambro MR: Griffith's 5-Minute Clinical Consult. Philadelphia, Lippincott Williams & Wilkins, 2005.

Eke T, Morrison DA, Austin DJ: Recurrent symptoms following traumatic corneal abrasion: Prevalence severity and the effect of a simple regimen of prohylaxis. Eye 13:345-347, 1999.

FIRST Consult. Available at: www.firstconsult.com

Flynn CA, D'Amico F, Smith G: Should we patch corneal abrasions? A meta-analysis. J Fam Pract 47:264-270, 1998.

Gorbach SL, Falagas M: 5-Minute Infectious Diseases Consult. Philadelphia, Lippincott Williams & Wilkins, 2001.

Harris DR, Grafstein E, Hunte G: Topical non-steroidal anti-inflammatory drugs for treating traumatic corneal abrasions. Cochrane Collaboration, vol 4, 2005. Available at: www.cochrane.org

Hulbert MF: Efficacy of eyepad in corneal healing after corneal foreign body removal. Lancet 337:643, 1991.

Janda AM: Ocular trauma: Triage and treatment. Postgrad Med 90:51-52, 55-60, 1991.

Kaiser PK, Pineda IR, An B, et al: A study of topical nonsteroidal anti-inflammatory drops and no pressure patching in the treatment of corneal abrasions. Ophthalmology 104:1353-1359, 1997.

Kaiser PK: A comparison of pressure patching versus no patching for corneal abrasions due to trauma or foreign body removal. Ophthalmology 102:1936-1942, 1995.

Kirkpatrick JN, Hoh HB, Cook SD: No eye pad for corneal abrasion. Eye 7:468-471, 1993.

Lima-Gomez V, Cornejo-Mendoza AM: Value of ocular hypotony as a predictor of open-globe injury in patients with ocular trauma. Cir Cir 72:177-181, 2004.

McGwin G, Owsley C: Incidence of emergency department-treated eye injury in the United States. Arch Ophthalmol 123:662-666, 2005.

Michael JG, Hug D, Dowd MD: Management of corneal abrasion in children: A randomized clinical trial. Ann Emerg Med 40:67-72, 2002.

Moeller JL, Rifat SF: Identifying and treating uncomplicated corneal abrasions. Phys Sportsmed 31:15-17, 2003.

Ophthalmology, Cornea. Available at: http://www.emedicine.com/oph/CORNEA.htm

Patterson J, Fetzer D, Krall J, et al: Eye patch treatment for the pain of corneal abrasion. South Med J 89:227-229, 1996.

Roberts JR: Myths and misconceptions: An eye patch for simple corneal abrasions. In Roberts' Practical Guide to Common Medical Emergencies. Philadelphia, Lippincott-Raven, 1996, pp 41-62.

Solomon A, Halpert M, Frucht-Pery J: Comparison of topical indomethacin and eye patching for minor corneal trauma. Ann Ophthalmol 32:316-319, 2000.

Tierney LM, McPhee SJ, Papadakis MA: Current Medical Diagnosis and Treatment. New York, McGraw-Hill, 2005.

Weicherthal L: Corneal abrasion and foreign bodies. In Wolfson AB (ed): Harwood-Nuss' Clinical Practice of Emergency Medicine, 4th ed. Philadelphia, Lippincott Williams & Wilkins, 2005, pp 123-126.

WEBSITES

Ophthalmology Teaching Website, Faculty of Medicine, University of Toronto: Lectures, 2005. Available at:
http://eyelearn.med.utoronto.ca/lecture05-06.htm

Ophthalmology Teaching Website, Faculty of Medicine, University of Toronto: Slit lamp techniques, 2004. Available at:
http://eyelearn.med.utoronto.ca/ClinicalSkills/SlitLamp/01Outline.htm

Pramanik S: Assessment of Ocular Trauma, 2005. Available at:
http://webeye.ophth.uiowa.edu/eyeforum/trauma.htm

Chapter 34

Endometrial Biopsy

Martha Petersen

PROCEDURE GOALS AND OBJECTIVES

Goal: To obtain a high quality sample of endometrial tissue for histology while observing standard precautions and with minimal risk to the patient.

Objectives: The student will be able to …

- Describe the rationale, indications, and contraindications for performing an endometrial biopsy.

- Identify common complications associated with the performance of endometrial biopsy.

- Describe the essential anatomy and physiology associated with endometrial biopsy.

- Identify necessary materials for performing endometrial biopsy and their proper use.

- Demonstrate the correct and safe technique for obtaining an adequate sample of endometrial tissue.

- Describe post-procedure care and patient education and counseling following endometrial biopsy.

BACKGROUND AND HISTORY

Endometrial cancer is the most common invasive gynecologic cancer in women in the United States, with abnormal uterine bleeding (AUB) being the primary presenting symptom. The mean age at diagnosis is 60 years, making it essentially a postmenopausal condition. Mortality is low because the disease is usually diagnosed at an early stage, when women seek medical attention for unexpected bleeding. In perimenopausal women, 70% of gynecologic office visits are due to AUB, which often requires ruling out endometrial cancer. In women younger than 30 years of age, AUB is never an endometrial malignancy (Paraskevaidis, 2002).

Before 1935 the procedure of choice for the evaluation of AUB and the endometrium was dilation of the cervix and curettage (D&C) of the endometrial lining. The use of suction as opposed to scraping was introduced with the Novak curette. In addition to the Novak curette, there are other choices of instruments, such as the flexible Pipelle aspirator or Tis-U-Trap. Suction is provided by a syringe attached directly to the insertion device or by an external pump (Mounsey, 2002).

INDICATIONS

The only true screening indication for endometrial biopsy (EMB) is in women at high risk for endometrial cancer secondary to a history of hereditary nonpolyposis colorectal cancer. The current American Cancer Society guidelines recommend screening via endometrial biopsy starting by age 35, and performed annually thereafter. Otherwise, EMB is used in the assessment of the lining of the uterus for causes of AUB, possible malignancy, infertility, and monitoring of hormonal therapy. Sensitivity of EMB is as high as 96% in detecting endometrial abnormalities (Albers, 2004; Smith, 2005). Indications for EMB are summarized in Table 34-1.

CONTRAINDICATIONS

The contraindications for EMB are summarized in Table 34-2.

POTENTIAL COMPLICATIONS

- Vasovagal reaction: The most common complication of EMB is a transient vasovagal reaction. This reaction is strongest and seen more frequently in women on β-blocker medications.

- Uterine perforation: If sound or cannula passes greater than 12 cm in normal-sized uterus, perforation must be suspected. Stop the procedure and monitor the patient for 1 hour in the office. If in-office ultrasound is available, evaluate for bleeding into the cul-de-sac. If present, refer the

Table 34.1	**Indications**
Monitor	Abnormal uterine bleeding (AUB) with adjuvant therapy with tamoxifen citrate
	Endometrial response to progesterone therapy for adenomatous hyperplasia
Evaluation	Prior to initiating estrogen therapy in women at risk for endometrial cancer due to: low parity, family history of endometrial, breast, ovarian cancer; liver failure; hypothyroidism; hirsutism; alcohol abuse; unopposed estrogen
	Enlarged uterus (as confirmed by ultrasound)
	AUB: Postmenopausal bleeding, with hormonal replacement therapy, possible hyperplasia
Malignancy	Atypical glandular cells of undetermined significance (AGUS) on Pap screening
	"Endometrial cells" or "estrogen effect" on Pap report in postmenopausal women
	Endometrial stripe > 5 mm on transvaginal sonography (TVS) in a postmenopausal woman

Adapted from Albers (2004), Mounsey (2002), Stenchever (2001), and Zuber (2001).

Table 34.2	**Contraindications***
Absolute	During menses
	Possibility of pregnancy
	Uncooperative patient
	History of unstable angina
Perform in hospital setting	Moderate to severe cervical stenosis
	Coagulation disorder or on anticoagulant or antiplatelet therapy
	Morbid obesity

*Rule out cervicitis and pelvic inflammatory disease prior to biopsy in all patients.
  Adapted from Albers (2004), Mounsey (2002), and Stenchever (2001).

patient to the emergency room. If no bleeding is seen, the patient can be discharged home. Be certain the patient has someone to monitor her at home for the next 24 hours, and instruct the patient to call with any fever, excessive pain, or blood loss. Wait 6 to 8 weeks for uterine healing before attempting biopsy again.

■ Inadequate sample: If specimen is reported as inadequate, repeat the procedure or use another method of evaluation, such as D&C, hysteroscopy, or transvaginal sonography (TSV), or a combination.

■ Infection: Post-procedure infection is rare if the procedure is performed properly and there is no pre-existing infection. Patients should notify the office immediately if fever or pain develops. Antibiotic prophylaxis for endocarditis is considered unnecessary (Mounsey, 2004), but patients at risk may be treated with tetracycline (500 mg bid for 4 days) following the procedure, at the clinician's discretion (Zuber, 2001).

FIGURE 34-1. Anatomy of the uterus and surrounding structures.

REVIEW OF ESSENTIAL ANATOMY AND PHYSIOLOGY

ANATOMY

Figure 34-1 illustrates the anatomy of the uterus and its surrounding structures.

PHYSIOLOGY AND PATHOPHYSIOLOGY

The endometrium consists of two layers, the stratum basale and the stratum functionale. The stratum functionale cells proliferate under the influence of estrogen and desquamate at the time of menses. The thickness of the endometrium varies throughout the menstrual cycle from 1 to 2 mm at the time of menses to 4 mm in the early proliferative (follicular) phase, to about 12 mm at ovulation, and maintaining 12 mm during an appropriate secretory (luteal) phase. Hyperplasia is defined as the abnormal proliferation of endometrial cells usually caused by estrogen unopposed by the action of progesterone. The presenting symptom is AUB. Endometrial hyperplasia is described as mild, moderate, or complex and in histological terms such as cystic, adenomatous, or glandular. The major findings on endometrial biopsy sample are as follows (Canavan, 1999):

- Proliferative, secretory benign or atrophic endometrium

- Simple or complex (adenomatous) hyperplasia without atypia

- Simple or complex (adenomatous) hyperplasia with atypia (considered precancerous)

- Endometrial carcinoma

PATIENT PREPARATION

The EMB is a safe and quick procedure. Clarify the procedure completely to the patient and discuss possible alternative techniques. Endometrial evaluation can be achieved by a variety of methods, so it is important that the patient understands the choices and reasons for the chosen procedure. Obtain informed consent.

Explain to the woman that she may experience slight cramping during and after the biopsy, but it is not painful. The patient may take a non-steroidal anti-inflammatory drug (NSAID) 1 hour before the biopsy to reduce any discomfort. The patient can expect to remain in the office for about 1 hour after the procedure, but she may then drive and resume normal daily activities.

■ Materials Utilized for Endometrial Biopsy

The choice of equipment depends on the reason for the biopsy and clinician preference. The smaller the canula type, the more comfortable for the patient but less tissue will be obtained. Conversely, the larger curettes acquire more tissue sample but produce more discomfort. For evaluation of possible malignancy, the biopsy should be preceded by endocervical curettage (ECC).

For endometrial sampling, the choices include:

■ Novak curette: This is a nondisposable rigid canula made of stainless steel that attaches to a syringe plunger for suction. The tissue sample is drawn through the canula into the syringe.

■ Pipelle aspirator: This is a disposable device made of clear, flexible polypropylene sheath, 23 cm in length with a small opening in the distal end. It has an inner plunger that when pulled back provides suction. It is marked so that the uterus cavity can be measured and biopsy performed in one step.

■ Tis-U-Trap set: This is a sterile plastic disposable device that requires external suction. It consists of a clear plastic tissue collection chamber with a flat filter and one of several types of curettes. Endometrial tissue is collected directly into the collection chamber, thereby eliminating the need to transfer the tissue sample into another container.

■ Tao Brush: This is a narrow polypropylene brush covered by a clear protective sheath. After insertion into the uterine cavity, the sheath is pulled back to allow for sampling with the brush. The sheath is then replaced over the brush, trapping the tissue sample (Figs. 34-2 and 34-3).

■ Suction: Suction is created by a syringe or internal piston system. An external source, such as a wall or portable pump providing 25 to 27 inches Hg of negative pressure, is needed.

FIGURE 34-2. Endometrial biopsy setup (**from top**): anesthetic, tenaculum, Novak curette, and cervical dilators.

FIGURE 34-3. Instruments (**left to right**): uterine sound, Novak curette, Tis-U-Trap, and Pipelle.

- General equipment:
  - Absorbent material to go under the patient
  - Disinfectant material of choice for cleansing the cervix
  - Topical or injectable lidocaine or benzocaine for the cervix
  - Labeled tissue containers with appropriate preservative (not needed if sampling device has container attached, such as the Tis-U-Trap)
  - Sanitary napkins for post-procedure hygiene
  - Fluid-proof gown and protective eyewear
  - Unsterile gloves
- Sterile equipment:
  - Gloves
  - Speculum
  - Uterine sound (depending on type of biopsy instrument used)
  - Endocervical curette (if ECC is to be performed)
  - 4 × 4-inch gauze pads
  - Ring forceps
  - Tenaculum
  - Cervical dilators (two types are available): Mechanical (unopened but available if needed)—sterile rigid metal or plastic curved rods in graduated thicknesses; Medical (particularly useful for the postmenopausal cervix)—either laminaria (sizes 2 mm through 10 mm), a natural osmotic cervical dilator made from seaweed and packaged as narrow tampon, which is inserted into the cervix 2 to 12 hours prior to the procedure to soften and open the cervix, or synthetic laminaria (Dilateria, Lamicel, Dilapan), an absorbent polyvinyl acetal sponge, impregnated with less than 500 mg of magnesium sulfate (Epsom salt) and compressed and inserted into the cervix 2 to 12 hours prior to the procedure to absorb fluid and gently open the cervix
  - Anesthetic (optional)—one of the following: 2% lidocaine with epinephrine, 5 mL injected into the cervix before procedure or 0.5% to 1% lidocaine without epinephrine; 20% benzocaine spray or gel applied to cervix

Procedure for Endometrial Biopsy

1. Put on a gown and protective eyewear.

2. Review the specific directions for equipment and sampling device being used and be certain all parts are in working order before beginning the procedure. Place the patient in the lithotomy position with her legs in stirrups and drape appropriately. Perform a bimanual examination with unsterile gloves to evaluate size and position of the uterus and the uterocervical angle. Palpate the adnexa to rule out tenderness that may indicate infection.

3. Change to sterile gloves.

4. Using a vaginal speculum, inspect the cervix for discharge, stenosis, or other abnormalities. Using ring forceps holding cotton or gauze, wipe the cervical os with water-based antiseptic.

5. Perform ECC if indicated (see later, "Supplementary and Alternative Procedures")

6. Apply or inject anesthetic to the cervix 5 to 10 minutes prior to starting procedure.

- Spray or apply gel *or*

- Inject lidocaine at 4 o'clock and 8 o'clock positions

7. Grasp the anterior lip of the cervix with the tenaculum in a horizontal position and lock in place. To avoid lacerating the cervix, grasp enough tissue. The tenaculum is used to stabilize the cervix and uterus during the procedure. Apply gentle traction on the tenaculum to straighten the uterocervical angle.

8. Measure the depth of the uterine cavity with the uterine sound. Document uterine depth.

Note: This step is optional if biopsy device is marked for measurement.

- Using moderate pressure, insert the sound through the os until gentle resistance is encountered, usually at a depth of 6 to 9 cm. Note the measurement of the uterine cavity and remove the sound.

- Use dilators if it is difficult to pass the sound through the internal os. Start with the smallest dilator, progressing to the next size until the os is opened enough for the sound to pass. (This is unnecessary if medical dilators are used prior to the procedure.)

9. Collect the endometrial sample (Figs. 34-4 and 34-5).

10. Steady and straighten the cervix with slight traction on the tenaculum.

11. Insert the sampling cannula through the os being careful to avoid touching vulvar or vaginal tissue that would cause contamination.

12. Rotate the sampling cannula device between the thumb and forefinger as it passes through the os. Apply gentle pressure until it reaches the fundus, as indicated by previous measurement or by resistance, then withdraw very slightly.

13. Stabilize the sampling cannula with one hand while activating suction with the other.

- If using a syringe sampling device, steadily withdraw plunger in one smooth motion, being sure not to advance the cannula or to let the plunger slide forward.

- If using external suction, activate suction according to manufacturer's instructions.

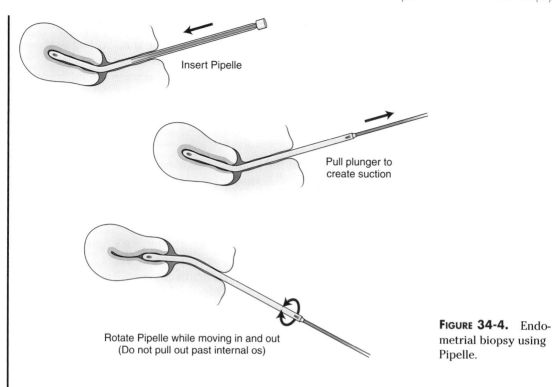

Insert Pipelle

Pull plunger to
create suction

Rotate Pipelle while moving in and out
(Do not pull out past internal os)

FIGURE 34-4. Endo-
metrial biopsy using
Pipelle.

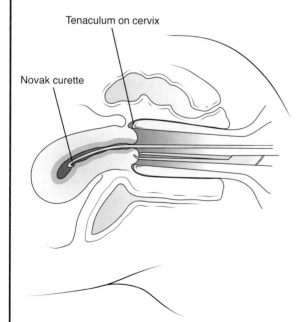

Tenaculum on cervix

Novak curette

FIGURE 34-5. Endometrial biopsy using Novak
curette.

14. Gently pull the cannula toward the
internal os and then push it back into
the uterine cavity at least four times,
being careful not to withdraw past the
internal os. Rotate the cannula
consistently in a clockwise direction
several times, and then counterclockwise,
while performing the movement in all
four quadrants of the endometrial cavity
in a systematic fashion in a vacuuming
type pattern.

15. Release suction pressure and remove the
cannula.

16. Deposit the sample into an appropriate
labeled and fixative-filled specimen
container. With the Pipelle, use sterile
scissors to cut off the tip to expel the
sample.

Note: This step is not necessary with the
Tis-U-Trap.

continued

17. Remove the tenaculum.

18. Cleanse the vagina and cervix gently with gauze.

19. Remove the speculum.

20. Dispose of equipment according to standard biohazard precautions.

FOLLOW-UP CARE AND INSTRUCTIONS

The patient should remain in the examination room for 15 minutes and in the office for another 30 minutes. A vasovagal reaction typically occurs within the first 10 minutes after the procedure, if at all. The patient should be instructed that slight spotting and cramping is considered normal. The patient may drive after discharge from the office.

Patient may be advised to take NSAIDs as needed for cramping after the biopsy, as these provide the additional benefit of antiprostaglandin activity. Acetaminophen is an acceptable option for discomfort. The patient should use sanitary napkins only and report if bleeding is heavier than her normal menses or if a fever develops. It is recommended that women refrain from sexual activity until the bleeding has stopped.

SUPPLEMENTARY AND ALTERNATIVE PROCEDURES

- Endocervical curettage is *always* indicated prior to endometrial biopsy if any malignancy needs to be ruled out. ECC samples must be deposited into a separate container.

- Hysteroscopy can be used with or without concurrent biopsy.

- Transvaginal sonography may be used to assess endometrial thickness, with an endometrial stripe ≤ 4 mm having 96% sensitivity in ruling out endometrial cancer (Mounsey, 2002).

- Saline infusion sonography involves filling the uterine cavity with saline prior to ultrasound and allows for visualization of endometrial thickness and polyps.

REFERENCES

Albers J, Hull S, Wesley R: Abnormal uterine bleeding. Am Fam Physician 69:1915-1926, 2004.

Canavan T, Doshi N: Endometrial cancer. Am Fam Physician 59:3069-3077, 1999.

Katz V: Diagnostic procedures. In Stenchever M, Proegemeuller W, Herbst A, Mischell D (eds): Comprehensive Gynecology, 4th ed. St. Louis: Mosby, 2001, pp 232-233.

Mounsey A: Postmenopausal bleeding: Evaluation and management. Clin Fam Pract 4:173-192, 2002.

Paraskevaidis E, Kalantaridou SN, Papadimitriou D, et al: Transvaginal uterine ultrasonography compared with endometrial biopsy for the detection of endometrial disease in perimenopausal women with uterine bleeding. Anticancer Res 22:1829-1832, 2002.

Smith RA, Cokkinides V, Eyre HJ: American Cancer Society guidelines for the early detection of cancer, 2005. CA Cancer J Clin 55:31-44, 2005.

Zuber T: Endometrial biopsy. Am Fam Physician 63:1131-1135, 2001.

BIBLIOGRAPHY

American College of Nurse-Midwives: Clinical Bulletin No. 5, Endometrial Biopsy, 2001. Accessed 6/2/2005: http://www.acnm.org/pubs/Clinical_Bulletin_5.pdf

Schwayder JM: Pathophysiology of abnormal uterine bleeding. Obstet Gynecol Clin North Am 27:219-234, 2000.

Chapter 35

Foot Examination of the Patient with Diabetes

Nikki Katalanos

PROCEDURE GOALS AND OBJECTIVES

Goals: To perform a thorough routine foot examination on the patient with diabetes.

Objectives: The student will be able to …

- Describe the indications, contraindications, and rationale for performing a routine foot examination on the patient with diabetes.

- Describe the essential anatomy and physiology associated with examination of the foot of the patient with diabetes.

- Describe the logical order of steps used to perform a foot examination of the patient with diabetes.

- Describe normal and abnormal findings associated with examination of the foot of the patient with diabetes.

- Describe foot self-care information to be provided to the patient with diabetes for the prevention of future complications.

Table 35.1	**Categories of Diabetes Mellitus**

Type 1 diabetes: results from β-cell destruction, usually leading to absolute insulin deficiency
Type 2 diabetes: results from a progressive insulin secretory defect in a background of insulin resistance
Diabetes due to other causes: genetic defects, diseases of the exocrine pancreas, drug or chemical induced
Gestational diabetes: diagnosed during pregnancy

From American Diabetes Association: Standards of medical care in diabetes. Diabetes Care 28:S4-S36, 2005.

Table 35.2	**Criteria for the Diagnosis of Diabetes**

Symptoms of diabetes plus casual plasma glucose concentration ≥ 200 mg/dL. Casual is defined as serum taken without regard to time of last meal.
or
Fasting plasma glucose ≥ 126 mg/dL. Fasting is defined as no caloric intake for at least 8 hours.
or
2-hour post load glucose ≥ 200 mg/dL during an oral glucose tolerance test (not recommended).
Confirm by repeat testing on a different day.

From American Diabetes Association: Standards of medical care in diabetes. Diabetes Care 28:S4-S36, 2005.

BACKGROUND AND HISTORY

Diabetes mellitus is a group of diseases that are characterized by higher than normal levels of blood sugar. The disease is a result of defects in insulin production or insulin action, or both (Table 35-1). The Centers for Disease Control and Prevention (CDC, 2004) estimates that the prevalence (existing cases) of diabetes across all ages is 18.2 million Americans, including 13 million diagnosed and 5.2 million undiagnosed cases. The incidence (new onset) is 1.3 million people per year. Regardless of type, the morbidity from this ubiquitous disease is quite costly, with total costs for direct care reaching $92 billion and costs for indirect care, which would include time lost from work, disability, and early death, adding another $40 billion.

Lifestyle changes and early detection (Table 35-2) can delay or prevent many of the complications from diabetes. Estimates of the number of people with nervous system damage, ranging from mild to severe, directly caused by diabetes, is as high as 60% to 70%. As a result, the person with diabetes often has sensory or pain impairments in their hands and feet. In the United States, more than 60% of all nontraumatic amputations of the lower limb are among people with diabetes. According to the CDC (2004), aggressive foot care can reduce amputation by as much as 45% to 85%.

INDICATIONS

The most common sequelae of diabetic neuropathy are foot ulceration, infection, and, ultimately, amputation. Early recognition and aggressive management of foot care can prevent or delay the associated morbidity. The longer the person has diabetes, the greater the risk for ulcerations of the foot. Evidence indicates that these events are strongly related to poor glucose control and/or vascular co-morbidities.

Risk factors that increase the potential for ultimate foot damage that may lead to amputation include the following:

- Peripheral neuropathy

- Increased pressure on the foot

- Deformities of the foot or toenails

- Peripheral vascular disease

- Previous history of foot ulcers (or amputation)

- Acute or chronic infection of the foot or toenails

- Poor foot hygiene

The patient with diabetes should be asked at each routine visit whether he or she has pain, numbness, or tingling sensations of the extremities. The patient should also be asked if he or she has any problems or leg cramping with walking. Any positive response to these questions warrants a comprehensive foot examination. In addition, note how far the patient can comfortably walk, and if the patient's shoes are a comfortable fit.

The value of the foot examination in a person with diabetes is well documented. The American Diabetes Association (2005) recommends that a comprehensive foot examination be performed annually on the low-risk patient and that a visual examination be conducted at each routine visit. Patients with any of the above-mentioned risk factors should be closely examined on a quarterly basis, at minimum.

CONTRAINDICATIONS

There are no medical contraindications to the examination of the foot in a person with diabetes. In some cultures, however, the foot is considered unclean and should be the last part of the body that is examined.

POTENTIAL COMPLICATIONS

There are no reported complications to this examination when the procedure is performed as described. The medical-legal concerns are that the clinician performs the examination incorrectly and too infrequently. It is essential that the method and tools used for examination be fully documented in the medical record. Many facilities use a diabetes flow chart for routine examinations.

REVIEW OF ESSENTIAL ANATOMY AND PHYSIOLOGY

In order to perform the foot examination, an understanding of the anatomy of the vascular system is needed. Figure 35-1 shows the basic anatomy of the foot and the vascular supply of the lower extremities.

PATIENT PREPARATION

After the diagnosis of diabetes has been made, the patient needs time to adjust and accept that many lifestyle changes will need to be made. The first visit is usually best spent discussing the disease itself and answering any questions the patient may have. The patient should be encouraged to view this as a partnership, one in which he or she will make many of the actual decisions with regard to self-care and treatment. A thorough history and physical examination should then be performed if time permits, or, at a minimum, at a timely follow-up visit. A foot examination, as described later, should be included in this initial evaluation.

The diagnosis of diabetes, in particular type 2 diabetes, brings with it many preconceived notions and fears. Often there are family members with diabetes who have had bad experiences. Patients have heard stories of blindness, amputations, dialysis, and early death. The patient is often already conditioned to fear the disease and its consequences; therefore, it is essential that the initial approach to the patient with diabetes be reassuring and optimistic. Above all, the patient (or parents) should not be led to feel at fault for having developed diabetes.

After the first visit, the preparation of the patient should include having the patient remove his or her shoes and socks before the examiner enters the room.

Materials Utilized for Performing the Diabetic Foot Examination

- Semmes-Weinstein monofilament 5.07 (10 g) (Fig. 35-2)
- 128-Hz tuning fork

FIGURE 35-1.   **A,** Arterial system of the lower extremity. **B,** Venous system of the lower extremity. **C,** Anatomy of the foot.

FIGURE 35-2.   Semmes-Weinstein monofilament.

Procedure for Performing the Diabetic Foot Examination

The comprehensive foot examination entails visual inspection, palpation, and tests for sensation.

 ## Visual Inspection

The foot should always be examined with the shoes and socks off. The foot should be visually inspected at each routine visit for the following:

1. Color: Pale, bluish, or dusky coloration of the feet may mean poor perfusion. Erythema may indicate an area of excessive friction or it may be evidence of an ongoing or new infection. Yellow toenails may indicate a long-standing fungal infection.

2. Callus: Look for areas of skin thickening, particularly corns, callus, and over bunions. There may be an infection beneath the build-up. Evaluate the cause of the callus. Do the shoes fit well?

3. Fissures: Tears in the skin, particularly between the toes, are easy access to future infection. It may be a sign of a fungal infection or excessive moisture.

4. Ulcers: Look for signs of old or healing ulcerations. New ulcerations need to be immediately evaluated.

5. Maceration: Signs of excessive sweating, skin breakdown, or tinea pedis may also open avenues for infection.

6. Lack of hair: A possible indication of vascular disease—or is it just where the socks rub?

7. Toenails: Look for signs of fungal infections or injury. Are the toenails solidly adhered to the nail bed? Are they thickened or "flaky" looking?

8. Appearance: Look for misshapen feet that may forewarn of potential problems, such as bunions, hammertoes, "rocker" bottoms, or other soft tissue and bony deformities. Is the skin of the foot thin looking or shiny? Note hygiene as well.

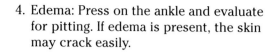

9. Shoe wear: Evaluate the shoes for signs of excessive pressure or friction on the feet. Are the shoes capable of protecting the foot from punctures or injury? Do they support the foot properly?

10. Socks: Do they fit the foot well? Are there areas of wear or holes?

Palpation

The foot should be palpated for the following:

1. Temperature: A cool or cold foot may mean poor perfusion. A warm foot, especially if the heat is localized, may be a sign of infection.

2. Pulses: Evaluate the pedal pulses. They should be strong (2+) and equal in both feet.

3. Perfusion: Press on the toenail and observe the capillary filling. A healthy foot reperfuses in 3 seconds or less. Greater than 5 seconds is an indication of poor perfusion.

4. Edema: Press on the ankle and evaluate for pitting. If edema is present, the skin may crack easily.

Tests for Sensation

The tests for sensation allow the practitioner to evaluate for the presence of neuropathy. A focused history and physical examination should help to establish both the presence and degree of the neuropathy. Pain or temperature may also be checked, using great care, as part of the sensory evaluation.

1. Vibration: Press the vibrating tuning fork against the bony prominence of the first (big) toe on the dorsal-lateral aspect. Ask the patient to tell you when he or she feels the vibration start and when it stops.

2. Pressure: Press the monofilament lightly against the specified areas of the foot until it bows (Fig. 35-3). Record the presence or absence of sensation for each area tested.

Right foot

Left foot

FIGURE 35-3.
Demonstration of monofilament testing and areas of the foot that should be tested.

SPECIAL CONSIDERATIONS

Consideration should be given to previous pathology (e.g., foot ulcers, deformities, tinea pedis). Tinea pedis can be very difficult to eradicate in any patient, but it is especially difficult in the patient with diabetes. Tinea pedis, minor infections, and shallow ulcerations can often be treated in the office. More severe cases and most deformities are best referred to podiatry, or in the case of infection, to an infectious disease consultant.

FOLLOW-UP CARE AND INSTRUCTIONS

Patient education is critical in the prevention of future morbidity. There are many prepared handouts available, and a few of these resources are listed at the end of the chapter.

General advice to the patient:

- Check your feet every day. Look for cuts, sore spots, red spots, and blisters. A mirror can be used to see the bottom of the feet. A good way to use it is to mount it on the lower wall.

- Wash your feet everyday. Use only warm water and a mild soap. Check the temperature of the water before getting into the tub or shower. Use the back of your hand. Clean carefully between the toes and dry the foot thoroughly. Apply a mild lubricating ointment to the heels and any dry areas. Do not use lotion between the toes.

- Keep the toenails trimmed. Be sure to trim straight across. Gently file the edges. Do this twice a month. Women should take off any toenail polish before being checked at the office.

- *Always* wear shoes and socks. Make sure the shoes are a good fit and do not pinch anywhere. Closed-toe shoes are safer, but sturdy sandals are fine. Check your shoes for foreign objects before putting them on. Socks should fit well, be without holes, and be kept clean and dry. Never, ever walk barefoot! Not even at the beach, where the sand can be hot enough to burn you.

- Check your blood sugar regularly. The best prevention of foot problems is well-controlled blood sugar.

REFERENCES

American Diabetes Association: Standards of medical care in diabetes. Diabetes Care 28:S4-S36, 2005.

Centers for Disease Control and Prevention. National diabetes fact sheet: General information and national estimates on diabetes in the United States, 2003, Rev. ed. Atlanta, Ga: U.S. Department of Health and Human Services, Centers for Disease Control and Prevention, 2004.

BIBLIOGRAPHY

American Podiatric Medical Association: Available at:
http://www.apma.org/s_apma/index.asp
Feet Can Last a Lifetime: A Health Care Provider's Guide to Preventing
Diabetes Foot Problems: An excellent resource for the practitioner
that includes flow sheets and management plans for foot care.
Available at: http://www.diabetic.com/education/feet/feet2/index.htm
Habershaw GM: Management of the diabetic foot. In Leahy JL, Clark NG,
Ceflu WT (eds): Medical Management of Diabetes Mellitus.
Philadelphia, Saunders, 2000, pp 479-498. Slightly out of date, but still
one of the best overall books on diabetes care.
McCullock DK: Evaluation of the diabetic foot. Up To Date online
14.2.2006. Available at: www.utdol.com

Chapter 36

Procedural Sedation

Tony Brenneman

PROCEDURE GOALS AND OBJECTIVES

Goal: To minimize patient discomfort while attempting to maintain spontaneous respirations and airway-protective reflexes in order to facilitate appropriate medical care.

Objectives: The student will be able to ...

- Differentiate between *conscious sedation* and *procedural sedation*.

- Describe current JCAHO sedation care standards.

- Identify indications and contraindications for procedural sedation.

- Describe potential complications and techniques that may be employed to avoid or treat problems during sedation.

- Describe the essential anatomy and physiology associated with administration of procedural sedation.

- Identify the materials necessary for the administration of procedural sedation.

- Identify the agents used in procedural sedation, dosing methods, and discharge criteria.

BACKGROUND AND HISTORY

Procedural sedation provides a way in which clinicians can perform diagnostic tests and clinical procedures that are sometimes painful or highly anxiety provoking in a manner that prevents or minimizes patient discomfort. Historically this method has been labeled *conscious sedation*, but this term has now become antiquated and imprecise, as all sedation causes some type of change in consciousness. The current accepted phrase is *procedural sedation*, which more accurately reflects the goal behind the process. Procedural sedation then refers to the techniques of managing a patient's pain and anxiety to facilitate appropriate medical care in a safe, effective, and humane fashion (Brown, 2005), with the main goal being to minimize patient discomfort while attempting to maintain spontaneous respiration and airway-protective reflexes. Procedural sedation is currently used in inpatient, emergency services and most outpatient settings. Practitioners must be aware of current guidelines and terminology in order to provide procedural sedation.

The move to procedural sedation intimates that there is a continuum of sedation for the patient no matter the amount of sedative used. There also has been a lack of objective measures in levels of sedation. Based on this, criteria have been established to help define goal levels for procedural sedation. In 2001, the revised Joint Commission on Accreditation of Healthcare Organizations (JCAHO) sedation care standards replaced the term "conscious sedation" with "moderate sedation/analgesia" and attempted to provide clearer definitions of what this meant. The difficulty remains that this is still a subjective process and that each clinician must always be aware of how the patient is responding to the sedatives and dissociatives that he or she is being given. The JCAHO sedation guidelines provide qualitative goals for each practitioner while conducting procedural sedation, but ultimately we must strive to maintain safety by minimizing risks and ensuring safe discharge.

DEFINITIONS

The progression from mild sedation to general anesthesia is a continuum, and definitions of sedation are evolving. Useful definitions include the following:

- Analgesia—Relief of pain without intentionally producing a sedated state. Altered mental status may be a secondary effect of medications administered for analgesia.

- Anxiolysis—A state of decreased apprehension concerning a particular situation; in this state, the level of awareness does not change.

The continuum of and definition of levels of sedation/analgesia according to the American Society of Anesthesiologists include:

- Minimal sedation (anxiolysis)—A drug-induced state during which the patient responds normally to verbal commands. Cognitive function and coordination may be impaired, but ventilatory and cardiovascular function are unaffected.

■ Moderate sedation/analgesia (conscious sedation)—A drug-induced depression of consciousness during which the patient responds purposefully to verbal commands either alone or accompanied by light tactile stimulation. No interventions are required to maintain airway and adequate ventilation. Cardiovascular function is usually maintained.

■ Deep sedation/analgesia—A drug-induced depression of consciousness during which the patient cannot be easily aroused but responds purposefully following repeated or painful stimulation. The ability to independently maintain ventilatory function may require assistance in maintaining a patent airway and adequate ventilation. Cardiovascular function is usually maintained.

■ General anesthesia—A drug-induced loss of consciousness during which the patient cannot be aroused, even by painful stimulation. The ability to independently maintain ventilatory function is often impaired. The patient often requires assistance to maintain a patent airway, and positive-pressure ventilation may be required because of depressed spontaneous ventilation or drug-induced depression of neuromuscular function. Cardiovascular function may be impaired.

(Developed by the American Society of Anesthesiologists [ASA] and approved by the ASA House of Delegates, October 13, 1999. Referenced http://www.asahq.org/publicationsAndServices/sedation1017.pdf; accessed 07/15/05 at 1545.)

INDICATIONS

Sedation/analgesia provides two general types of benefit: (1) sedation/analgesia allows patients to tolerate unpleasant procedures by relieving anxiety, discomfort, or pain; and (2) in children and uncooperative adults, sedation/analgesia may expedite the conduct of procedures that are not particularly uncomfortable but that require the patient not move (ASA, 2002). Ultimately, the goals of procedural sedation and analgesia are to alleviate anxiety, minimize physical pain and discomfort, minimize negative psychological responses to treatment, maximize amnesia, control behavior to expedite performance of procedures, maintain safety by minimizing risks, and ensure safe discharge (Hsu, 2005).

CONTRAINDICATIONS

Patients should be evaluated prior to the procedure for their suitability for sedation. From this a decision must be made if there are contraindications for sedation or anxiolytic medication use. Allergies to possible medications used in the procedure may exclude the patient unless alternative medications may be substituted. Previous reactions to sedation or general anesthesia should be noted and may contraindicate the use of procedural sedation depending on the outcomes of prior use. Food ingested within the past 6 hours or clear liquids within the past 2 hours would preclude the patient from sedation unless there was an emergency situation involved, and then the benefits of the procedure must be weighed against the potential of aspiration.

Absolute contraindications are uncommon, but the practitioner should consider comorbid illness or injury and the ability to manage the patient's airway. Patients with significant comorbid cardiac, hemodynamic, or respiratory compromise should be approached with caution, as should patients who may be difficult to intubate or manually ventilate. If the patient is classified as a Class IV or V, as defined by the ASA physical status classification system, a nonanesthesiologist should not provide moderate sedation or anesthesia for that patient, but should refer the patient on to an anesthesiologist who may recommend general anesthesia or other treatment course (Table 36-1).

Ultimately, the largest contraindication may be the practitioner. If the practitioner does not have the understanding of the medications administered, the ability to monitor the patient's responses to the medications given, or the skills necessary to intervene in managing all potential complications, he or she should be excluded from performing the procedure with procedural sedation or anxiolytics. Practitioners also need to be in compliance with the institution's requirements, whether special credentials and privileges are

Table 36.1 American Society of Anesthesiologists (ASA) Physical Status Classifications

PATIENT CLASSIFICATION	EXAMPLE
ASA 1: A normal, healthy patient. The pathologic process for which surgery is to be performed is localized and does not entail a systemic disease.	An otherwise healthy patient scheduled for a cosmetic procedure
ASA 2: A patient with systemic disease, caused either by the condition to be treated or other pathophysiologic process, but which does not result in limitation of activity	A patient with asthma, diabetes, or hypertension that is well controlled with medical therapy, and has no systemic sequelae
ASA 3: A patient with moderate or severe systemic disease caused either by the condition to be treated surgically or other pathophysiologic process, which does limit activity	A patient with uncontrolled asthma that limits activity, or diabetes that has systemic sequelae such as retinopathy
ASA 4: A patient with severe systemic disease that is a constant potential threat to life	A patient with heart failure, or renal failure requiring dialysis
ASA 5: A patient who is at substantial risk for death within 24 hr and is submitted to the procedure in desperation	A patient with fixed and dilated pupils status post head injury
E: Emergency status—added to the ASA designation only if the patient is undergoing an emergency procedure	A healthy patient undergoing sedation for reduction of a displaced fracture, classified ASA 1E

required, or if there are particular state, professional association, or regulatory body requirements to perform procedural sedation.

POTENTIAL COMPLICATIONS

Complications to procedural sedation include, but are not limited to, vomiting, respiratory depression, hypoxia, hypotension, and cardiac arrest. The most serious complication is respiratory failure from airway obstruction or hypoventilation. Advanced airway management skills are a mandatory prerequisite for performing these techniques. Cardiac depression also may occur and must be rapidly recognized to avoid cardiac arrest or death.

Complications are most likely to occur within 5 to 10 minutes after administration of intravenous medication and immediately after the procedure when procedural stimuli are removed (Krauss, 2000). Thus, monitoring should be especially close during these periods. These complications are less likely to occur when using alternative routes of administration, such as oral, nasal, rectal, or intramuscular, but these routes do not preclude them from occurring.

Intravenous sedative/analgesic drugs should be given in small, incremental doses that are titrated to the desired end points of analgesia and sedation (ASA, 2002). Sufficient time must elapse between doses to allow the effect of each dose to be assessed before subsequent drug administration. When drugs are administered by nonintravenous routes (e.g., oral, rectal, intramuscular, transmucosal), allowance should be made for the time required for drug absorption before supplementation is considered. Because absorption may be unpredictable, administration of repeat dosing of oral medications to supplement sedation/analgesia is not recommended.

As a practical consideration, unnecessary stimulation, such as inflation of a blood pressure cuff, may hinder the induction of sedation in a young or anxious child or adult. Once a complete set of vital signs has been obtained, deflate the cuff and monitor the patient visually until the drugs have begun to take effect. At this point, monitoring of pulse oximetry and heart rate, at a minimum, should be initiated. This could avoid additional doses of sedatives being given to the patient and pushing the patient into a much deeper level of depression than intended when the cuff is deflated or removed.

Hepatic or renal abnormalities may impair drug metabolism and excretion, resulting in increased drug sensitivity and longer duration of drug action. This does not preclude the patient from procedural sedation, but the patient should be monitored closely.

Medications that the patient is currently taking may interact with the sedatives and analgesics. Checking for specific drug interactions prior to starting the procedural sedation is recommended. Alcohol or illicit substance abuse may increase a patient's tolerance to sedatives and analgesics. In addition, if the patient has been using these substances prior to sedation, the addition of sedatives/analgesics may be additive or synergistic and may require intubation earlier than anticipated with normal dosing of medications.

Tobacco use can increase the risk of airway irritability, bronchospasm, and coughing during sedation, requiring additional airway monitoring.

PATIENT PREPARATION

Identify the patient by armband identification as well as verbal questioning. Be sure to ask the patient what procedure he or she is there for and that it is the correct procedure. Prior to giving any anxiolytic or analgesic medication, get consent for both the procedural sedation as well as the procedure that the patient is to undergo. The patient should be told of any risks involved with either the procedure or the sedation that is going to be used, as well as any post-sedation side effects to be expected.

A directed history taking and physical examination should precede sedation (Krauss, 2000). Underlying medical problems should be assessed, and information about medication use, allergies, previous adverse experiences with sedation or general anesthesia, and the time and nature of the last oral intake should be obtained.

Auscultation of the heart and lungs should be performed, vital signs taken, and the airway evaluated. Patients who have stridor, significant snoring, sleep apnea, advanced rheumatoid arthritis, dysmorphic facial features, Down's syndrome, upper respiratory infections, or an abnormal airway examination (including Class III or class IV oral examination) should be considered to be at increased risk for airway obstruction during sedation. Also, these patients potentially have a difficult airway to manage if mask ventilation or intubation becomes necessary.

REVIEW OF ESSENTIAL ANATOMY AND PHYSIOLOGY

A normal airway examination should consist of the following:
- Opens mouth normally (Adults: greater than 2 finger widths or 3 cm)

- Able to visualize at least part of the uvula and tonsillar pillars with mouth wide open and tongue out (patient sitting)

- Normal chin length (Adults: length of chin is greater than 2 finger widths or 3 cm)

- Normal neck flexion and extension without pain/paresthesias

An abnormal airway examination can consist of the following:
- Small or recessed chin

- Inability to open mouth normally

- Inability to visualize at least part of uvula or tonsils with mouth open and tongue out

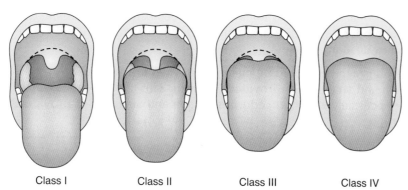

Class I   Class II   Class III   Class IV

FIGURE 36-1. The progression of diagrams from left to right suggests increased difficulty in airway management during sedation (Hata, 2005). (Referenced May 9, 2005: http://www.vh.org/adult/provider/anesthesia/ProceduralSedation)

- High arched palate
- Tonsillar hypertrophy
- Neck with limited range of motion
- Low-set ears
- Significant obesity of the face and neck
- Class III or Class IV oral examination (Fig. 36-1)

Materials Utilized for Procedural Sedation

Although rare, procedural sedation and analgesia may result in an allergic reaction, respiratory arrest, or cardiopulmonary arrest (Godwin, 2005). The incidence of complications is dependent on the drugs used, rate and dose of administration, and patient sensitivities. Although the literature is mixed regarding what specifically needs to be at bedside, there is clear agreement that pulse oximetry be performed. In addition, if the patient has a history of cardiac disease, ongoing monitoring with electrocardiography should be performed.

Other equipment that must be immediately available, but not necessarily at bedside, includes:

- Pharmacologic antagonists and appropriately sized equipment for establishing a patent airway and providing positive-pressure ventilation with supplemental oxygen

- Suction, advanced airway equipment, and resuscitation medication, which should be immediately available and in good working order

■ A functional defibrillator for whenever deep sedation is administered and when moderate sedation is administered to patients with mild or severe cardiovascular disease

Intravenous access should be maintained when intravenous procedural sedation and analgesia is provided (Godwin, 2005). Intravenous access may not be necessary when procedural sedation and analgesia is provided by other routes.

MONITORING

Monitoring the patient during sedation involves visual observation for ventilatory function, response to verbal commands (unless they are unable to respond in a meaningful way [e.g., very young children]), and determination of vital signs at regular intervals. Monitoring of exhaled carbon dioxide should be considered for all patients receiving deep sedation and for patients whose ventilation cannot be directly observed during moderate sedation.

Vital signs should be recorded at specific and regular intervals. At a minimum this should include before starting the procedure, after administration of the drug, when the procedure is complete, during early recovery, and when recovery is completed and patient is ready for discharge. Capnography, or monitoring of exhaled carbon dioxide, is becoming increasingly available and may be useful in assessing ventilation during sedation and analgesia. Capnometry is a technique used to monitor end tidal CO_2 and, therefore, may detect early cases of inadequate ventilation before oxygen desaturation takes place (Godwin, 2005). This is currently not required by any of the literature but has been indicated as useful when ventilatory monitoring is impaired or if the patient is unable to respond to verbal stimuli during the procedure itself.

AGENTS FOR PROCEDURAL SEDATION

The appropriate choice of agents and techniques that are used for sedation or analgesia is practitioner dependent and reflects the comfort level and experience that he or she has with administering the particular medication. It also is dependent on the constraints imposed by the patient, supervising physician, type of procedure, and the facility. Once these constraints are identified, the choices of analgesics/sedatives may be more limited. The following are common medications used in sedation and analgesia to achieve minimal to moderate sedation. However, one must keep in mind that all of these drugs have the potential to push the patient into deep sedation, requiring airway management, reversing agents, cardiac dysfunction, and need for additional airway support. Therefore, the practitioner should be able to rescue patients whose level of sedation becomes deeper than initially intended.

Multiple agents and various combinations of agents can be used to provide sedation and analgesia. Opioids are used primarily when analgesia is required. Sedation is often an added benefit for the patient's comfort during the procedure, but it is not the primary indication for administration. Benzodiazepines and other sedatives, such as barbiturates and chloral hydrate, are useful medications when achieving anxiolysis and amnesia. They are best given just prior to a procedure or during the procedure itself. When considering the selection of an agent, it is important to consider the properties of the agent as well as the type of procedure that is being performed (painful or nonpainful). This can dictate using only one medication as opposed to multiple medications and possibly drug-drug interaction. However, if the procedure is painful and the patient would benefit from an anxiolytic, it is appropriate to use a combination of opioids and benzodiazepines, recognizing that there is an additive/synergistic effect of these medications and that additional monitoring will be required. These medications are listed in Tables 36-2 and

Table 36.2	**Opioids**				
AGENT	ROUTE	USUAL DOSAGE	ONSET/PEAK	DURATION	COMMENTS
Fentanyl	IV—Adult	Start with 0.5-0.1 µg/kg over 2 min			Analgesia, reversible with naloxone
		Titrate 0.25-0.5 µg/kg every 5 min to a maximum of 4-5 µg/kg	1-2 min/3-5 min	30-60 min	Respiratory depression increased with other respiratory depressants, cardiacarrhythmias increased
	IV—Peds	Start with 0.5 µg/kg over 2 min Titrate 0.25-0.5 µg/kg every 5 min			
Morphine	IV—Adult	Initial dose 3-4 mg over 2 min	2-5 min/20 min	4-5 hr	Analgesia, reversible with naloxone
		Titrate 1-2 mg every 5 min			Respiratory depression increased with other respiratory depressants, hypotension possible
	IV—Peds	Initial dose 0.05 mg/kg over 2 min Titrate 0.02-0.05 mg/kg every 5-10 min			
Meperidine	IV—Adult	Start with 25-50 mg over 2 min			
		Titrate 10-15 mg every 5 min to a maximum of 150 mg total	5 min/20 min	2-4 hr	Analgesia, reversible with naloxone, produces generalized CNS depression and increased respiratory depression with additional agents
	IV—Peds	Start with 0.5 mg/kg over 2 min Titrate 0.25-0.5 mg/kg every 5 min			

CNS, central nervous system; IV, intravenous; Peds, pediatric population.

Table 36.3	**Benzodiazepines**				
AGENT	ROUTE	USUAL DOSAGE	ONSET/PEAK	DURATION	COMMENTS
Midazolam	IV—Adult	Initial dose 0.02 mg/kg or 0.5-2 mg over 2 min Titrate by 0.5 mg every 5 min to a maximum of 5 mg total	1-3 min/3-5 min	<2 hr	Requires another agent for analgesia Causes respiratory depression, hypotension Prolonged sedation may occur in elderly
	IV—Peds	Initial dose 0.05 to 0.1 mg/kg over 2 min Titrate by 0.025 mg/kg every 5 min, not to exceed a cumulative dose of 0.6 mg/kg			
	PO—Peds	0.25-0.75 mg/kg	10-20 min/ 20-50 min		
Diazepam	IV—Adult	Initial dose 2.5-5 mg over 5 min Titrate by 2.0-2.5 mg every 5 min *Note:* Not recommended for pediatric patients due to long duration	1-5 min/5-8 min	6-8 hr	Requires another agent for analgesia Causes respiratory depression, hypotension Prolonged sedation in elderly Not used in pediatric population
	PO—Adult	5-10 mg	30-60 min/ 30-90 min		
Lorazepam	IV—Adult	Initial dose 0.5 mg to 2 mg over 5 min Titrate to a maximum dose of 4 mg	5 min/15-20 min	6-8 hr	Same as diazepam
	PO—Adult	Initial dose 2 mg May repeat times once after 20-30 min *Note:* Not recommended for pediatric patients due to long duration	20-30 min/ 60-90 min	6-8 hr	

IV, intravenous; Peds, pediatric population; PO, oral.

36-3. The gold standard remains fentanyl and midazolam in combination due to their fast onset, short duration of action, ease in titration, and favorable cardiovascular profile.

Reversing agents for the opioids is naloxone, and flumazenil for the benzodiazepines. These are dosed as indicated in Table 36-4. If the patient has received both medications and is in respiratory distress, encouraging deep breathing or bag-mask device assistance may be all that is required. However, if this is inadequate and a reversing agent is indicated, always use naloxone as the first agent of choice.

Table 36.4	**Reversing Agents**				
AGENT	ROUTE	USUAL DOSE	ONSET/PEAK	DURATION	COMMENTS
Naloxone	IV—Adult	0.04-0.1 mg for first dose for partial reversal of opioid-induced respiratory depression. May repeat every 2 min until arousal level is obtained			
		May give up to 0.4-2 mg for first dose if apnea has developed but with concern for increased side effects (see drug label)			
		May repeat every 2-3 min to maximum of 10 mg			
		Note: If patient is on opioids prior to additional sedation (as in cancer pain), initial dosing should be started at 0.04 mg and instilled every 2 min until arousal occurs to avoid withdrawal syndrome	2 min/5-15 min	Variable; monitor patient closely	May be cleared faster than opioid. Monitor closely for resedation. Use with extreme caution in elderly or those with cardiac conditions. Acute withdrawal syndrome may also be seen
	IV—Peds	0.01 mg/kg for children <20 kg			
Flumazenil	IV—Adult	0.2 mg over 15 sec			
		May repeat every 60 sec with additional 0.2 mg to a maximum of 1 mg	1-2 min/ 6-10 min	30-90 min but variable; monitor patient closely	Benzodiazepine reversal use is discouraged; potential for benzodiazepine withdrawal or status epilepticus
	IV—Peds	0.01 mg/kg for children <20 kg over 15 sec			Limited efficacy in reversing respiratory depression
		May repeat every 60 sec with additional 0.01 mg/kg to a maximum of 1 mg or 0.05 mg/kg, whichever is lower			

Procedure for Procedural Sedation

1. Confirm patient identity by two methods prior to procedure or sedation.

2. Obtain consent for the procedure and sedation and discuss with the patient the risks involved with both the procedure and sedation.

3. Have a family member (or whoever will accompany the patient home) present when discussing post-procedure sedation side effects, especially when using amnestic medications.

4. Obtain a thorough history to ascertain any prior history of allergic reaction to

continued

anxiolytics or analgesics. Avoid use of these medications if indicated.

5. Perform a physical examination, including the heart, lungs, vital signs, and visualization of the oral airway, prior to sedation.

6. After the patient has been examined, prepare the room for any need that may arise during the procedure. At a minimum, the patient should be monitored by pulse oximetry, and, if he or she has a history of cardiac arrest, with electrocardiography as well.

Note: A minimum of two people is needed in the room during the administration of sedation and the procedure. This ensures that one person can monitor airway, ventilation function, and responsiveness while the other performs the procedure.

7. Make available a cart containing intubation kits, antagonists, and suctioning equipment in case the patient should develop apnea or slip into deep sedation, requiring intubation. The airway assessment prior to sedation is of utmost importance in determining which intubation kit to use.

8. Administer the sedative/amnestic as indicated by prior consent. If oral, these typically are given 20 to 30 minutes prior to the procedure being performed with someone present to monitor the patient. If given intravenously, these can typically be given 5 to 10 minutes prior to the procedure, again with physically present monitoring.

9. Monitor during sedation through visual observation for ventilatory function and response to questioning.

Note: If patient is unresponsive to questioning or the observed ventilatory function decreases anytime following the

dosing of sedation, monitor oximetry. If O_2 saturations decrease below 92%, initiate oxygen, consider reversing agents and ventilatory support, call for support, and initiate respiratory support as indicated.

10. Record vital signs, at minimum, before starting the procedure, after administering the drug, after the procedure is completed, during early recovery, and immediately prior to discharge.

Note: If at any time during this monitoring the patient appears to need support, start oxygen immediately, call for support and initiate respiratory support as indicated by patient's oxygen saturation and responsiveness to questioning.

11. Monitor the patient until near-baseline levels are obtained and he or she is no longer at risk for cardiopulmonary depression. Drowsy patients should not be left unattended, or in areas in which ventilation cannot be adequately observed.

12. Give aftercare instructions to both the patient and whoever accompanies him or her, because it is not unusual for the patient to forget information heard when still partially sedated. Remind both the patient and whoever accompanies him or her that after the use of sedative medications the patient should not drive or make legally binding decisions for 24 hours following the procedure.

13. Discharge the patient home with instructions on when to call if side effects or complications develop. Inform the patient and person accompanying him or her that if nausea or vomiting develops, to change to a clear liquid diet until it resolves.

DISCHARGE CRITERIA

Patients recovering from procedural sedation must be monitored until they are near baseline levels and are no longer at risk for cardiopulmonary depression. Vital signs should be monitored and be stable and at baseline prior to discharge. This includes checking pulse oximetry until they are no longer at risk for hypoxemia. Drowsy patients should not be left unattended or in areas of the facility that may not have adequate observation available.

Prior to undergoing procedural sedation, the patient and family member should be instructed that when sedation is used, whether it includes amnestics or not, that they may have impaired cognitive ability for a prolonged period. They should plan to avoid driving, operating machinery, or making legally binding decisions for at least 24 hours following the procedure.

Written instructions must accompany the patient due to the potential of impaired ability to remember. Post-procedure instructions should include signs and symptoms of potential adverse outcomes and complications. Contact information that includes a 24-hour contact number is advisable in case an emergency does arise. The patient should be instructed to switch to a clear liquid diet until symptoms resolve if he or she develops nausea or vomiting. Generally this is short lived and diet can be advanced as tolerated.

REFERENCES

American Society of Anesthesiologists Task Force on Sedation and Analgesia by Non-Anesthesiologists: Practice guidelines for sedation and analgesia by non-anesthesiologists. Anesthesiology 96:1004-1017, 2002.

Brown TB, Lovato LM, Parker D: Procedural sedation in the acute care setting. Am Fam Physician 71:85-90, 2005.

Godwin SA, Caro DA, Wolf SJ, et al: Clinical policy: Procedural sedation and analgesia in the emergency department. Ann Emerg Med 45:177-196, 2005.

Hata T, Nickel E, Hindman B, Morgan D: Procedural Sedation Resource Center: Guidelines, Education, and Testing for Procedural Sedation and Analgesia. Accessed May 9, 2005: http://www.vh.org/adult/provider/anesthesia/ProceduralSedation/

Hsu DC: Procedural Sedation and Analgesia in Children. Accessed April 19, 2005: http://utdol.com/application/topic.asp?file=pedi_em/10221&type=A&selectedTitle=5~13

Krauss B, Green S: Primary care: Sedation and analgesia for procedures in children. N Engl J Med 342:938-945, 2000.

BIBLIOGRAPHY

Bahn EL, Holt KR: Procedural sedation and analgesia: A review and new concepts. Emerg Med Clin North Am 23:503-517, 2005.

Chudnofsky CR, Lozon MM: Sedation and analgesia for procedures. In Marx JA, Hockberger RS, Walls RM (eds): Rosen's Emergency

Medicine: Concepts and Clinical Practice, 5th ed. St. Louis, Mosby, 2002, pp 2578-2587.

O'Donnell JM, Bragg K, Sell S: Procedural sedation: Safely navigating the twilight zone. Nursing 33:36-44, 2003.

Chapter 37

Patient Education Concepts[*]

Richard D. Muma

GOALS AND OBJECTIVES

Goal: To perform effective patient education.

Objectives: The student will be able to …

- Describe why patient education is a worthwhile effort.
- Identify and describe Cole's suggestions for enhancing the patient education process.
- Identify and describe the proposed factors that influence patient education.
- Identify several sources for patient education materials.

[*]This chapter was adapted from Muma R, Lyons BA, Newman TA, Carnes BA (eds): Patient Education: A Practical Approach. New York, McGraw-Hill, 1996.

BACKGROUND AND HISTORY

This chapter summarizes recommendations as originally proposed by Collier and colleagues in *Patient Education: A Practical Approach* (Cole, 1996; Muma, 1996). Cole points out that there have been dramatic changes in the number of providers, advances in medical technology, and the understanding of disease, as well as striking developments in various methods to treat these problems. The goal of these advancements in health care delivery is to be able to provide better patient treatment, working toward the goal of effecting a healthy outcome. The chief means to accomplish this goal is through an interactive educational process. Whether it involves asking an individual to take medication or to make substantial lifestyle changes to promote better health, providers must be able to communicate, educate, and motivate the patient effectively.

Various approaches to patient education have been outlined over the years. All emphasize the importance of providing accurate information and encouraging patients to assume more responsibility for their own treatment. Many of the techniques used to accomplish such education share common characteristics. For example, explanations need to be given in simple terms, avoiding jargon that might be confusing. Also, the health care provider must assess the patient's understanding of the information in case further explanation is necessary to clarify questions or reduce confusion. Careful attention must also be given to patients' emotional responses to a particular diagnosis or treatment method, as these reactions can have a significant impact on outcome.

Effective patient education should be duly recognized as an integral building block in the entire health delivery process, of equal importance to clinical and technologic advancements in the field. Good patient education provides the following benefits (Greenberg, 1989):

- Enables patients to assume greater responsibility for their own health care

- Improves patients' ability to manage acute and chronic illness

- Provides patients with opportunities to choose healthier lifestyles and practice preventive medicine

- Improves compliance with medication and treatment regimens

- Increases patients' satisfaction with their medical care and thus reduces the risk of liability

- Attracts patients to your practice

- Leads to a more efficient, cost-effective health care system

COLE'S SUGGESTIONS FOR ENHANCING THE PATIENT EDUCATION PROCESS

PAY ATTENTION TO USING GOOD INTERVIEWING TECHNIQUES

Helping patients deal successfully with medical problems involves being able to both educate and motivate for change. This requires the use of skillful interpersonal techniques. One needs to be attuned to both verbal and non-verbal aspects of the interaction. With time and practice, one develops a sense of when it is best to be silent and listen to a patient and when to provide specific educational information or support. Being prepared and organized beforehand (e.g., having laboratory work on the chart, pulling together handouts, having a treatment plan written out specifically for the patient) facilitates the entire process and will likely improve understanding and compliance.

PRESENT INFORMATION THROUGH SEVERAL CHANNELS

Do not rely solely on direct verbal communication to ensure a patient's understanding. For some individuals, verbal learning is not as successful as visual learning. Some individuals may understand and retain information better if they are able to view a handout or chart or follow an explanation concerning a radiograph. Also, some patients may benefit from the opportunity to meet and talk with others who have dealt with a certain problem or are currently undergoing treatment for a particular medical condition. Such peer support can be an effective tool in motivating an individual to comply with treatment.

ALWAYS SUPPLEMENT THE EDUCATIONAL PROCESS WITH PATIENT EDUCATION RESOURCES

The patient education process can be overwhelming because so much information may need to be covered. It is therefore recommended that patients be provided with brochures, handouts, medication inserts, an outline of the treatment plan, listing of internet sites, or other materials that will permit later perusal to reinforce what was covered during the actual interview.

INVOLVE FAMILIES OR SIGNIFICANT OTHERS WHEN POSSIBLE

Remember that patients are part of a larger family system. Most often, these family members are concerned about the health of their loved one, and involving them in the treatment process can be useful. Indeed, such involvement may in some cases ensure compliance with a treatment plan. Ask how the patient is going to explain a particular health problem to his or her family. Invite family members to attend a follow-up appointment so that they, too, can hear about the situation and learn how they can help.

BE SURE TO RAISE THE SENSITIVE ISSUES

There are certain subjects that tend to be highly sensitive, and some patients may have underlying concerns or fears that they may not openly voice. Topics such as sexuality or death and dying often fall into this category. Because these topics may produce embarrassment or feelings of despondency, a patient may be reluctant to inquire about them. Therefore, it is critical for the health care professional to initiate such discussion when it is clearly pertinent to the treatment plan (e.g., medications that might interfere with sexual functioning, the need for a patient to recognize that the treatment options for a particular condition may be only palliative). Raising these issues signals that it is all right to talk about more sensitive matters and allows the patient to express his or her underlying fears and concerns openly.

BE ATTUNED TO EMOTIONAL REACTIONS

As already noted, patients experience emotional reactions to learning of a particular illness and the need to follow a course of treatment. Providing comprehensive health care requires exploring these emotional topics. Whether the patient is expressing fear, anger, anxiety, or depression, unless the health care professional inquires about such reactions and takes steps to address them, treatment outcome may be in jeopardy. Allowing the patient to express feelings and offering him or her support are viewed as an integral part of the patient education process.

DO NOT FEEL THAT ONCE THE TOPIC IS COVERED IT IS COMPLETELY RESOLVED FOR THE PATIENT

For some individuals, providing education about a disease or treatment plan is enough to motivate them to go forward and carry out the prescribed treatment. For others, however, there may be lingering confusion or questions after the interview that need to be addressed at a later time. In addition, certain aspects of the treatment plan that are more difficult for a patient to deal with (e.g., making lifestyle changes such as smoking cessation or weight reduction) need to be reviewed and re-encouraged at a later appointment. It is always prudent to review a patient's treatment plan at each subsequent follow-up visit, offering praise for the accomplishments and noting areas that need additional attention.

PROPOSED FACTORS THAT INFLUENCE PATIENT EDUCATION

There are many parts to the concept of health, including how one thinks about disease and its cures. Health care in the United States is based primarily on treating acute, well-advanced disease processes, using an infectious disease paradigm. However, the causes of poor health and serious disease processes are linked to multiple factors, particularly behavioral and cognitive habits, along with specific social and physical environments. Patients often react to illness and its management in ways learned from others, according to their cultural norms, and according to their own perception of the severity of the illness. Before engaging in a patient education session, one must realize that every patient responds differently, and several variables or factors play a role in that response. Some of those factors identified for discussion in this chapter include age, ethnicity, family issues, socioeconomic status, and the chronicity of illness.

AGE

Although an obvious consideration, age is not always reflected in patient education materials and is often overlooked in the patient education counseling session. One must remember that the range of care starts with infants and ends with the elderly. Let us start with children. They are not small adults, and their wants, needs, thinking process, and emotional and physical status differ from those of an adult. For example, small children often view hospitalization as a punishment, not as a means of getting well (Anderson, 1990). This belief is further reinforced when parental figures make statements such as, "If you go outside without a coat you may get sick and have to go see the doctor." This type of belief often leads to false perceptions about clinicians and to a child's difficulty in accepting medical advice or treatment. Infants, although not directly involved in patient counseling sessions, have special needs and respond to touch and nonverbal communication (Anderson, 1990). As children grow older, however, one must keep in mind the current fads, language, and norms that exist. For example, teenagers often believe themselves to be experts in every area, and in some cases do not heed advice. Furthermore, certain instructions given to teenagers regarding prevention of illness may not be "cool" or in line with the thinking of their peer group.

Adults are more mature and have concerns that are different from those of adolescents. For instance, young adults (ages 20 to 40) are at a point in life in which multiple activities (e.g., college, relationships, children) keep them busy (Anderson, 1990). These patients need practical approaches to education; approaches that are not time-consuming and unrealistic in relation to their lives. As adults grow older (ages 41 to 60), they become more conscious of the possibility of health problems and in most cases are willing to follow a patient education prescription. However, some may lack self-confidence, which can cause avoidance of the risk of failure in learning anything new (Anderson, 1990). Adults older than 65 years are similar to middle-aged adults in their willingness to learn new ideas, but the provider must be aware of individuals' past experiences, involve them in the learning process, and motivate them to learn (Anderson, 1990). Elderly patients may feel that it is hardly worth the effort to learn new information and skills because they think their life is nearing an end (Anderson, 1990).

ETHNICITY

Before we discuss ethnicity, it is important to define the adjective *ethnic*. Ethnic is defined in the 1982 edition of *The American Heritage Dictionary of the English Language* as "of or pertaining to a social group that claims or is accorded special status on the basis of complex, often variable traits including religious, linguistic, ancestral, or physical characteristics." *Ethnicity* is defined as the condition of belonging to a particular ethnic group. Examples of ethnic groups in the United States include African American, Asian, white, Hispanic, and Native American. There are at least 106 ethnic groups, including more than 170 Native American groups, in the United States (Thernstrom, 1980). Ethnic groups should not be confused with minority groups, as the latter are seen as different from the majority group of which they are part. However, some ethnic groups are also classified as minorities (e.g., African Americans in the United States). One can see that the phenomenon of ethnicity is complex, ambivalent, paradoxical, and elusive (Senior, 1965). As clinicians, it is important to be aware of the ethnic backgrounds of patients. The differences in language and culture each group exhibits certainly influence the way patient education is communicated. For example, some think that human immunodeficiency virus (HIV) infection prevention literature is not communicated effectively to African-American populations. HIV prevention programs are hampered because of the presence of culturally specific attitudes and beliefs, including those pertaining to the roles of males and females (Lyons, 1994).

FAMILY

Although consideration of the individual is important in patient education, the patient's family is also of central importance if teaching is to be effective (Falvo, 1985). How a family functions influences the health of its members as well as how an individual reacts to illness. Including the family members and significant others in patient education sessions facilitates adherence, understanding of the disease process, and the confidence needed to perform specific skills. Hence, the health care professional should capitalize on what family members can do for the patient and work with them in encouraging the patient in tasks that may be difficult. For example, when educating a patient with diabetes mellitus who requires insulin injections, involvement of the family in teaching sessions that demonstrate insulin injections most likely will improve adherence. Family members can also serve as troubleshooters when the patient has difficulty performing complex tasks. However, not all patients have family or significant others available for support. This is frequently seen in cases of HIV infection. Patients are often isolated from others after their diagnosis is made known. These patients are often on complex medical regimens involving the use of intravenous catheters. Lack of support sometimes leads to poor care, missed doses, and increased morbidity and mortality.

The health care professional can do much to facilitate the effectiveness of patient teaching by fostering discussion among significant others. A professional who has continued contact with the patient and his or her significant others may check on the progress of the patient when necessary and appropriate, and identify any new problems that may interfere with optimal care.

SOCIOECONOMIC STATUS

The socioeconomic status of the patient should be carefully considered when initiating education sessions. Individuals in lower socioeconomic groups are less likely to seek treatment; if they seek treatment they tend to access health care later in the course of their illness, and they die sooner than do individuals in higher socioeconomic classes. Hence, the clinician should be aware of the patient's personal income, living arrangements, and employment status but should also have an increased awareness of the patient's health. Lower socioeconomic status has been linked to the development of disease states, the most noted being coronary artery disease (Marmot, 1978; Morgenstern, 1980). For example, the provider clearly cannot erase poverty and improve access to health care for all; however, he or she can exert a positive impact on lower socioeconomic groups by working with their members to promote healthier lifestyles (Lyons, 1994). Some individuals often do not know what resources are available. The provider should point individuals to local resources that provide services and, if that is not possible, attempt to arrange for those services for the patient.

CHRONICITY OF DISEASE

Finally, acute illnesses present differently from chronic ones and cause a variety of reactions among patients. Health care providers must be aware of the illnesses that require extra emotional support and possible psychiatric intervention when preparing for patient education sessions. Furthermore, it is not enough to simply inform a patient of his or her medical condition without time for an initial reaction. Patients require time to react to a new diagnosis. The perceived seriousness and natural course of a disease help determine how a patient will respond. For instance, the patient diagnosed with acute pharyngitis may feel really terrible during the illness but knows that it is a curable disease and usually self-limiting. Hence, this patient may have fewer emotional problems and require less counseling. Conversely, the patient diagnosed with stage IV breast cancer, in which the long-term prognosis is known to be poor, may have an emotional response that needs further intervention involving a psychiatrist, social worker, or nursing care.

SOURCES OF PATIENT EDUCATION

Finally, as pointed out by many (Lyons, 1996), patient education draws on a broad-based set of materials that can help explain a spectrum of topics. Traditionally, patient education has been accomplished with fact sheets; pamphlets; disease picture books; magazines; anatomic pictures; audiovisual materials such as videotapes, interactive video, computer-assisted instruction, laser disk technology, and the internet; and verbal instructions or materials of a practitioner's own creation (Graber, 1999; Lyons, 1996). The internet has become a ready source of educational materials, but clinicians should be cautious because much of this material is not written at a level that is comprehensible to many of our patients (Graber, 1999). Further investigation of these resources is necessary by the clinician or others knowledgeable about patient education materials before referring patients to these internet sites. Particular attention should be paid to readability and accuracy of the information. Many of the chapters in this text refer to appropriate sites for patient education, and the reader should refer to those chapters for specific website addresses.

REFERENCES

Anderson C: Patient Teaching and Communicating in an Information Age. Albany, NY, Delmar, 1990, pp 76-102.

Cole CM: An approach to patient education. In Muma RD, Lyons BA, Newman TA, Carnes BA (eds): Patient Education: A Practical Approach. New York, McGraw-Hill, 1996, pp 3-9.

Falvo DR: Effective Patient Education. Rockville, Md, Aspen, 1985, pp 99-109.

Graber MA, Roller CM, Kaeble B: Readability levels of patient education material on the World Wide Web. J Fam Pract 48:58-61, 1999.

Greenberg L: Build your practice with patient education. Contemp Pediatr September, 85-106, 1989.

Lyons BA, Valentine P: Prevention. In Muma RD, Lyons BA, Borucki MJ, et al, (eds): HIV Manual for Health Care Professionals. Norwalk, Conn, Appleton & Lange, 1994, p 257.

Lyons BA: Selecting and evaluating sources of patient education materials. In Muma RD, Lyons BA, Newman TA, Carnes BA (eds): Patient Education: A Practical Approach. New York, McGraw-Hill, 1996, pp 15-21.

Marmot MG, Adelstein AM, Robinson N, et al: Changing social-class distribution of heart disease. Br Med J 2:1109-1112, 1978.

Morgenstern H: The changing association between social status and coronary heart disease in a rural population. Soc Sci Med 14A:191-201, 1980.

Muma RD: Factors influencing patient education. In Muma RD, Lyons BA, Newman TA, Carnes BA (eds): Patient Education: A Practical Approach. New York, McGraw-Hill, 1996, pp 11-12.

Senior C: The Puerto Ricans: Strangers Then Neighbors. Chicago, Quadrangle Books, 1965, p 21.

The American Heritage Dictionary of the English Language. New York, Dell, 1982, p 247.

Thernstrom S: Harvard Encyclopedia of American Ethnic Groups. Cambridge, Mass, Belknap Press of Harvard University, 1980, p vii.

BIBLIOGRAPHY

Bickley LS, Szilagyi PG: Bates' Guide to the Physical Examination and History, 8th ed. Philadelphia, JB Lippincott, 2002.

Bernstein L, Bernstein RS: Interviewing: A Guide for Health Professionals, 4th ed. Stamford, Conn, Appleton & Lange, 1985.

Coulehan J, Block M: The Medical Interview: Mastering Skills for Clinical Practice, 4th ed. FA Davis, 2001.

Guckian J (ed): The Clinical Interview and Physical Examination. Philadelphia, JB Lippincott, 1987.

Henderson G: Physician-Patient Communication. Springfield, Ill, Charles C Thomas, 1981.

Sherilyn-Cormier L, Cormier W, Weissen RL: Interviewing and Helping Skills for Health Professionals. Monterey, Calif, Wadsworth Health Sciences Division, 1984.

Stevenson I: The Diagnostic Interview, 2nd ed. New York, Harper & Row, 1971.

Chapter 38

Outpatient Coding

Lynn E. Caton

GOALS AND OBJECTIVES

Goal: To increase understanding of the coding process as applied to outpatient medical services for financial reimbursement and to provide clinicians with a systematic framework to assist in the accurate coding of outpatient activities.

Objectives: The student will be able to ...

- Explain the history, purpose, and importance of outpatient coding.

- Describe the mechanism for coding the components of the patient history.

- Describe the mechanism for coding the components of the physical examination.

- Describe the mechanism for coding the components of clinical thinking in diagnosis and treatment within a patient encounter.

BACKGROUND AND HISTORY

The coding of medical diseases is not a recent undertaking. In England, about the time of Sherlock Holmes and Dr. Watson, a list of diseases began with the *London Bills of Mortality*, 1845. The tracking of births and deaths actually began in the 1500s to provide details of the infamous bubonic plague epidemics. The "Great Plague" killed nearly 25% of Londoners from 1563-1665 (*London Bills of Mortality* from uuhsc.utah.edu). In 1874 the Registration Amendment Act required medical practitioners to formally issue death certificates, and failure to do so incurred a penalty. In 1881 William Ogle set up an inquiry system in an attempt to cut down on ambiguously worded death certificates. Shortly thereafter, the Royal College of Physicians established the revised nomenclature for causes of death classifications (Beacon Healthcare Solutions, 2000-2003).

In 1900 the *International Classification of Diseases, Clinical Modification* (ICD-CM) codes were introduced and have been used to classify diseases since then. In 1977 the Ninth Revision (ICM-9-CM) was published by the World Health Organization and has attained widespread recognition and use. The United States Congress passed the Medicare Catastrophic Coverage Act in 1988 and, even though the Act was later repealed, the mandate for use of ICD-9-CM remained a requirement for each Medicare Part B claim submitted for payment. The Centers for Medicare & Medicaid Services (CMS) has published guidelines that have been put into effect in each state, and the most recently published guidelines in use are from 1997 (CMS, 1997; Beacon Healthcare Solutions, 2000-2003).

The current procedural terminology (CPT) system (American Medical Association, 2005) is a method of describing and coding the components of a patient encounter, including medical, surgical, and diagnostic services. CPT was developed by the American Medical Association (AMA) and first published in 1966. CPT is maintained and updated by an editorial panel of physicians and advised by two committees of physicians and other health care professionals (Rose, 2001).

Documentation Guidelines for Evaluation and Management Services provides CPT codes that identify a service rather than a procedure (E/M codes). E/M codes are a subset of CPT as developed by the AMA. There are two sets of guidelines for E/M codes, one published in 1995 and another published in 1997. Although the 1997 version is more complex, it is most widely used by physicians, probably because the 1997 guidelines are less ambiguous.

The most difficult components of CPT to understand are related to documentation of the patient encounter. These components are history, physical examination, medical decision making, and surgical and diagnostic procedures. Tables and examples included in this chapter will clarify CPT E/M components and their application to documentation and coding.

PURPOSE OF MEDICAL RECORD DOCUMENTATION AND CODING

Medical records should be complete and legible and describe each patient encounter in the patient medical record, including electronic communications (see Chapter 39).

Documentation should include the following:

- Reason for encounter (chief complaint)

- Relevant history, physical and diagnostic tests

- Assessment, diagnosis, and plan for care and treatment

- Date of encounter and identity of provider

- Rationale for ordering diagnostic tests and other services

- Past and present diagnoses for future reference

- Identification of risk factors

- Patient progress and success of treatments or revisions of treatment and diagnoses

Documentation of treatment success and disease remission is an important component of coding the complexity of a patient encounter. Therefore, noting that diabetes or hypertension, for example, is controlled or uncontrolled is helpful in monitoring a patient's condition and an element of medical decision making.

Documentation should support the CPT and ICD-9-CM codes used for billing insurance companies (CMS, 1997).

How to Code

The first step is to select the ICD-9-CM code that best defines the diagnosis. Once the diagnosis code is selected, then the CPT E/M code is selected based on the criteria outlined in following sections and summarized in Table 38-1.

Effective coding requires using the elements that are part of any good history and physical examination, applying the ICD-9-CM numbering system to the diagnosis, and then fitting the information documented in the medical record to the proper CPT E/M service level and including any CPT codes for procedures performed during the patient encounter. The next step is to use the above information to appropriately generate a billing statement.

IMPORTANCE OF DOCUMENTATION AND CODING

It is important to provide an accurate evaluation of each patient encounter and record a well-documented report of the history, examination, and diagnostic and treatment plans. This ensures that each patient's medical treat-

Table 38.1 Criteria for CPT Evaluation and Management Coding

HISTORY			EXAM	MEDICAL DECISION MAKING		
HPI	ROS	PFSH	EXAM AREAS/ SYSTEMS	DIAGNOSTIC AND MANAGEMENT	AMOUNT OF DATA	RISK
Location	Constitutional	**Past:**	General appearance	Status of problems	Test ordered or performed	Comorbidities
Quality	ENT	Prior illness	Eyes	Diagnoses under investigation	Test reviewed	Decision to perform urgent and/or invasive procedures
Severity	Cardiovascular	Surgery	ENT	Begin or change of treatment	Decision to obtain old records	
Duration	Respiratory	Hospital	Neck	Additional workups	Discussion with physicians	
Timing	Gastrointestinal	Medications	Respiratory	Referrals	Review of test by physicians	
Context	Genitourinary	Allergies	Cardiovascular			
Moderating factors	Musculoskeletal	Dietary status	Chest			
Associated symptoms	Skin	**Family:**	Abdomen			
	Neurologic	Current health	Genitourinary			
	Psychiatric	Causes of death	Lymph			
	Endocrine	Hereditary	Musculoskeletal			
	Lymphatic	**Social:**	Skin			
	Allergy	Marital status	Neurologic			
		Employment	Psychiatric			
		Occupation				
		Drugs, alcohol, tobacco				
		Education				

ENT, ears, nose, mouth, and throat; HPI, history of present illness; PFSH, past family and/or social history; ROS, review of systems.

ment is available for review by other health care professionals on subsequent visits as well as documentation of the progression, remission, or resolution of acute and chronic diseases. The accurate coding of the diseases contributes to the ability of medical professionals to provide detailed communication to their peers and enhances population-based medical research. The most important impact of excellent documentation is improved patient care.

The use of documentation and coding should be primarily to provide continuity of appropriate and necessary preventive, diagnostic, and therapeutic services, not just a task oriented to billing for medical services and satisfying insurance claims.

The following patient example has an E/M code, an ICD-9-CM code and a CPT procedure code for the throat culture. The elements are marked for each section of the note. Summary of the documentation elements is as follows:

History Types
- Problem Focused
- Expanded Problem Focused
- Detailed
- Comprehensive

Elements of Patient Clinical History
- HPI—history of present illness
- PFSH—past, family, social history
- ROS—review of systems

Example A

Chief complaint (CC): "Sore throat for five days" *(required of all E/M levels)*

Subjective (S): This patient is a 25-year-old nonsmoking male in for acute onset of sore throat 5 days ago. *(HPI-Duration, one element)* He has had a fever, measured at home at 103° F and chills. *(Associated symptoms, second HPI element)* He denies cough, ear pain, nasal congestion, or eye itching or drainage. His neck has been sore and it is painful to swallow. *(Location and severity of pain, third HPI element)* He denies nausea, vomiting or diarrhea. He takes no medications regularly and has no known allergies to medication. He has been taking fluids and eating soft foods. He missed work today as an accountant and didn't sleep well last night. *(Fourth HPI context element)*

The HPI also includes ROS of the eyes, ears, nose, throat, neck, respiratory, allergies, and gastrointestinal systems, or six systems.

Past medical history positive for appendectomy at age 14.

Objective (O):

General appearance (GA): A fatigued appearing 25-year-old male in no distress. VS: BP 136/88, P 92 regular, Respirations 12, T: 101.4° F orally. Wt: 155 lbs, Ht: 70".

HEENT:

Eyes: clear, without discharge or erythema, conjunctivae are clear, PERRLA

Ears: Pinna normal and nontender, external auditory canal patent without erythema or cerumen, TM's dull without fluid levels or inflammation.

Nose: clear, minimal clear discharge, septum deviated to the left, no lesions noted.

Throat: Inflamed with 2+ tonsils and large amount of exudates bilaterally.

NECK: Thyroid normal, smooth without masses, 3+ anterior change adenopathy tender to palpation.

HEART/LUNGS: normal, no murmurs, rubs: Lungs clear to auscultation and percussion anteriorly, posteriorly, and laterally.

Because the ears, nose, mouth, and throat (ENT) examination is considered by CPT as one examination, the number of systems examined and documented is five in this example.

Quick Strep positive for strep CPT code 87060 is the code for bacterial culture of the nose/throat.

Assessment (A): Strep Throat—ICD-9-CM code is 034.0

Plan (P): Pen Vee K 500 mg four times a day (qid) for 10 days

---

The considerations for determining the CPT E/M service code for the above example are as follows:

■ HPI—four elements

■ ROS—six, PFSH—three elements

■ Examination—seven systems

■ Decision making and risk exists since prescription drugs were used, the problem is acute, and the problem is an undiagnosed new one. There is a moderate differential diagnosis and minimal data to review.

■ Time—generally around 15 minutes for this problem

The E/M code for Example A is a level four based on the information included in the HPI, ROS/PFSH and the prescribing of medication.

OVERVIEW OF CODING

The CPT/ICD-9-CM process begins with a patient encounter. The clinician performs a history and physical examination, determines a diagnosis, and formulates a plan, which may include diagnostics, therapeutics, and patient education (counseling). Working backward in this scenario, the first step is to select the ICD-9-M code that best defines the diagnosis. ICD-9 is not unlike the Dewey decimal system, with three numeric places to the left of the decimal and two places to the right, further defining the diagnosis. For example, the ICD-9 code for sore throat is found under pharyngitis, not sore throat. The code for pharyngitis is 462 if the problem is acute. The number is 472.1 if the problem is chronic. If the diagnosis is tonsillitis, the code is 463, and if the etiology were streptococcal, the code would be 034.0. Once the diagnosis code is selected, then the CPT E/M code is selected based on the criteria outlined in following sections and summarized in Table 38-1.

PATIENT HISTORY

The levels of history are coded as one of four types. Each type of history includes all or some of the following elements. The extent of obtaining and recording the various types of history depends on the clinical situation, nature of the presenting problem (chief complaint), and the clinical judgment of the health care professional.

It is important to note here that the CPT guidelines have not reinvented the basic medical history that all physicians use to guide the evaluation of each and every patient. The history types may be less recognizable terms, but the elements of a clinical history will be very familiar to all clinicians. CPT has taken the universal language of medicine and added some quantifiable terminology and a numerical classification system for reproducibility.

HISTORY DEFINITIONS

Chief Complaint (CC)

This is a statement of the reason for the encounter, usually in the patient's own words.

History of Present Illness (HPI)

The HPI is a chronological description of the patient's present illness. The CPT definition and elements are not different from the standard medical history. It is important for coding that the questions that typically are asked in the history of present illness be recorded to validate the thought process of the history taker. These elements are also part of a standard HPI.

Elements
1. Location
2. Quality
3. Severity
4. Duration
5. Timing
6. Context
7. Modifying factors
8. Associated signs and symptoms

Table 38.2	**Elements of CPT E/M Levels of Service**		
99212 LEVEL II CPT E/M Service *Brief Problem Focused*	99213 LEVEL III CPT E/M Service *Brief Problem Expanded*	99214 LEVEL IV CPT E/M Service *Extended Problem Detailed*	99215 LEVEL V CPT E/M Service *Extended Problem Comprehensive*
1 HPI	1 HPI	4 HPI	4 HPI
0 ROS	1 ROS	2 ROS	10 ROS
0 PFSH	0 PFSH	1 PFSH	3 PFSH
1 Exam	2-4 Exam	5-7 Exam	8+ Exam
Straight DM	Low DM	Moderate DM	High DM
10 minutes	15 minutes	25 minutes	40 minutes

DM, decision making; HPI, history of present illness; PFSH, past family and/or social history; ROS, review of systems.

Review of Systems (ROS)

Review of systems coding is the classic history taking of all body systems. This review is based on a series of questions asked of the patient about various signs and symptoms related to organ systems. A complete review of systems includes all 14 or 16 components, depending on your method of inclusion or exclusion. The E/M guidelines note 14 systems and include skin/breast and allergic/immunologic together rather than separately. The appropriate ROS is based on the problem. Either the problem requires a pertinent ROS with just those systems related to the problem reviewed or an extended ROS in which additional systems possibly related to the chief complaint and HPI are reviewed. The complete ROS is all systems pertinent to the CC and HPI plus all other systems reviewed and documented. This documentation must specifically note patient responses, positive or negative. These responses must be individually documented (Table 38-2; see also Table 38-1).

Past, Family, and/or Social History (PFSH)

Past medical history includes history pertinent to the CC and HPI, and at least one item from each of the three areas (Past, Family, Social) is required for a detailed report of a comprehensive patient encounter. Logically the PFSH should be complete for a new patient encounter. See Table 38-1 for examples of what must be included for each PFSH area.

CODE LEVELS AND ELEMENTS OF HISTORY, EXAMINATION AND DECISION MAKING

Examinations

The coding of the physical examination uses the same nomenclature as the E/M coding of the history. The four categories are brief problem focused, brief problem expanded, extended problem detailed, and extended problem comprehensive (see Table 38-2). The types of examinations described by CPT are general multisystem or a complete examination of a single organ system. The single organ system examination may also document the examination of other symptomatic or related organ systems.

Both the multisystem and the single organ system codes are open for use by any health professional in any specialty area of medicine. This includes consultation codes.

CODE LEVELS AND ELEMENTS OF HISTORY AND EXAMINATION

The elements of each examination required by CPT increase with the E/M code level. In Table 38-2 the E/M level for an extended visit or code 99215 requires that eight or more elements of the physical examination be documented. In addition, the physical findings need to be described if there is an abnormality. It is not sufficient to examine an organ system or body area and describe it as abnormal without elaboration of the physical findings (see Example B).

 Example B _____

S: The patient is a 25-year-old male in for acute onset of sore throat 5 days ago. He has had a fever, measured at home at 103° F and chills. He denies cough, ear pain, nasal congestion or eye itching or drainage. His neck has been sore and it is painful to swallow. He denies nausea, vomiting or diarrhea. He has been taking fluids and eating soft foods. He missed work today as an accountant and didn't sleep well last night.

   O:

GA: A fatigued appearing 25-year-old male in no distress.

VS: BP 136/88, P 92 regular, Respirations 12, T: 101.4° F orally. Wt: 155 lbs, Ht: 70″.

   HEENT: Normal except for an abnormal appearing throat and tonsils.

(This description would be unacceptable by CPT)

   NECK: Normal, no masses, thyroid smooth and nontender.

   HEART/LUNGS: Normal, no murmurs, rubs or abnormal lung sounds.

   A: Strep Throat

   P: Pen Vee K 500 mg qid for 10 days

However, when describing an area of the body or organ system that is normal or negative for physical findings, the term normal or negative is sufficient (see above example for the examination of the neck).

The elements of a general multisystem examination as well as the single organ system examination are outlined in Table 38-3. It should be noted that an examination of the eye constitutes a single organ examination for CPT purposes and the examination of the ears, nose, mouth, and throat (ENT) is also one organ system.

Table 38.3 **Coding Elements for the Physical Examination**

SYSTEM/BODY AREA	ELEMENTS OF EXAMINATION
Constitutional	Measurement of any three of the following seven vital signs: (1) sitting or standing BP; (2) supine BP; (3) pulse rate and regularity; (4) respirations; (5) temperature, (6) weight, (7) height
	General appearance of patient (e.g., development, nutrition, body habitus, deformities, attention to grooming)
Ears, nose, mouth, and throat (ENT)	Inspection of the external ears, nose (overall appearance, lesions, masses, or scars noted).
	Otoscopic examination of the external ear and tympanic membrane
	Hearing assessment (whisper test, finger rub, or tuning fork)
	Inspection of nasal mucosa, septum, and turbinates
	Inspection of lips, teeth, and gums
	Examination of the oropharynx: oral mucosa, salivary glands, hard and soft palate, tongue, tonsils, and posterior pharynx
Eyes	Inspections of the lids and conjunctivae
	Examination of the pupils and irises (PERRLA)
	Ophthalmoscopic examination of the optic discs (full funduscopic examination)
Neck	Examination of the neck for masses, symmetry, tracheal position, and crepitus
	Examination of the thyroid
Chest (breasts)	Inspection of the breasts
	Palpation of the breasts and axillae
Respiratory	Assessment of respiratory effort (e.g., intercostals, retractions, use of accessory muscles, diaphragmatic movement)
	Percussion of the chest
	Palpation of the chest (e.g., tactile fremitus)
	Auscultation of the lungs (e.g., breath sounds, adventitious sounds, rubs)
Cardiovascular	Palpation of the heart (location, size, thrills)
	Auscultation of the heart with notation of abnormal sounds and murmurs
	Examination of carotid arteries, abdominal aorta, femoral arteries, pedal pulses
	Extremities for edema and/or varicosities
Gastrointestinal (abdomen)	Examination of abdomen with notation of masses of tenderness; liver and spleen; presence or absence of hernia; when indicated, anus, perineum, and rectum, including sphincter tone, presence of hemorrhoids, and rectal masses
	Obtain stool sample for occult blood test when indicated
Genitourinary	Male:
	Examination of scrotal contents, with notation of hydrocele, spermatocele, tenderness of cord, testicular mass; penis; digital rectal, with notation of size, symmetry, modularity, tenderness of the prostate
	Female:
	Pelvic examination with or without collection for smears and cultures, including examination of external genitalia; vagina; urethra; bladder; uterus; adnexa, for masses, tenderness, organomegaly, modularity
Lymphatic	Palpation of lymph nodes in two or more areas: neck, axillae, groin, other
Musculoskeletal	Gait and station
	Inspection and/or palpation of digits (e.g., clubbing, cyanosis, inflammation, petechiae, ischemia, infections, nodes)
	Examination of joints, bones, and muscles of one or more of the following six areas: head and neck; spine, ribs, and pelvis; right or left upper extremity; right or left lower extremity
	The examination is to include the following for each area: inspection and/or palpation noting misalignment, asymmetry, crepitation, defects, tenderness, masses, effusions; assessment of range of motion, noting pain, crepitation, or contracture; assessment of muscle strength and tone with notation of atrophy or abnormal movements
Neurologic	Cranial nerves with notation of deficits
	Deep tendon reflexes noting pathology
	Sensation (sharp, dull, vibrations, proprioception)
Psychiatric	Description of patient's judgment and insight
	Mental status: orientation to time, place, and person; recent and remote memory; mood and effect
Skin	Inspection of skin and subcutaneous tissues (rashes, lesions, or ulcers)
	Palpation of skin and subcutaneous tissues (for indurations, nodules and tightening)

Single Organ System Examinations

The single organ system examination (SOSE) is the same as the multisystem examination (MSE) except that the single systems are more detailed. For example, the E/M documentation for a comprehensive examination would include at least nine organ systems or body areas. The single organ system examination would include all the elements specified for that organ system.

These elements are very specific to each organ system. The examination elements that must be documented for a SOSE of the cardiovascular system for a comprehensive examination code include additional specified examinations of the vital signs and respiratory, cardiovascular, gastrointestinal, and neurologic systems. These elements are primarily related to differential diagnoses of cardiovascular diseases. See the complete 1997 E/M guidelines for details.

CLINICAL THINKING IN DIAGNOSIS AND TREATMENT

Medical Decision Making

Medical decision making in coding is one of the most confusing areas for clinicians to understand and code appropriately. The terminology can be misleading, so instead of medical decision making, think of the clinical thinking process of differential diagnoses and evaluation of patients with extensive medical histories and several comorbidities. If the chief complaint generates a long list of differential diagnoses with a large amount of diagnostic data to review, and a high risk of mortality or morbidity could result from either the treatment or disease itself, the clinical thinking is usually complex and the code for the decision making is likely to be high complexity. See Table 38-4 for a summary of E/M code levels and elements of medical decision making. To qualify for a given type of decision making, two of the three elements outlined in Table 38-4 must be met or exceeded. For high complexity criteria to be met, two of the elements listed below must be extensive or high to qualify.

There are four types of medical decision making:

■ Straightforward

■ Low complexity

Table 38.4 **Types of Medical Decision Making**			
CLINICAL THINKING	DIFFERENTIAL DIAGNOSES	AMOUNT AND COMPLEXITY OF REVIEWED DATA	RISK OF COMPLICATIONS, MORBIDITY AND MORTALITY
Straightforward	Minimal	Minimal/None	Minimal
Low complexity	Limited	Limited	Low
Moderate complexity	Multiple	Moderate	Moderate
High complexity	Extensive	Extensive	High

Table 38.5 **Documentation Requirements for New Patient Office Visits, New Patient Codes**

CODE LEVELS, 1-5	HISTORY	EXAMINATION	MEDICAL DECISION MAKING	TYPICAL FACE-TO-FACE TIME (min)
99201	Problem Focused	Problem Focused	Straightforward	10
99202	Expanded problem focused	Expanded problem focused	Straightforward	20
99203	Detailed	Detailed	Low	30
99203	Comprehensive	Comprehensive	Moderate	45
99205	Comprehensive	Comprehensive		60

- Moderate complexity

- High complexity

Elements of medical decision making:
- Number of diagnoses or management options

- Amount and/or complexity of data to be reviewed

- Risk of significant complications, morbidity and/or mortality

Example A (see earlier) reflects a CPT coding level four (see Table 38-2). This patient encounter would be coded a level five if the ROS included 10 systems reviewed and the notation that all other systems were negative when coding an established patient visit. (See later for the definition of new patients.)

Counseling

Documentation of a patient encounter that is primarily related to counseling or coordination of care requires a face-to-face encounter with the patient in the outpatient setting where the time spent is the primary factor qualifying the documentation of the E/M services. See Table 38-5 for details of documenting an E/M code based on counseling and face-to-face time as part of the new patient encounter. The documentation requirements for established patients are similar.

New Patient Visits

The new patient visit is coded differently than an existing patient visit. In most medical encounters this is because of the amount of time required to obtain a complete history from the patient. Therefore, all the E/M levels are adjusted and have different documentation requirements than for the previously seen patient. It should be noted here that a new patient is defined by the location of service and not by the provider of service. In other words, the patient must be establishing care and a medical record for the initial encounter in the medical practice. Table 38-5 describes the E/M codes and the elements of history and physical examination required for each level. The terminology and definitions remain the same as for established patient visits. The definition of a new patient, which is coded at a higher level, is a patient who has not received any professional services from the health professional or another health professional of the same specialty who belongs to the same group practice within the last 3 years.

SUMMARY

Many clinicians view coding as just part of billing; however, as noted earlier, it should be regarded as part of the documentation process and good patient care. Usually, once medical professionals understand the process and begin documenting what has occurred in the examination room, all the positive aspects of good documentation are realized in patient care and reimbursement.

REFERENCES

American Medical Association: CPT 2005: Current Procedural Terminology, Standard Edition. AMA, 2005.

Beacon Healthcare Solutions. ICD.9.CM—Diagnostic and Surgical Procedures Codes. Copyright 2000-2003. Available at: www.beaconllc.com/hcref/cclookup/icddescription.htm

Centers for Medicare & Medicaid Services: Documentation Guidelines for Evaluation and Management Services. CMS, 1997.

London Bills of Mortality 1660-1700. (http://uuhsc.utah.edu/dfpm/epi/section2_London_Bills_of_Mortality.pdf)

BIBLIOGRAPHY

Hill E: Understanding when to use the new patient E/M codes. Fam Pract Manag 10:33-36, 2003.

Oregon Health & Science University, Department of Family Medicine (www.ohsu.edu/som/fammed/) progress notes and coding templates.

Rose JS, Fisch BJ, Hogan WR, et al: Common medical terminology comes of age, Part Two: Current code and terminology sets—strengths and weaknesses. J Healthc Inf Manag 15:319-330, 2001.

Chapter 39

Documentation

David P. Asprey

GOALS AND OBJECTIVES

Goal: To provide clinicians with the knowledge and skills necessary to accurately and successfully document clinical procedures.

Objectives: The student will be able to ...

- Describe the purpose of documenting clinical procedures.
- Discuss the importance of documenting clinical procedures in the medical record.
- List the components of a standard clinical procedure note.

BACKGROUND AND HISTORY

The medical record is a repository of information that is compiled by many individuals regarding a single patient. The information includes history and physical examination findings, data, interpretation of data, and descriptions of medical acts that were performed. The record serves many different audiences, which may include the clinician, other health professionals involved in the patient's care, the patient, supervisors, clinical investigators, and administrators.

Many of the clinical procedures discussed in this text warrant or require the clinician involved in performing the procedure to prepare and record a clinical note for the medical record that documents and describes the performance of the procedure and the associated findings. Performing a procedure without documenting it in the clinical note can result in loss of critical information affecting patient care or the ability of the health care system to receive reimbursement for the care provided. Documentation of procedures that have been performed in the medical record can serve several purposes. These purposes include the following:

- **Memory aid:** The medical record originally served as a vehicle for recording information that may otherwise be forgotten about the patient's medical condition. However, the patient's complete medical database is a combination of the clinician's written information and thought processes. Documentation of the clinical procedure and its findings can serve to assist the clinician in recalling important findings, techniques used, or complications encountered while performing a procedure.

- **Communication device:** The medical record also functions to communicate information about a procedure performed and its findings to other clinicians and health professionals. Because medicine is a team function, many others will access the information recorded in a patient's medical record as they provide care to the patient. Because many others will use the same medical record, following an established standard for the manner in which this information is recorded is very important.

- **Quality assurance instrument:** Individuals and organizations involved in providing patient care need to monitor the quality of the care provided. A key component of this process involves medical record review by peers. The medical record is assessed for thoroughness, accuracy, and documentation of essential elements of a procedure. Record review can serve as a source of feedback that helps to ensure that the clinician is following established standards of care.

- **Risk reduction aid:** One of the best defenses against malpractice litigation is a detailed, concise, and accurate medical record that demonstrates the rational and systematic approach the clinician used in performing a procedure. The medical record serves as a legal document and may be used in court as evidence.

■ **Reimbursement aid:** Most third-party payers require chart review in assessing reimbursement or reimbursement levels. In performing clinical procedures, it is essential to document all aspects of the history, physical examination, indications, and findings to support the charges for which reimbursement is being requested. The medical record is used to verify that the procedure performed was indicated and performed appropriately. In view of this, it becomes critical to carefully document all the associated activities involved with performing the procedure. The perspective that the third-party payer may use is: *If it is not recorded, it was not done.* Chapter 38, Outpatient Coding, provides a review of the importance of documentation related to the billing and coding process.

■ **Evaluation tool:** Documentation of clinical procedures may be used in evaluation. Virtually all medical systems have a mechanism of quality control that includes evaluation of all clinicians' charts by peer review or quality control boards. Write-ups by students and others in training are evaluated, and performance is monitored by their supervising faculty and staff. Developing strong documentation skills is an important competence for clinicians in training to obtain.

■ **Research tool:** The medical record also serves as a data source for clinical research in some cases. Retrospective chart reviews are commonly used in clinical epidemiology studies. Data must be carefully and accurately recorded for it to be useful in research studies.

OTHER POINTS FOR CONSIDERATION IN RECORDING CLINICAL PROCEDURES

■ **Record all the pertinent data:** Both positive and negative findings from an examination or procedure findings may contribute directly to assessment and differential diagnosis. Any diagnosis made or problem identified should be clearly spelled out in the record. When other aspects of the history or physical examination suggest that an abnormality might exist or that it should be ruled out, be sure to include this information, even if the abnormality is absent or the finding is a pertinent negative. Another clinician should be able to read your account and be able to determine the rationale for your conclusion.

■ **Data not recorded are data lost:** Regardless of how vividly you may recall the detailed information associated with your patient and the procedure performed, it is highly improbable that you will be able to remember it clearly in a few weeks or a few months. Unless you record the presence and absence of findings and the specific steps completed in performing the procedure, you are at risk of being unable to answer questions regarding the activities associated with that procedure in the future. The fact that something is not present in the medical record does not mean that it was not done or not observed (absence of evidence is not evidence of absence), but it does allow for this to be an equally plausible explanation.

■ **Be objective:** The clinician recording the data in the medical record needs to take great care to ensure that only objective information is recorded. Statements that can be interpreted as judgmental or condescending have no place in the medical record. Although it is important to remain objective, doing so should not be misconstrued to mean that clinical impressions should not be recorded; rather, there should be a rational basis for your conclusions or impressions.

■ **Consider the use of diagrams:** Diagrams can sometimes provide a better description than words alone. Diagrams used to identify topographic locations of lesions or techniques used in performing a procedure or to illustrate clinical findings can be powerful tools. Clinicians who learn to use diagrams can help improve the accuracy of their record and improve their efficiency. Clinical procedures often have findings that warrant the use of a diagram to document findings or techniques used in the procedure.

■ **Avoid the use of nonstandard abbreviations:** Although abbreviations may prove useful in some limited instances to provide a measure of efficiency in making entries into the medical record, they have significant potential for error and confusion on the part of those who read and interpret them. This same principle is true of acronyms and symbols; exercise caution in electing to use any of these tools in a medical record. *When in doubt, spell it out.*

■ **Make sure the record is legible:** If your record is not legible to others, it will not serve its purpose well as a communication tool, nor will it serve you well as a legal document. Follow the conventional rules used in making entries into the medical record.

CLINICAL PROCEDURE NOTES

Entries made into the medical record specifically regarding clinical procedures performed constitute a unique format. Although they may be incorporated into a subjective, objective assessment and plan (SOAP) note format in some instances, the more significant procedures often warrant a separate entry specific to the procedure performed. Each time that an entry is made into the medical record regarding a clinical procedure, a conventional format should be used to help ensure that the essential and important aspects of the procedure are included and to aid others who access the record in finding the important information. One such format is listed in the following section. A sample note is presented in Figure 39-1.

Demographic data:
  Name: Mary Smith, ID# 123-45-6789, **Age**: 48 years, **Date**: 08/09/01, **Time**: 1:45 pm,
  Location: Procedure room W139, outpatient clinic.
Procedure performed:
  Incision and drainage of abscess in perirectal area
Primary indications for performing the procedure:
  Treatment of localized skin infection and relief from associated pain
Contraindications:
  None, patient reports no known allergies
Consent:
  Informed consent was obtained and form signed and filed in medical record before
  performing the procedure.
Personnel:
  Procedure was performed by Jane Doe, PA, with assistance from Sara Shoe, RN.
Anesthesia:
  A regional field block was performed using 8 mL of 1% lidocaine without
  epinephrine.
Description of the procedure performed:
  The patient was positioned in a dorsal recumbent position and the skin of the
  perianal area was cleansed using povidone-iodine (Betadine). A regional field
  block was performed with 1% lidocaine. The patient was then draped, and an
  elliptic incision was performed parallel to the skin tension lines in the skin overlying the abscess. The abscess was explored with a sterile cotton-tipped applicator,
  and cultures were obtained and sent to the laboratory. A sterile, blunt hemostat was
  then used to disrupt loculations in the skin comprising the abscess with blunt
  dissection technique. The area was massaged to facilitate the expression of purulent
  material from the depths of the abscess. The wound was irrigated with 300 mL of
  normal saline solution. The wound was then packed with iodoform gauze. The wound
  was covered lightly with an absorbent bandage.
Findings:
  The abscess margins were approximately 1.5 cm deep $\times$ 2.0 cm wide. Moderate
  amounts of purulent material were expressed from the abscess with no unusual odor
  noted. Multiple loculations were present within the abscess, and they were disrupted
  with blunt dissection. The depths of the abscess were explored with no evidence of
  rectal fissure formation, and the abscess appeared to be limited to the subcutaneous
  fat layer of the skin. No foreign bodies or matter were noted in the abscess.
Description of any important physical examination findings, after the procedure:
  No evidence of rectal fissure formation was noted on reexamination of the abscess
  after drainage.
Complications, including blood loss, side effects, and adverse reactions:
  No complications were encountered. Estimated blood loss was 5 mL.
Instructions and follow-up plans:
  The patient was instructed about the proper technique to pack the abscess with
  iodoform gauze and bandage the wound. Patient was advised to repack the wound
  twice daily. Patient was educated regarding signs of advancing infection and
  instructed to contact our office or return to the clinic if they occur. A prescription for
  Tylenol No.3—to be taken 1 to 2 tablets PO every 6 hours during the next 48 hours
  "total of 16 tablets"— for pain relief was given. The patient was advised not to drive or
  operate equipment while taking this medication. Patient was advised to schedule
  a return appointment in 10 days.
Time procedure completed and condition of patient:
  The procedure was completed in 20 minutes, and the patient was released to travel
  home with her spouse in good condition.

FIGURE 39-1.   Sample procedure note.

CLINICAL PROCEDURE NOTE FORMAT

If the clinician performing the procedure determines that a separate note is warranted, the format proposed in this section may be used to record the essential information.

1. Demographic data (patient name and identification number, age, date, time, and location)
2. Name or description of procedure performed
3. Primary indication or indications for performing the procedure
4. Contraindications, including potential allergies to medications that may be used in performing the procedure
5. Consent (if obtained)—indicate that informed consent was obtained and that forms were signed and filed in medical record before performing the procedure
6. Personnel—indicate the clinician who performed the procedure and any attendants who assisted with the procedure
7. Description of any important physical examination findings before performing the procedure. This should include vital signs prior to initiating the procedure.
8. Anesthesia (specific agent, quantity used, and route administered), if applicable
9. Description of the procedure performed (include description of equipment used and any variations to the technique); diagrams may be useful in documenting the location of lesions, and so on
10. Description of the relevant findings associated with the procedure, including abnormal structures, pending laboratory tests, or specimen samples sent for examination; diagrams may be useful in recording pertinent findings
11. Description of any important physical examination findings after the procedure (e.g., vascular supply intact distally, neurologic examination findings, functionality of joint or adjacent structures). Documentation of vital signs post procedure is important.
12. Complications, including blood loss, side effects, and adverse reactions
13. Instructions and follow-up plans
14. Time that procedure was completed and the condition of patient at that time

CONCLUSION

Documentation of the clinical procedure in the medical record is an essential component of any complete procedure. Exercising care to be certain that the entry into the medical record follows a conventional format and is thorough helps avoid potential problems associated with incomplete entries.

BIBLIOGRAPHY

Bates B: A Guide to Physical Examination and History Taking, 6th ed. Philadelphia, JB Lippincott, 1995.

Coulehan JL, Block MR: The Medical Interview: Mastering Skills for Clinical Practice, 5th ed. Philadelphia, FA Davis, 2006.

Suggs K, Meehan A, Rahr RR: Patient record. In Ballweg R, Stolberg S, Sullivan EM (eds): Physician Assistant: A Guide to Clinical Practice, 3rd ed. Philadelphia, WB Saunders, 2003, pp 157-180.

Chapter 40

Giving Sad and Bad News

F. J. Gianola

GOALS AND OBJECTIVES

Goal: To give sad or bad news consistently and with minimal anxiety or stress.

Objectives: The student will be able to …

- Define sad and bad news.
- Describe the goals for giving sad and bad news.
- Describe the principles of SPIKES, the six-step approach for giving sad and bad news.
- List the six steps in the SPIKES protocol.

> *An expert in breaking bad news is not someone who gets it right every*
> *time—she or he is merely someone who gets it wrong less often, and who*
> *is less flustered when things do not go smoothly.*
>
> Robert Buckman, 1992

BACKGROUND AND HISTORY

For the past 3,000 years, physicians have had an exquisite ability to describe disease processes. Their ability to observe, diagnose, prognosticate, and treat disease—in a manner appropriate for the time—is well documented (Simon, 1999). But truth-telling to the patient was not the norm. In 1951 Kline and Sobin described methods to avoid giving information (Kline, 1951). A 1961 paper in *JAMA* (Oken, 1961) reported that 90% of physicians would not choose to let their patients know of a diagnosis of cancer. This was done in good faith and in the spirit of beneficence, based on the belief that the truth would shatter patients' hope and hasten their deaths.

By 1971 there was a sea change in attitudes. By that time, 97% of physicians would tell their patients of a cancer diagnosis (Novack, 1979). However, sharing bad news with a patient is difficult and causes significant stress, as discussed in an extensive review (Fallowfield, 2004). A major cause of this stress is the lack of proper training and evaluation for providers. Lack of training and subsequent inappropriate communications can result in long-term devastating effects to both patients and providers. For the most part, patients want to know the truth even if it is sad, bad, or difficult (Benbassat, 1998). The principle of autonomy (Beauchamp, 2001) requires this level of information in order for patients to make informed decisions about their care. A decision *not* to know is also a choice that is discussed later in this chapter. A mutually responsive patient-clinician relationship is crucial for productive, secure, and successful therapeutic encounters, and giving sad news is often part of the interaction.

INDICATIONS

Many of the clinical procedures within this text provide practitioners with diagnostic data. For example, the patient-clinician relationship (involving either the primary care provider or the specialist consultant) can create an expectation that test results will be shared. In any procedure, preparations must be made; instruments must be obtained and set up. In many cases, a step by step method for a procedure has been planned with the knowledge that normal anatomic variation may change some of the steps. The procedures are done in a case-based manner, and both the provider and the patient should be aware of the contraindications and potential complications. This is also true of breaking difficult news to patients. The most powerful instrument for this procedure is your words. Words soothe, words cause wars, and words can bring peace. In the medical profession, words can change the course of peoples' lives. When giving sad or bad news, providers must think before they speak.

What is "bad" news? In Buckman's paper "Breaking bad news: Why is it still so difficult?" it means "any news that drastically and negatively alters the patient's view of his or her future" (Buckman, 1984). Despite the passage of time, breaking bad news is still difficult. Sad, bad news is not necessarily news of fatal illness. The information can be any chronic disease that changes a patient's life, such as diabetes, hypertension, macular degeneration, progressive hearing loss of unknown origin, or multiple sclerosis. Sometimes we diagnose these so often that it becomes commonplace. However, for the patient the diagnosis is new and can be both life-changing and life-threatening. The choice of words and how we present them may well change the patient-clinician relationship forever in either a positive or negative manner. The name given an illness can alter the patient's personal, family, and societal life (Wood, 1991). In the majority of instances when the clinician states and confirms a life-changing diagnosis, the patient does not hear anything else during the encounter.

PREPARING TO SHARE BAD NEWS

In preparing to give sad or bad news, one should think about the content of the message. Confidence is built on a foundation of competence. Cultural sensitivity and awareness and language should be part of your initial considerations. Remember that sharing the information is a dialogue with the patient, not a monologue by the provider. Silence is not an enemy; it can provide needed time for the patient to comprehend the information. An empathetic, caring, comforting, and pleasant manner is crucial in giving this news (Larson, 2005). Yet the situation is often so tense that being empathetic and caring can be very difficult. Many times the news creates an emotionally explosive reaction and the bearer of the news gets the blame. To remain calm and reassuring requires preparation and experience. Experience comes only with time and multiple encounters with such situations.

As stated earlier, with any other procedure, having your instruments set out properly is the first step. Just as procedures are not exactly the same every time, bringing sad or bad news requires individualized consideration. Different approaches are required. Just as experience builds a provider's confidence and ability in history-taking or performing physical examinations, the provider's approach to sharing bad news may change with time, and frequency will help build confidence. Following are some guidelines for this process. Interviewing skills should incorporate the Buckman recommendations (Buckman, 1992).

■ Nonverbal communication: make eye contact, lean forward, give encouraging looks, and nod (when appropriate).

■ Questions should be simple and brief, open-ended progressing to focused, and closed questions should be used only if necessary to obtain specific information.

- Summarize information periodically and ask clarifying questions to obtain a fuller understanding of the history.

- Engage in active listening, including restatement and summarization, which indicates you have heard the patient.

- Listen with empathy, reflect back to the patient empathetically what the patient has said. Respond to the mood and feelings of the patient.

A PROCEDURE FOR SHARING BAD NEWS

Robert Buckman was one of the first to develop guidelines for sharing bad news. The guidelines are meant to "be practical and useful in daily clinical situations based on some consistent and coherent principles, intelligible, teachable, and, most important, learnable" (Buckman, 1992).

SPIKES

The SPIKES approach (Baile, 2000) to sharing bad news consists of the following elements:

- **S**etting up: **S**etting up the interview

- **P**erception: assessing the patient's **P**erception

- **I**nvitation: obtaining the patient's **I**nvitation

- **K**nowledge: giving **K**nowledge and information to the patient

- **E**motions: addressing the patient's **E**motions with empathetic responses

- **S**trategy: **S**trategy and summary

Setting Up

In setting up the interview there are five areas to be aware of in planning a strategy. Some may seem obvious but should not be overlooked. *Arrange for privacy* in an office or private room; if this is not obtainable, create some privacy in the patient's room. Have a member of the patient's family or a close friend of the patient be present. The *patient should not be alone* for this information. *Sit down* so it conveys to the patient you are not in a rush to leave. Sitting puts you at eye level with the patient and creates a more supportive impression. Eye contact can *establish a connection* with the patient; however, being culturally aware in this situation is fundamental. Showing common courtesy and respect and not appearing rushed go a long way toward a successful discussion. Address the patient by his or her surname unless you know him or her well and have used the first name in the past. Depending on the comfort level of the patient, touching the patient on the arm or shoulder may help make this connection. Set your pager or cell phone on silent mode and schedule *sufficient time* for sharing this infor-mation. If there are any issues with time let the patient know so it is not a surprise if you must leave. Arrange for no interruptions.

Perception

Assess the patient's perception. How does the patient perceive the medical situation? How much does the patient know about the illness? The choice of words in the opening question is important. They should be your words so that you feel comfortable with them. The content in such questions can be as follows:

- *Do you know why you had this procedure?*

- *What have you been told about your condition?*

- *Have you been very worried about this …?*

- *When these symptoms first started, what did you think it was?*

- *How worried have you been about yourself?*

- *Have you been worried about this being serious?*

- *What do you think is going on with …?*

Asking open-ended questions not only helps gauge how much the patient knows but also may reveal the patient's expectation of treatment, concerns, or denial of the present illness. The answers may help the provider find a starting point. They also allow the provider to correct misconceptions or misinformation. Listen for the emotional content of the patient's responses to learn both what he or she wants to talk about and does not want to talk about. Body language can provide a considerable amount of information if the patient moves away, wrings the hands, or is tearful. Seemingly happy, nonchalant, or blasé body language and attitude can also give you an indication of the patient's emotional state.

Invitation

Obtain the patient's invitation for sharing the data acquired from the procedure. Providers must obtain permission from the patient before divulging the sad or bad news. Most patients want to know the diagnosis, prognosis, and any available treatment. Some do not. Health care decisions may be made or shared with family or community leadership (Mitchell, 1998). If the patient does not want to know specifics, offer support and an appointment to talk again in the future. With the patient's permission, talking to a family member or close friend can be arranged. Again, the style and exact words to use should be your own. Following are some examples of the content:

- *Would you like me to tell you the specifics of your condition, or is there someone else you would like me to have a word with?*

- *How much do you want to know if your condition is serious?*

- *If this condition turns out to be serious, would you like to know specifically what the situation is?*

- *Some folks would like to hear the treatment plan first without knowing the full details of what is wrong. Is that what you would be more comfortable with?*

- *Would you like me to summarize your condition or do you want to know precisely what we are dealing with?*

<u>K</u>nowledge

Provide knowledge and information to the patient. There are two parts to this section. First, provide understandable information to the patient. Second, offer a therapeutic conversation in which you listen, hear, and respond to the patient's reaction to the information. Before starting this section of the paradigm, it is imperative to know the purpose or goals of the interview. The goals should incorporate four key components: diagnosis, plan of treatment, prognosis, and support. Although the content of each component is case-based and specific for each patient, you are obliged to have a goal for the interview. Your goal and the patient's may differ, but they may be brought closer together by the end of the interview. The patient has the right to accept or reject the information, as well as the treatment or diagnosis. The patient has a right to respond in any (lawful) way he or she may choose. Medical providers must be prepared to accept these responses.

By this point in the dialogue, the patient has given consent to the provider about the amount of information he or she is willing to hear. The process of imparting knowledge to the patient is a true dialogue. This process must be assessed frequently by observing the patient's responses to the information. Sharing the information should be gentle, consistent, and at the patient's pace. Information should be given in small digestible portions. The clinician can assess whether the information is being comprehended by asking questions such as these:

- *Can I clarify anything?*

- *Does this information make sense to you?*

- *This can be confusing, but do you follow me so far?*

If there is a gap between the patient's expectations and the data being presented, the following statement may be included:

- *This condition is much more serious than ...*

The patient requires the information in order to make an informed choice. When providing the information, start at the level of the patient's understanding and terminology. For example, instead of saying "demyelination," say "damage to the insulation covering of the nerve"; instead of saying "metastasize," use the word "spread." Clarify to make sure your understanding and the patient's understanding of the words are the same. To do this, ask the patient to repeat the general meaning of what has been said. Repeat the essential portions. People hearing sad or bad news have limitations in processing information when facing serious illness. An empathetic response may be as follows:

- *I know it is hard to hear and remember all the specifics at once …*

The use of simple handwritten illustrations or flow charts can be helpful, and including your name and office number can bring a very personal feeling to the situation. This handwritten aid may help the patient remember more of the encounter. Pamphlets and educational materials should also be used.

Listen for the patient's concerns while proceeding through the sharing of information. Ask about worries and fears, because many times they stem from rumors or inaccurate information. The patient may have concerns about the effects of the treatment or quality-of-life issues. By listening and acknowledging the patient's concerns, you can address them then or at a future appointment. Sometimes patients ask questions while the clinician is talking. These are often important questions and should be addressed carefully. Finish the sentence, then ask the patient to repeat the question. Many times these questions are the heart of the discussion and can be very productive. Not infrequently, as the interview is drawing to an end, the patient wants to restart a portion of it again. This is not necessarily obstinate behavior, but rather is an indication that the patient is afraid and anxious. Sit down for a moment to reassure the patient, acknowledge the concern, and set up another time to talk further about the issue. A short moment may save significant anguish for the patient and illustrates your concern. Demonstrating concern by listening allows the clinician to accommodate the patient's perspective. These actions can help bring together the provider's and patient's goals and objectives to create a stronger patient-provider relationship.

Emotions

Addressing the patient's emotions with an appropriate empathetic response can determine the outcome of breaking sad or bad news. Emotional reactions by the patient are often the cause of considerable trepidation for the provider. Experience is the one thing that addresses the anxiety of the unknown. Each encounter decreases the number of unexpected reactions to sad and bad news. The reactions are as varied as the patients; however, there are some general categories and behaviors to be expected.

Patient reactions can include disbelief, shock, denial, displacement, fear and anxiety, anger and blame, anger against specific entities, guilt, depression, overdependency, crying and tears, "why me," threats, humor, seduction, bargaining, awkward questions, and the search for meaning. Not all of these reactions can be addressed here, but those that are seen most frequently are identified. Additionally, there are specific issues related to breaking sad or bad news to children, whether the bad news is about themselves or others. Although these issues are not discussed in depth in this chapter, it is important to be aware of the different needs that younger patients have.

Disbelief

Disbelief is a frequent response, especially if the news is not expected. This reaction is not meant to create tension with the provider; it highlights the difficulty of taking in the news. The issue is not about factual disagreements, and the provider needs to focus on acknowledging the patient's difficulty in acceptance. Consider the following responses:

■ *News about this serious illness must come as a shock, especially when you are feeling so good.*

■ *How does this make you feel?*

Shock

The common meaning of shock is alarm, distress, or terror. This reaction is not difficult to identify. The provider's response is much more difficult. How can you console and support this reaction? This reaction shows a failure to function and an inability to make decisions. It is most commonly expressed in silence, with an inability to speak or respond to your questions. Occasionally there can be more dramatic expressions of wailing and deep anguish by pacing around the room or falling to the floor inconsolably. Allowing the patient to express very deep feelings is okay. Questions that may help are as follows:

■ *Are you okay?*

■ *What are you thinking now?*

For both disbelief and shock, try:

■ *This news must be overwhelming for you.*

Denial

When experiencing denial, the patient has a sincere conviction that the news is incorrect or a mistake. The patient may ask you to recheck results because he or she is sure there was a mix-up in the laboratory. In a more subtle form, the patient may start talking about long-term plans (e.g., planning to build a house, a year-long sailing excursion) when the news is such that the probability for these plans to be fulfilled is unrealistic. The provider's reaction to the patient's denial may be defensive, reacting to the perception that the provider is viewed as incompetent. Denial is a protective response to protect the self from harm and to view the future self intact. Denial is a normal response to overwhelming information that threatens the future existence of the person. Questions to ask the patient should include the following type of information:

■ *What is it that makes you believe information is inaccurate?*

■ *Accepting this news must not be easy.*

Denial in the initial period of hearing sad and bad news is normal. Denial that continues for an extended period of time will increase the patient's distress, needs to be addressed cautiously, and requires comprehensive negotiation.

Fear and Anxiety

Fear and anxiety are often used interchangeably; however, they are different entities. A specific object or event or the thought of a specific object or event often prompts fear. Fear is acute, with a quick response to the prompt and a quick fade when the prompt is removed. Anxiety is chronic. It may come on rapidly and often takes longer to resolve after the prompt has been removed. Identify the cause or source of the fear or anxiety by listening adequately to the patient's feelings. Trying to reassure the patient without discovering the source will be ineffective and will not decrease the intensity of anxiety or fear. Acknowledge the patient's feelings. Identifying and acknowledging the patient's feelings may reduce the fear or anxiety in some cases. Provide as much detailed information as seems appropriate to the case. See what happens when the information is provided. If providing it reduces the fear or anxiety, you have succeeded in this area. You may continue to give information as the patient requests it. If the information does not appear to help, stop giving it, because the patient will not accept the information. If the patient's fears and anxiety are severe or prolonged, get help and consider referral to a mental health professional. Following are some empathetic questions for patients with anxiety or fear:

- *With all this news, what worries you the most?*

- *Have you been thinking about what might happen to you? That must be quite stressful for you.*

- *Could you tell me your main worries? Endless worry about (recurrence) must be dreadful.*

Finally, with anxious or fearful patients, the greater their anguish, the greater your urge to over-reassure them. Over-reassurance creates a greater distance from the reality of the situation, which is counterproductive for both the provider and patient.

Anger and Blame

Anger and blame are the emotions that are most often directed at the health care provider. Understanding the anger a patient may feel is useful and can prepare you for using specific techniques to address it rather than being overwhelmed by it. Knowledge and recognition of the types of anger will make it easier for you keep hold of the situation and sustain a sense of composure to support the patient during the interview. Being judgmental in this situation is not helpful. Buckman has identified "rough and ready" classifications of a patient's anger (Buckman, 1992):

- Abstract anger (appropriate or inappropriate)

    - Against the disease—symptoms, disability, freedom, "death sentence"

    - Against loss of control and powerlessness—determination of lifestyle, movements; dependency on others

    - Against loss and potential—loss of hopes and aspirations: career, relationships, family, life fulfillment

- Against laws of nature/randomness—random biologic events, unfairness (why me?)

■ Anger against specific entities (appropriate or inappropriate)

- Against self—causal anger (if patients feel they are causing their own disease), body for failing, opportunities missed, own attitude

- Against friends and family—own health, "residual anger from old family rifts or feuds," receiving advice, charity, sympathy; causal anger may be appropriate (e.g., believes friends caused disease through passive smoke) or inappropriate (abandonment or distancing)

- Against medical and other health professionals—"blaming the messenger" for the news, loss of control (now is with medical team), medical team members who are healthy, communication gaps (not listening, uncaring), management decisions (should have diagnosed earlier and treated differently)

- Against "outside forces"—workplace, occupation, environment, home, socioeconomic or political forces

- Against God—"abandonment (he has forsaken me) ... perceived vindictiveness (divine retribution) ... poor return on faith and religious observances over many years" (Buckman, 1992)

Appropriate questions may be as follows:
■ *You are angry. What other feeling do you have?*

■ *You sound very angry that this was not picked up earlier.*

Open-ended questions and acknowledging anger seem simple but can cause an explosive outburst. Remember that you are in control of the situation and usually will not be the target of anger. An empathetic question removes the provider as the target and does not escalate the patient's anger. Often the conversation can move on to the present situation.

An interesting note: "Human beings seem to be programmed to decrease their anger when it meets a submissive response. Body language that moves away from counteraggression helps to diffuse a patient's anger. When a patient is angry it is worth trying to keep your head lower than the patient's. A useful technique is to have the patient seated upright on the examination couch, while you sit on a chair or stool. It is interesting to note how difficult it is to maintain anger when the target of it is sitting below you." (Buckman, 1992).

Guilt

Guilt appears to have three components. It is a self-focused or directed emotion. There is self-blame, and there is an aspect of sorrow or regret. Rarely are any of these components helpful to the patient. In most cases guilt about an illness is maladaptive. An empathetic content comment may be:
■ *Thinking this (condition) is your fault must be very painful.*

Depression. Situational depression is not an uncommon reaction to sad and bad news. The diagnostic criteria are well-known: depressed mood, irritability, weight change, difficulty sleeping or difficulty getting up from sleep, fatigue, feelings of worthlessness, recurrent thoughts of death or suicide, decreased ability to think, concentrate, or make decisions. If the symptoms are present and a diagnosis is made, be prepared to treat. The patient will usually feel significant relief after the provider has identified the depression for the patient, reviewed the symptoms, and explained that it is treatable and resolvable.

Crying and tears. Crying and tears are not an emotion but a symptom of anger, fright, rage, sadness, frustration, despair, and others. Tears come easily to some and rarely for others. It is odd that in this Western culture, although tears signal that one is upset, we are uncomfortable comforting strangers who are crying. Some fairly straightforward actions can help the provider cope and comfort. Move closer to the patient. Often people who are crying feel alone. Offer a tissue or handkerchief. Make sure there are tissues in place when you are giving sad or bad news. Offering a tissue gives the patient evident permission to cry, gives the patient something to dry the tears and clean a runny noise (it is very difficult to continue a conversation without this accommodation), gives the provider something to do, and brings the provider and patient closer together. Try touching the patient on the shoulder, elbow, or arm to try to identify the emotion causing the tears and offer an empathetic response. If the cause is not obvious, simply ask:

■ *Can you tell me what is causing you to cry?*

Awkward question. Two questions that many providers find thorny are *How long have I got?* and *Am I terminal?*. *How long have I got?* is probably the most common question asked when hearing bad news. It is also difficult to provide a single answer to cover all the possibilities. However, there are three principles to keep in mind. Assess what the patient thinks the situation is at the moment. Ask the patient what he or she has been thinking about this question. Clarify what the patient is truly asking. Assume nothing. You can inquire:

■ *Are you asking me how long you have to live?*

Give the patient some type of answer that is close to the clinical data. Remember the power of words and that the answer will be remembered for a long time, even if it is inaccurate. Give hard data, if possible, because the outcome is patient-specific. Statements could include the following:

■ *It could be several months or a small number of years, but probably not many.*

■ *This condition is very serious, maybe several weeks or a few months.*

Uncertainty is difficult and unpleasant. People are unique organisms who know they are going to die sometime, yet the exact time and date are always uncertain. It is very difficult to make a genuine heartfelt empathetic statement. Simply offer a comforting acknowledgement, such as:

■ *It must be very difficult not knowing what will happen next or when it will happen.*

When the patient asks *Am I terminal?*, be sure to clarify what terminal means to the patient. Providing an answer to the question you assume is being asked can be very embarrassing and may be less than endearing. The content of your response could include the following:

■ *Your question is very important and I will attempt to answer it. But could you tell me what you are thinking when you ask about being terminal?*

Sad and bad news presented to children. Breaking sad or bad news to children about themselves or others requires a unique skill set and a high-quality delivery. There is much literature on this subject, including books and new guidelines developed by the American Academy of Pediatrics. It is generally thought that early knowledge of a life-threatening diagnosis and not suppressing or concealing it is associated with healthy psychological adjustment for the child (Slavin, 1982). Providing this information is normally done with the help of a skilled specialist counselor, but there could be times when it may need to be done without a counselor. Buckman has identified five principles for delivering sad and bad news to children (Buckman, 1992):

■ The closest adult family member should always be present and an agreed-upon approach to the interview should be followed. The family member may request participation. Family members often have helpful insights that can help avoid unexpected surprises. Only in the most ominous, urgent situation should you attempt to discuss these issues without a close relative present.

■ Review frequently with the child his or her understanding of the information you are providing. A child's perception of what you are saying can be very different from what the child is hearing. Provide the information in a language that reflects the questions that the child is asking.

■ It is common for the same question to be asked repeatedly, to go over the same information. It is the normal manner in which children process information they have been told so they can be sure they have understood correctly what has been said.

■ Many children believe that if they think something, then it will happen. If they are angry with someone who later becomes seriously ill, children may believe their anger toward the person caused the illness. This is called "magical thinking." If a child is asked repeatedly by a parent to perform a task such as putting toys away and the child does not remember to perform the task, the child may feel guilty and responsible if the parent then becomes ill. (*If only I had picked up my toys papa would not be so sick*). This type of thinking is not obvious; however, one way to assuage the child's potential guilt is to say directly:

   ■ *Sometimes people get ill for no apparent reason.*

   ■ *It's not your papa's fault he is ill, it's not our fault, and it definitely is not your fault. Sometimes these things just happen.*

■ If you are inexperienced or uncertain, find assistance as soon as possible. Find an expert or a more experienced team member. You may be asked to be in further interviews with the child if a bond has been created or you know the family well.

Strategy

Contemplate a strategy for the case. By this point in the interview, depending on the sad or bad news, the patient may feel isolated and uncertain. The patient will be looking to you to help make sense out of the uncertainty. Knowing the patient's perspective on the illness and how much he or she knows about the situation and combining the patient's goals and your modified goals, expresses an alliance with the patient in creating a plan for the near future. The medical treatment plan forms the initial element of the patient's support strategy.

Help the patient identify his or her best coping skills and what type of support system can be created. Engaging the patient in some responsible action can be empowering. The concept of support does not mean doing everything possible for the patient. That is impractical and impossible. Active, effective listening is the initial step in support. Listen in a non-judgmental manner to what the patient says. Help the patient identify the observed emotions and behavior and support the patient, especially if you may not agree personally with the other point of view. Summarize the discussion to include the patient's condition and the plan for the future. In the plan it is helpful to provide the patient with the sequence of coming events, including tests, treatment or palliative care, and the next appointment time frame. Writing these down for the patient provides a reminder of the events to come and the personal interaction that is needed in giving sad and bad news. Finally, ask the patient in your style and words:

■ *Is there anything we missed or other questions you would like to ask?*

CONCLUSION AND FURTHER THOUGHTS

This process may appear arduous, complex and time-consuming. It is not. As with any procedure, experience improves and bolsters confidence. It does not necessarily make it easier.

Clinical empathy as an element of emotional labor can provide the clinician more professional satisfaction (Larson, 2005). When giving sad and bad news, remember that we have two things in common with all human beings on earth. We are born and we die. We are the only species that is aware of life's limitation. Between birth and death is commentary. As medical providers we have the honor of witnessing the commentary and listening to our patients' stories. Providing sad and bad news is part of our commentary.

References

Baile WF, Buckman R, Lenzi R, et al: SPIKES—A six-step protocol for delivering bad news: Application to the patient with cancer. Oncologist 5:302-311, 2000.

Beauchamp T, Childress JF: Principles and Practices of Biomedical Ethics, 5th ed. New York, Oxford University Press, 2001.

Benbassat J, Pilpel D, Tidhar M: Patients' preferences for participation in clinical decision making: A review of published surveys. Behav Med 24:81-88, 1991.

Buckman R: Breaking bad news: Why is it still so difficult? Br Med J (Clin Res Ed) 288:1597-1599, 1992.

Buckman R: How to Break Bad News: A Guide for Health Professionals. Baltimore, Md, The Johns Hopkins University Press, 1992.

Fallowfield L, Jenkins V: Communicating sad, bad, and difficult news in medicine. Lancet 363:312-319, 2004.

Kline NS, Sobin J: The psychological management of cancer patients. JAMA 146:1547-1551, 1951.

Larson EB, Yao X: Clinical empathy as emotional labor in the patient-physician relationship. JAMA 293:1100-1106, 2005.

Mitchell JL: Cross-cultural issues in the disclosure of cancer. Cancer Pract 6:153-160, 1988.

Novack DH, Plumer R, Smith PL, et al: Changes in physicians' attitudes toward telling the cancer patient. JAMA 241:897-900, 1979.

Oken D: What to tell cancer patients: A study of medical attitudes. JAMA 175:1120-1128, 1961.

Simon SR: Moses Maimonides: Medieval physician and scholar. Arch Int Med 159:1841-1845, 1999.

Slavin LA, O'Malley JE, Koocher GP, Foster DJ: Communication of the cancer diagnosis to pediatric patients; impact on long-term adjustment. Am J Psychiatry 139:179-183, 1982.

Wood ML: Naming the illness: The power of words. Fam Med 23:534-538, 1991.

Bibliography

Beauchamp T, Childress JF: Principles and Practices of Biomedical Ethics, 5th ed. New York, Oxford University Press, 2001.

Buckman R: How to Break Bad News: A Guide for Health Professionals. Baltimore, Md, The Johns Hopkins University Press, 1992.

Fallowfield L, Jenkins V: Communicating sad, bad, and difficult news in medicine. Lancet 363:312-319, 2004.

University of Washington School of Medicine: Ethics in medicine: Breaking bad news. Accessed 12/01/05: http://eduserv.hscer.washington.edu.offcampus.lib.washington.edu/bioethics/topics/badnws.html

Index